AGGRESSIVE HEALTH

AGGRESSIVE HEALTH

RECLAIM YOUR ENERGY
AND CHARGE AT LIFE

Mike Nash
www.aggresivehealth.co.uk

DISCLAIMER

The information within these pages is not intended to replace medical advice or be a substitute for a physician. But remember, doctors are not robots. I'm sure you've had bad experiences with some doctors and good experiences with others. Find a helpful one. Find one that wants you to succeed and cares about your health. Find one that is knowledgeable in the area of nutrition, health and exercise. That's your responsibility.

If you are currently taking a course of prescription medication, you should never alter your eating habits without consulting your doctor or specialist because dietary changes usually affect the metabolism of prescription drugs, especially if you are taking medication for a diabetic condition. Because there is always some risk involved, the author, publisher, and/or distributors of this book are not responsible for any adverse detoxification effects or consequences resulting from the use of any suggestions or procedures described hereafter.

Some of the devices/mind-machines and procedures described in AGGRESSIVE HEALTH are experimental. Conclusive studies of the long and short-term effects of some of these devices/mind-machines and procedures have not been performed. None of the information contained in this book should be construed as a claim or representation that these devices are intended for the use in the diagnosis, cure, treatment, or prevention of disease or any other medical condition. The use of some of these devices may be dangerous for those who are not in sound mental and physical health. For example, the light and sound devices that use flickering light may produce seizures in those subject to photo-induced epilepsy. Anyone taking or withdrawing from prescription or recreational drugs should be aware that drug use may affect his or her perceptions and responses to the stimuli of some of these devices. Some of the devices are restricted by law to use under medical supervision only. Before using these instruments consult your physician and check with your federal, state and local regulatory agencies for general advice.

Published by Raw Perfection Ltd. Milton Keynes, England
Copyright ©Raw Perfection Ltd 2005
Produced in England by Print Solutions Partnership, Surrey, England
Photography by Lee Warren Photography
Cover design by Eatsleepthink Design Ltd
www.eatsleepthink.co.uk Tel: +44 (0) 1780 759059   Mobile: +44 (0) 7711 062706
Clubbells®, Circular Strength Training™, Body-Flow™, Warrior Wellness™ are all trademarks belonging to RMAX.tv Productions.

ISBN 0-9542271-1-5

British Library Cataloguing in Publication Data.
A catalogue record for this book is available from the British Library.

This book is dedicated to Alan Austin-Smith, friend, mentor and founder of Take Control and the Success Scholarship. Without his commitment to helping others realise their full potential, this book would never have been written. Thank-you Alan.

TABLE OF CONTENTS

The secret to mastering AGGRESSIVE HEALTH...the importance of Vision in achieving your dreams...A powerful N.L.P. technique for creating a laser like focus...the power of incremental improvements... the one law that separates those who succeed from those who fail...the ONLY question you need to ask to guarantee you succeed...how to unleash the power of your reticular activating system... the most powerful prescription know to mankind... why YOU are the only one that matters.

PART I – HOW TO BUILD AN UNSHAKEABLE FOUNDATION THAT GUARATESS EXPLOSIVE HEALTH FOR A LIFETIME

The dangers of cooking EVERYTHING... the enemy of enzymes, vitamins and minerals ...why transfatty acids can kill your sexuality...the most significant 'raw food vs. cooked food' experiment...the ONLY foundation your health can be built on... why digestive leukocytosis can drain your immune system and how to avoid it...why 900 cats answer the most challenging health questions...how to select the most nutrient dense foods and make them taste delicious... the ultimate formula for radiating more energy... unlocking natures pharmacy...how to excrete more calories...optimise hormonal communication for magnificent health... how to minimise cell loss...how to speed up digestion.

An anti-cancer food recommended by Dr. Arthur Robinson...a 50 year old secret behind cancer prevention...how to rebuild your blood for exceptional health...natures answer to anaemia...how to save money on useless supplements...the cheapest answer to unrivalled bowel, liver and intestinal health...anti-ageing with SOD... freedom from damaging super oxides...the AGGRESSIVE HEALTH master juice formula...the super food choice behind 5 of the worlds best athletes... simple solutions for brain health and neurotransmitter equilibrium...how to balance EEG readings with no drugs...a powerful B12 superfood that should be at the heart of your health regime.

Why chewing on 'life force' is critical for explosive health...epileptic seizures gone and driving licence reinstated... the cheapest most effective food for 'keeping you full' and boosting your 'life force'... Dr Charles Shaw highlights the most potent anti-cancer foods... 7 reasons why sprouted foods should be at the heart of your diet... 5 reasons why sprouted beans are my No.1 food...banish enzyme inhibitors safely and effortlessly... why lecithin is critical in your diet...why enzymes are the key to turbo-charge your health...the power behind Vitalzym...the power of prayer ... where to turn to for zinc...why Dr Ernst Krebs, Jr recommends foods high in B17 (laetrile)... 7 reasons why hemp is the planets most superior food... 4 super nuts that provide unrivalled nutrition...

Why society has labelled fat as the bad guy...why the roaring oil trade is part responsible for the rise in heart disease...13 reasons why it's illegal to put transfatty acids in baby foods... why grinding flax seeds is superior to taking flax oil...say goodbye to constipation forever...the one almighty seed that supplies EVERYTHING... why protein and fat together create remarkable results... discover which fat has less calories than any other...boost your metabolism with this amazing food...unrivalled protection against viruses, bacteria and infections... a farmers lesson that he'll never forget...8 reasons to have extra virgin olive oil at your dinner table...7 lost secrets behind the avocado...why bee pollen is essential if you love high fat meals...32 reasons why essential fats are a must.

PART II – YOU'VE MASTERED THE BASICS, NOW PREPARE TO DIAL INTO THE HIGHEST STANDARDS OF AGGRESSIVE HEALTH

PART III – ELIMINATE UNWANTED STRESS *FOREVER*, USE MIND TECHNOLOGY TO SUPERCHARGE YOUR BRAIN AND CHARGE TOWARDS AN AWESOME EXISTENCE

weight on where it counts – your brain... the power of enriched environments... how to develop wisdom from the point of view of a neuro-scientist... why you should be helping your grandparents stay active both mentally and physically... why many people are suffering from brain shrinkage... the great news: it's never to late to regenerate you brain... discover what part of your body consumes over 20% of the oxygen available... discover how Body-Flow™ is your answer to simultaneous brain and body enrichment.

Why a focus on neurotransmitters is the key to brain health... Sarah Leibowitz, Ph.D. highlights a brain destroying diet... the unknown connection between refined carbohydrates and crime... Dr Elliot Blass teaches you the mechanism behind peoples sugar cravings... why drug abuse is a better option than food abuse... why mind technology and nutrition is a combination par excellence... how to simulate womb euphoria... 11 keys points to endorphin stimulation... the link between choline, bee pollen and hemp seeds for a turbo-charged memory... the dangers of the diet pills and the drug 'speed'... Why Ginkgo Biloba is essential for optimising brain health... the critical neurotransmitter axis: dopamine and serotonin... avoid the perils of Prozac... restore serotonin naturally with NO side effects... how the 'bus' analogy can help you manufacture meals to energise your brain... 7 reasons behind dopamine's power... why getting sweaty together is great for health... use the 'shotgun' approach and wave goodbye to mental decline... solid erections and moist love-making...the nuts that rev you up, the nuts that soothe your soul.

The safest alternative to Prozac... the unknown link between exercise and brain power... why combining play with exercise creates such amazing results... the power of nerve growth factor... how nerve growth factor and brain-derived neurotropic factor support neurons throughout your brain... how to achieve the tranquiliser effect though exercise... why jogging may be more powerful than psychotherapy... 7 reasons why exercise eliminates depression... how you can increase the brain related enzyme Co-enzyme Q10 naturally.

PART IV – EMBRACE AN UNLIMITED FUTURE AND PREPARE TO CREATE MIRACLES EVERY STEP OF THE WAY

A critical shift in your thinking for increased longevity... reaching out for your maximum lifespan... Dr Roy Walford sheds some light on the possibility of slow the ageing process...6 reasons why calorie restriction promotes longevity... 3 pivotal points of 'optimal minimum' eating... Discover why the Hunzas are a community of Centenarians... The Dagastanis give you yet more reasons to add greens to your diet... Dead Nutritionists lead by example – who was right vs. who was wrong... Discover Hippocrates simple answer to health.

Why www.biomedx.com are at the leading edge of the health revolution... Gods only mistake: Not giving us warning lights... why zeta potential is key for eliminating toxins and suspending nutrients... how Dr T.C Mcdaniel cured his own heart problem when cardiologists gave up... how zeta potential effects your every day life... are your core homeostatic processes balanced?... how a shift in awareness can reverse your biological age... visualisation for even better health... my final message to you... the ultimate AGGRESSIVE HEALTH evaluation.

Throughout AGGRESSIVE HEALTH, I talk of an exciting approach to nutrition, exercise and stress free living that could, in short, change your life. In order to succeed though, you need a new mentality. You need to begin staring at the world with an 'aggressive' look in your eye and an attitude that is committed to results. You need to be able to brush off everyday challenges that may try and halt your progress and focus on what you want with laser like intensity. Ultimately you want to charge towards your dreams and desires *as if* they were the only thing that mattered.

With statistics showing that 95% of diets fail, the ball is in your court. Do you join the 95% who flick through a few pages and wimp out because they don't believe in themselves? Or do you suspend your opinions and beliefs about what is possible and read AGGRESSIVE HEALTH from cover to cover, exposing yourself to the secrets that will allow you to become part of the elite 5%?

I wrote AGGRESSIVE HEALTH out of a desire to maximise my energy, alertness, brain function and body function and in the process saturate my body with pure undiluted pleasure. Nutrient rich food, physical mastery and mind technology are all part of this fascinating puzzle. The formula is simple: The more you apply the greater the rewards.

A word of warning though, AGGRESSIVE HEALTH is very powerful. Not only will you discover how to regain your health and move away from disease faster than you can imagine, but once you've read it in its entirety you'll realise it's a doorway to a more fulfilling existence.

The first approach to mastering AGGRESSIVE HEALTH is to dive straight in and try and do it all at once. It can be done, but I suggest you steer clear of this approach. My mother eliminated a potentially cancerous condition by applying every principle exclusively for 4 weeks, highlighting the power of an aggressive attitude and aggressive approach. But she had me by her side 24x7. If you decide to alter your eating patterns abruptly, tread carefully – you may invite the symptoms of severe detoxification.

The second approach is to make a gradual transition. I spent many years experimenting and found myself reverting back to old habits time after time. That's life! Embrace it, recognise it, and above all, welcome it! It will happen, you will have your 'off days' but by reading and understanding the principles of AGGRESSIVE HEALTH you'll have a proven plan to get back on the path to scintillating health... and stay there! Remember, you can't argue when you feel fantastic.

RAISE YOUR STANDARDS AND CHARGE TOWARDS UNRIVALED SUCCESS IN EVERYTHING YOU DO

When I began writing AGGRESSIVE HEALTH, it was my mission to seek out the most effective principles in the areas of health, nutrition and peak performance, and fuse them together to create an approach unlike any other. I wanted to create a program that delivered so many distinctions and nutritional wisdom it would raise the standards of health to a whole new level. In my mind, AGGRESSIVE HEALTH had to become the most powerful and effective system the world had ever seen! I wanted to help everyone from the individual striving to win Olympic gold to the millions of people wanting to lose a few pounds of unwanted flab.

Many authors claim that the process of writing a book is 20% inspiration and 80% perspiration. I couldn't agree more! In the five years it took to perfect what you're holding right now, I spent countless hours writing, researching, re-writing and editing.

Every writer knows how frustrating it can be to complete a chapter, or even finish a book. Many say that a book is never truly finished, but abandoned by the author when they've had enough of writing it! In my case this isn't true. I have made it my personal mission to bring to you the finest, most unique, tried and tested methods for producing revolutionary change on every level and now that it's complete, I'm more inspired about AGGRESSIVE HEALTH than ever before!

LET THE JOURNEY BEGIN...

AGGRESSIVE HEALTH leaves no stone unturned. In fact, I haven't yet found a book that delivers so much powerful information, on so many seemingly diverse subjects, and ties them together so beautifully. No other book that I've read combines the subjects of peak performance nutrition, pH balance and control, hormonal mastery, stress free living, movement sophistication, mind enhancing technology and longevity, as perfectly as the one you hold in your hands right now. It's a big claim, but once you've read it in its entirety, I'm sure you'll agree.

You've a lot to look forward to, so get excited. I'll share with you exactly what it takes to master AGGRESSIVE HEALTH and you'll soon realise, like many thousands before you, a few simple distinctions can truly change your life forever.

THE FIRST STEP TO AGGRESSIVE HEALTH:
A POWERFUL STATE OF MIND

I know you want to succeed, so pay close attention. The first step to your success is cultivating a burning desire that smoulders away inside of you and keeps you moving towards everything you deserve in life. With this ferocious intensity fuelling your resolve, you'll find it easy to read AGGRESSIVE HEALTH from cover to cover, exposing yourself to the most powerful life enhancing principles in existence.

The second step is making a commitment. A commitment to charge towards your dreams and desires. A commitment to tackle any challenges head on, and a commitment to do whatever it takes to succeed. Whether you want to maximise the electrical charge around each of your cells, create an amazingly efficient digestive system or control the key hormones that determine whether you gain weight or lose weight, AGGRESSIVE HEALTH delivers. In as little as 30 days, I'm convinced you'll be looking in the mirror at a 'new you', satisfied at how much you've learnt and applied, but hungry for more!

THE ONE KEY THAT MAKES ALL THE DIFFERENCE

A word of advice. If you remember one idea from this chapter remember this. If you really want to experience the unlimited freedom associated with AGGRESSIVE HEALTH today, tomorrow and for the rest of your life, you MUST create a compelling vision for yourself. You MUST create a clear concise image or sense of what it is you truly desire. Imagine looking through the eyes of ravenous carnivore as it stalks its victim. Imagine seeing your victim so helpless, it just drops its head and walks towards you knowing its fate. Now imagine seeing your dreams and desires from this perspective. So much so that they don't seem out of reach, but actually gravitate towards you. This is the first and most important step to AGGRESSIVE HEALTH.

Let me ask you a question. One year from now, where will you be? Will you be healthier or closer to disease and suffering? Will you look like the back end of a bus, or will you be in the best shape of your life? Will you be crackling with energy or run down like an old car battery? If you have a compelling vision, a clear concise image of what you want, you'll see yourself as fitter, healthier, stronger, more vibrant, charging at life with a new found freedom. Those who haven't made any decisions about their health may see themselves as fatter, more lethargic, less enthusiastic, and ready to throw in the towel and admit defeat.

BEGIN EXPERIENCING THE ULTIMATE EMOTION THAT GUARANTEES SUCCESS

Here's the key. With a compelling vision you begin to experience the ultimate emotion that guarantees your success. With this emotion oozing out of every pore of your being you'll feel propelled towards success. Armed with this emotion you'll never lose your desire to succeed! It's the difference between getting excited for a few weeks or making progress for a lifetime. Are you ready for it? The emotion I'm talking about is DRIVE! When you are driven to succeed, you might as well fasten your seat belt and enjoy the ride, because you *will* get what you want. With a compelling vision, you'll always be focused on taking the next step. Close your eyes now and let your deepest desires bubble to the surface and simmer in the forefront of your mind. See what you want in technicolor and let out a roar of excitement as if you were on the verge of making this part of your day to day reality. Feel this emotion pulsating through your veins, making the hairs on your arms stand up on end. Let it fill you with pure undiluted pleasure. Remember, a hungry predator with drool dripping from the corner of his mouth looks at the world differently than a timid little rodent scared to leave his tiny little hole.

IT'S TIME TO RE-IGNITE THE LONG FORGOTTEN DREAM

With a vision to guide you, and the drive, desire and commitment to succeed, your dream of having perfect health and a body and mind to match will soon become part of your daily reality. Remember, the quality of your health and the quality of your life isn't a question of capability; you are capable of incredible things. Sometimes however you may have failed to tap your full potential. It's my job to challenge you. First to take control of your immediate future by igniting your engines and secondly to help you condition the habits that create momentum and secure your success.

Just stop for a moment and think about your current eating habits. Do you jump out of bed in the morning and like a detective, seek out the foods that make you feel great, that make your body feel alive and your brain feel sharp and alert? Or... Do you lazily roll out of bed, stumble down the stairs and head straight for the coffee? Whatever your life is like at the moment, there is room for improvement. It doesn't matter if you want to lose 400lbs or 4lbs, whether you want to win Olympic gold or perform more energetically at the gym, if you make the decision to excel, everything you've ever dreamt of will be in your reach. Just remember one thing...

SUCCESS OR FAILURE DOESN'T HAPPEN OVERNIGHT

It doesn't matter how 'aggressive' your mindset is, success happens one step at a time, one day at a time, and is dependent on how committed you are to making incremental improvements. The same is true with the material in this book. **If you want success you must master each of the following principles individually until you are able to see how they create the ultimate approach I call AGGRESSIVE HEALTH.** Many approaches to health fail because the author concentrates on one principle alone, leading their followers into a false sense of certainty that 'their way is the only way'. You may read a book about balancing your pH and think that is all you need to focus on. You may read a book about controlling your hormones and think that is the secret to everlasting health. You may read a book about enzymes or hear a speaker talking about minerals, claiming they are the 'key to everything'. The reality is that no single approach works for everyone and I believe AGGRESSIVE HEALTH will set you free from such a limited mindset. AGGRESSIVE HEALTH will share with you key principles that have proven successful since the beginning of time and with advances in biological terrain testing and live blood microscopy, you can be certain of what it takes to reach the pinnacle of physiological functioning. It's up to you to then create YOUR daily habits that will determine YOUR success. I've had to discover what works for me and I'll give you many clues as to what is likely to work for you. Gradually you'll expand your mind and join the elite group of people who have waved goodbye to disease, have turned back the hands of time and who charge at life with a glint in their eye and a attitude to die for. Sound good? Well, there's one last thing to remember to complete this winning formula…

RESPONSIBILITY: THE ONLY WAY FORWARD

When you take responsibility, you stop wining like a little baby if things don't go your way and you stop blaming others for your misfortune. In short, you simply get down to business and make it happen. Maybe you'll book an appointment with your doctor before you begin to make powerful changes to your diet and your health. (If you take any drugs – prescription or non-prescription – or have been recently, I recommend you see your physician because dietary changes can affect the metabolism of prescription drugs). Maybe you'll book an appointment with me for a biological terrain analysis at www.aggressivehealth.co.uk. Maybe you'll read other books before you begin your quest to a more fulfilling life. Whatever your choice, as you take responsibility and let your vision guide you, you'll begin to make important decisions that will set in motion a chain of events that will ultimately shape your destiny.

THE AGGRESSIVE HEALTH MINDSET WILL SET YOU FREE

If you've ever asked the question 'How can I lose weight and keep it off?' you're reading the right book. But from now on, forget about weight loss and adopt the 'AGGRESSIVE HEALTH' mentality. What good is weight loss if your body isn't operating at its best? What good is weight loss if your brain isn't functioning more coherently? What good is weight loss if your bloodstream isn't crackling with electricity? What good is weight loss if you run your enzyme supply down to a level that can damage your health? What good is weight loss if you end up with weak joints, sagging muscles and multiple aches and pains? You'll understand more about these concepts later, for now, ask a different quality of question:

How can I begin today to make simple changes that guarantee UNRIVALLED HEALTH, OUTSTANDING LEVELS OF ENERGY AND BOTH PHYSICAL AND MENTAL MASTERY?

Your aim is to learn the most cutting edge strategies to get your body working as perfectly as possible. That is where we are headed. A word of warning though. To opt out of the eating habits of the herd does require a certain degree of self-discipline. Remember – Many people are being paid billions of dollars to advertise and market products that can destroy your health. Whether it is pharmaceutical drugs found at your local chemist, nutritionally deficient foods in supermarkets or just friends who want you to be like them, the opportunities to stray off course are everywhere. People will challenge you and your new habits for many reasons. It's up to you to develop momentum and hold on tight to your vision. As you do your life will never be the same again. Remember one thing. When you get it right – it's easy. That's where we're headed and changing the habits of a lifetime can be easy if you have enough reasons to begin. That is the power of AGGRESSIVE HEALTH. Each principle builds upon the last creating an almost magical approach to health.

With the right foods you unlock the door to more than just optimal health. Some people have talked about being so highly 'charged' with energy that they've felt more connected to their religion or spiritual path. Whether this happens to you or not remains to be seen, but the kind of energy I'm talking about can only be built on a foundation of superior eating habits and superior lifestyle choices…

UNLEASHING THE AWESOME POWER OF YOUR RETICULAR ACTIVATING SYSTEM (RAS)

If you maintain your focus on the principles of AGGRESSIVE HEALTH something magical will happen. You'll mysteriously find yourself gravitating towards anything and everything that can help you achieve your goals. Why? Because of a unique part of your brain called your Reticular Activating System (RAS). Your RAS simply determines what you notice and what you pay attention to. It is responsible for the screening of data into your mind. You see……even as you sit quietly……reading this book……there are countless pieces of information……you could focus on……you could focus on the temperature of your left toe……or the tightness of the clothes you are wearing ……or you could focus on the sounds around you…… and how they are affecting you……you may even focus entirely…… on the words you are reading……or the whiteness of the page……as you read.

You are constantly being bombarded by infinite amounts of data. Now, your conscious mind can only focus on a limited number of elements at any one time, whilst your brain decides what *not* to pay attention to. It does this by focusing on what you believe to be of importance, whilst ignoring the irrelevant. This is where your RAS comes in. If you buy a new item of clothing or a car for example, don't you find that you begin to see it everywhere! Do you think it didn't exist before? Of course not! The reality is that it probably did, you just weren't paying attention. Your RAS wasn't sensitised to its existence.

Now, when you focus exclusively on the compelling vision you have for yourself and being the best you can be, your brain will delete all the information that isn't necessary for the attainment of your goal, and highlight what you need to know in order to fully succeed. It's up to you to SPECIFY exactly what you want and activate your RAS. Think about it now. Start by making a mental image of what you'll look like and be like once you've achieved some of your goals. See yourself having finished reading AGGRESSIVE HEALTH. See yourself applying all the principles successfully and easily. See yourself the way you want. Make the picture big and bright and appealing so that you feel like charging at it right now. Feel a burning desire to do everything you can to become what you see. Tell yourself how much energy you want in a voice that is seductive and alluring. Let yourself know what time you want to wake up in the morning and how excellent you want to feel. Let yourself know that you want to squeeze the maximum amount of juice out of life whilst bathing in the pleasure of empowering emotions. The more appealing you make this image, the easier it will be for your brain to highlight what you need to do in order to achieve this kind of success. This is your vision! This is what creates the drive inside of you to succeed. Now back it up with a thunderous voice that reverberates through every cell of your being, "OK... Let the games begin!"

All you need now is that carnivorous look in your eye as you watch the image of your goals tuck their tail between their legs and walk towards their master. This is called a minor shift in perception! With a compelling vision you'll begin to notice everything around you that can assist you. People will start showing up that can assist you in your quest, articles in magazines may reinforce something you are about to learn and before long you may start meeting people that have also read this book and can share with you their own experiences. I know this may seem like a strange way of thinking, but by the time you've finished AGGRESSIVE HEALTH it'll make perfect sense.

WHAT YOU ARE ABOUT TO LEARN WILL CHANGE THE WAY YOU PERCIEVE FOOD FOREVER

Before long, a sprouted bean or seed won't be something you associate with a Chinese takeaway, but a source of 'live' enzyme rich nutrition that will help you take your health to a whole new level. An avocado won't just be something you can make guacamole from, but an insulin decreasing hormonal delight that can help you lose unnecessary fat. The hemp seed won't be something you associate to smoking 'dope' but a source of unrivalled nutrition that will supply you with the most absorbable form of protein known to mankind.

Your RAS is responsible for pointing you in the direction you want to go. Just take a look at the people who spend their whole life focusing on 'low fat' foods. When they go into the supermarket, that's all they're aware of! Their RAS is sensitised to them, but who says that low-fat food is healthy? Did you know that certain types of fat are as critical to your health as enzymes, vitamins and minerals? In fact, by not including certain fats in your diet, you immediately open the door to illness and disease. Many diets limit what you can eat, restricting your choice, but rather than taking anything away, AGGRESSIVE HEALTH gives you...

FREEDOM: EXPANDING YOUR CHOICE AND FLEXIBILITY

With AGGRESSIVE HEALTH you get to eat foods you never knew existed. With AGGRESSIVE HEALTH you get to experiment with ideas and concepts you never new existed. What you are about to learn is how food affects your body with laser-like precision. Once you've mastered a few simple concepts, you'll begin to learn about the power of Circular Strength Training™, kettlebell swinging and other peak performance approaches to exercise that will make you want to train, not just sit on your backside thinking about it. Then I'll open the doorway to the power of mind technology for stress free living and invite you in. Let me tell you something. Where you are headed is light years beyond anything you've experienced before. You may think this is all hype, but I can assure you that by the time reach the last few pages of AGGRESSIVE HEALTH, you'll know you've struck gold in buying this book. You'll be feeling so good, you won't want to make room for anything else. You'll know first hand how *you* function at *your* best.

FOOD: THE MOST POWERFUL PRESCRIPTION
KNOWN TO MANKIND

Every time you eat or drink something you give your body a very powerful set of highly specific instructions. Your biochemistry changes to accommodate what you've put in your system and your hormonal responses adjust accordingly. The same happens when you take a prescription from a doctor. When you swallow a pill or a medicine, your body has a response to the medication, just as it does to food.

Remember there is one prescription you must follow for the rest of your life if you want to thrive. Get plenty of sunlight, move your body regularly, breathe as much fresh air as you can, drink plenty of fresh filtered water and understand and use food as if it was the most powerful prescription in existence. Use the prescription wisely and you'll succeed beyond your wildest dreams. Use it sloppily and you may wake up one day in hospital, knocking at death's door, hoping that the reaper gives you another chance to make things right. It's that simple!

NO DIET SYSTEM IS PERFECT, BUT YOU ARE!

There's no such thing as a perfect diet, but there does exist a variety of foods that when eaten in the right proportions will make you feel better than you could possibly imagine. The good news is that it's easy.

Dr Roger Williams, author of Biochemical individuality found that the pepsin content of gastric juice among normal adults varied at least a thousand fold! A THOUSAND FOLD! This highlights the importance of finding the right diet for you, not just putting your faith in the next best-selling diet plan. Remember, until you've experienced exceptional health – you have no idea what it is. But once you find your own ideal personal fuel mix (which will be unique to you) you'll begin to thrive.

Remember, YOU are the only one who matters; YOU are the only one who knows when YOU feel excellent.

ARE YOU READY FOR THE CHALLENGE?

So there you have it. You make a decision, you make a commitment, you take responsibility, you create a vision that propels you forward, and you find yourself drooling with desire to achieve everything you want. All you need to do now is go for it. Two weeks of following the principles of AGGRESSIVE HEALTH should excite you. Take a look why:

1. Razor sharp thinking and pure mental clarity. As you begin to include a variety of superfoods in your diet and select the foods that maintain tight control of your blood sugar levels, you'll find yourself developing laser-like concentration as you wave good-bye to mental haziness and afternoon slumps.

2. Unlimited energy and vibrancy. As you begin to appreciate the role of chlorophyll-rich foods and their powerful balancing effects, you'll begin to rebuild your blood and rebalance your body. How would you like to feel more refreshed and alert in the morning and more energised throughout the day, EVERY DAY?

3. Look in the mirror with admiration as your shape changes before your very eyes. Don't expect to shed all of your excess weight in the first week! But do expect to lose about 1 to 2 pounds of fat and about 2 to 3 pounds of retained water. A week from now you could be 5 or more pounds lighter. You'll have control over your insulin levels (an excess of which can cause water retention) and be more balanced hormonally. Then it will only be a matter of time before you develop the body of your dreams!

4. Connect with your deepest feelings of wellbeing, joy and vibrancy. Electrolyte deficiencies can cause people to experience a whole host of problems. A week from now however, you can feel more balanced, more in control and more motivated. Why? Because you'll reintroduce powerful alkalising minerals into your body allowing you to function at your very best.

5. Eliminate cravings. AGGRESSIVE HEALTH will motivate you to eat nutrient dense super foods that are right for you. In the process you'll automatically experience less cravings as you meet all your nutritional requirements and optimise brain chemistry. Once you've taken care of that, you can concentrate on charging at life, spending time doing what you love!

6. Fine-tune your insulin levels. You'll learn shortly how the over-stimulation of insulin can destroy your body, leading to obesity, diabetes and heart disease. Fortunately, recent studies from Harvard medical school have shown that by eating in accordance with the principles of hormonal control, insulin-controlling benefits kick in almost immediately.

7. Rebuild your body with the most advanced exercises known to man. As you begin to learn about Circular Strength Training™, kettlebell training and the most effective body weight exercises known to man, you'll realise how quickly you can begin to sculpt you own body into something that not only looks better than ever, but also allows you to adapt to any environment. You will open the gateway to total body freedom as you master this critical piece of the AGGRESSIVE HEALTH puzzle.

8. Eliminate stress and develop a powerful mind. In the final section, once you've mastered the basics and find yourself crackling with energy and more motivated than you've ever been, you'll learn how to direct this energy in ways that enhance your brain and revolutionise your life. This is where the rubber meets the road. This is when you begin to EVOLVE at an accelerated rate. Prepare to sharpen your instincts and become systematic in your approach to health.

That's all I have to say for now. Let's get down to business and begin our journey into the realm of AGGRESSIVE HEALTH. Have fun, experiment like never before and maybe one day we'll get the chance to meet each other.

PART ONE

HOW TO BUILD AN UNSHAKABLE FOUNDATION THAT GUARANTEES EXPLOSIVE HEALTH FOR A LIFETIME

CHAPTER 1

SEND SHOCKWAVES THROUGH YOUR BODY BY HARNESSING THE MOST POWERFUL FORCE ON EARTH – NATURE

Sit back. Take a deep breath and relax. Imagine yourself in the future. You feel different. You feel more alive. You feel like you did when you were a child, full of zest and vitality, but the feeling is more powerful. You feel as if you've somehow been granted perfect health. You look in the mirror and notice a body that is slim and firm. You look closely at your skin and find it hard to find a single blemish. Your hair is rich and full. Your eyes twinkle and sparkle and you feel incredible!

As your bloodstream crackles with electricity, your immune system effortlessly destroys foreign invaders. Every part of your being is working beautifully and in harmony like the philharmonic orchestra. Your life seems effortless and blissfully joyful, and your mind is full of good humour and joy!

The future can be inspiring, can't it? But the future isn't somewhere you go, it is a place you create from the decisions you make every moment of every day.

ACCEPT NATURE'S LAW AND
ADOPT THE MINDSET OF A CHAMPION

Let's not pussyfoot around the subject anymore. If you want superior health, you must eat superior foods. Everything your body is made of was once the air you breathed, the water you drank, and most importantly the food you ate. Your body is programmed to turn matter into energy and energy back into matter. In simple terms, the colloidal mineral structure of your body is built out of the foods that have passed your lips. Any simple change to your nutrition habits will alter the look and function of your body and more importantly your brain. Hunt out and eat the finest foods available and you'll dramatically improve the foundation upon which your body is built. Finding the right fuel mix for your body is essential for success, but at the heart of true health is an understanding that must be embraced if you are ever to truly master AGGRESSIVE HEALTH.

COMMON SENSE SEPARATES TRUTH FROM FICTION

If you want to destroy something, set fire to it! If you want to destroy the vital elements within any food, cook it! The more heat - the more destruction!

♦   Temperatures of 118 degrees Fahrenheit or more destroy critical enzymes within food. The result: Digestion can suffer and food can travel, undigested, into your small intestine, where it putrefies, poisoning your blood. Enzymes are critical to life and need to be present within food for optimal digestion.
♦   Cooking leaches minerals out of food. Nobody has studied the effect of minerals as extensively as Dr. Joel Wallach. He has performed 17500 autopsies on 454 species and on 3000 humans and has proved they all died of some sort of mineral deficiency. He was nominated in 1991 for the Nobel Prize in Medicine.
♦   Cooking also destroys vitamins, which are needed to control the absorption and use of minerals.
♦   Whenever fat is cooked, transfatty acids are produced. Transfatty acids are one of the most destructive elements of any cooked food diet. They decrease testosterone, increase abnormal sperm, and interfere with pregnant animals. They are a major source of damaging free radicals and research shows that chefs who spend time wok or pan-frying have a higher incidence of lung cancer.
♦   When you eat cooked food, your body has to release copious amounts of enzymes in order to break down the food. Without enzymes, your food would never digest. According to Dr Edward Howell, your enzyme supply is limited and cooked food eventually runs it down to dangerously low levels.

Are you shocked? Do you immediately want to eliminate ALL cooked food from your diet? Well, you don't have to! This chapter is simply a wake-up call designed to open your mind and get you thinking in new directions. All you need to do for now is begin considering the importance of raw 'living' foods and superfoods (see appendix 1). As you'll soon learn, if they don't form the foundation of your diet, you'll have no foundation at all.

HUMANITY'S MOST IMPORTANT BATTLE:
RAW FOOD VERSUS COOKED FOOD

In their book, Goldot, Lewis E. Cook Jr. and Junko Yasui recount a very powerful study. The study was performed on three groups of rats and the results were fascinating. Take a look for yourself before you come to the same conclusions as the researchers.

GROUP ONE

From birth, the first group of rats were fed a raw diet of fruits, vegetables, nuts, and whole grains. As they grew they experienced every sign of good health. They grew fast. They had strong bodies. They were free from disease. They were also free from excess fat. They reproduced with vigour and enthusiasm and paved the way for their healthy offspring. They were vivacious, spirited, and very affectionate to one another. As soon as they reached the equivalent of 80 human years they were put to sleep and autopsied. Researchers found that every organ, every gland, and every tissue was in perfect condition. A diet of raw food prevented them from experiencing the 'normal' signs of ageing and degeneration.

GROUP TWO

From birth, this unlucky group of rats was fed a diet of cooked foods: Milk, meat, white bread, soda, sweets, cakes, vitamins and medicines. As they grew they experienced many of the same diseases that afflict people in present day society such as colds, fevers, pneumonia, poor eyesight, cataracts, heart disease, arthritis, cancer, etc. But it wasn't just their biological health that was on the line. Their emotional health was also very unstable as they constantly attacked each other. They gave birth to offspring that were constantly ill and aggressive. Death came prematurely to this group from diseases or various epidemics that swept through the entire colony. Autopsies revealed extensive degeneration to every organ, every gland, and every tissue of their bodies. The researchers had found a very impressive way to accelerate the speed in which the rats aged – by feeding them a diet similar to what most humans eat. The rats paid the ultimate price – early death from disease.

GROUP THREE

From birth, this group was fed the same foods as Group Two until they reached an equivalent human age of 40. They displayed behavioural characteristics identical to those in the previous group and had the same poor quality of health. At the end of this 'equivalent 40 year period' the rats were placed on a strict water fast for a number of days before being introduced to a 100% raw food diet, coupled with periods of fasting. The changes were dramatic. Within one month they began showing signs of exceptional health. They became affectionate, playful and more resilient to infection, showing no signs of illness or disease. At the end of an 'equivalent 80 year period', autopsies revealed that this group had completely reversed all biological signs of ageing. Every organ, every gland, and every tissue was in perfect condition.

WARNING: IF THE FOUNDATION OF YOUR DIET ISN'T BUILT ON RAW LIVING FOODS – THERE IS NO FOUNDATION

You hold in your hands a very powerful book, one that will shatter many illusions about health and the origins of disease. Be patient. Tread carefully. Learn. Discover. Digest. For every disciplined effort in life there is a multiple reward.

THE POWER OF ENZYME RICH RAW FOOD
AND THE PERILS OF ENZYME-LESS COOKED FOOD

In the 1930s, Dr Paul Kouchakoff demonstrated that after eating cooked food, there is an increase in the mobilisation of white blood cells in the body, a phenomenon called 'digestive leukocytosis'.

When faced with *too much* enzyme-less cooked food, your body will recruit white blood cells (leukocytes) to transport a large quantity of enzymes, for the task of breaking down food particles. In other words, when your body is unable to properly digest food, white blood cells will attack the food, in an effort to reduce it to usable components or eliminate it from the body. Until Kouchakoff's work, this was considered normal but Kouchakoff found that when foods are consumed in their raw state, digestive leukocytosis does not occur. Raw foods have just the right amount of natural enzymes/nutrients within them to allow them to perfectly self-digest within your digestive system. This leads to better digestion and assimilation. The message is simple:

♦   Processed food and cooked food reliably triggers off leukocyte mobilisation.
♦   Raw 'living' foods have no such effect.
♦   When you add raw 'living' foods to any meal you reduce leukocyte mobilisation dramatically.

WARNING: YOUR BODY FIGHTS
COOKED FOOD LIKE A DISEASE

F.M. Pottenger conducted a 10-year study on the effect of a cooked food diet on an animal's life cycle. Pottenger raised a colony of 900 cats placed on controlled diets. He fed them only meat and milk, either raw or cooked. Those fed on raw food produced healthy kittens every year without fail. Those fed on the cooked version of the exact same food developed the same diseases which afflict humanity, including heart disease, cancer, osteoporosis, sexual impotency, paralysis, pneumonia, glandular malfunctioning, kidney disease, arthritis, difficulty in labour and severe irritability. Take a look at what happened to each generation of cats fed on the cooked food diet:

1.   The first generation of kittens were ill and abnormal.
2.   The second generation was born either already diseased or dead.
3.   The mothers of the third generation were sterile.

Pottenger discovered that the damage created by cooked food requires four generations of raw foodism to correct. The faeces produced by the cats eating a cooked food diet caused plants to become stunted and weak. The faeces produced by the cats eating a raw food diet caused plants to grow normally. Cooked food addiction has a long-lasting effect on the future generation of our planet. As corny as it sounds, when you take responsibility for yourself, you begin to heal 'mother earth'.

WARNING: COOKED FOOD CAUSES YOUR ORGANS TO WORK FIVE TIMES THEIR NORMAL CAPACITY AND EXHAUST PREMATURELY

It's about time more and more people questioned the use of cooked food in their diet, including you. You don't have to eliminate it entirely, but it is no foundation on which to build superior health.

As you'll realise in the next few chapters, there exists a number of superfoods, that when consumed in their raw state have tremendous potential to maximise the electrical charge around each and every one of your cells. That's where we're headed.

Once you've experienced their true power you'll look at cooked food differently. You'll still want to eat certain foods, because they'll be critical in completing your own personal fuel mixture. When you do select these foods, you'll be doing so CONSCIOUSLY – not just because you are a victim of the sales and marketing tactics orchestrated to suck you in and part with your hard earned cash.

BEGINNING THE ULTIMATE BALANCING ACT

If raw plant foods are going to take pride of place in your diet, you're probably wondering where to start, how to keep variety in your diet and how to make it easy. The answer to all these questions will be presented to you in the next few chapters as you learn the organising principles of exceptional health. Whether you decide to overhaul your diet, modify your routine, or make some powerful yet minor changes, all will be revealed. For an immediate insight, go to Appendix 1.

LOOKING TO THE FUTURE WITH A GLINT IN YOUR EYE

It doesn't matter if your vision is to eat a 100% raw food diet, or to simply include a few of the finest raw superfoods in your diet. What does matter is that 'live' mineral rich foods become your No.1 priority. A diet plan can be as complicated as you want, but if the foundation isn't built on raw 'living' foods, eventually it will fail. This is what you have to look forward to:

♦ How to restore balance to an over-acidic system and guarantee explosive health, right from the word 'GO'!
♦ Which foods to select to supply maximum nutrition for all of your endeavours.
♦ How to balance the key hormones of your body to maximise fat loss.
♦ How to decrease stress hormones and enhance youth accelerating hormones.
♦ How to optimise neurotransmitter equilibrium within your brain, fostering a more alert, vibrant, ambitious state of mind.
♦ How to burn parasites out of your body and eliminate mucoid plaque.
♦ How to restore a balanced internal flora encouraging optimal digestion.
♦ How to prevent cravings and maximise the life and vitality of every cell in your body.

MAXIMISE NUTRIENT UPTAKE WITH RAW-GANIC FOOD

Never question the power of raw organic plant food! Back in 1993, Bob Smith, a trace minerals laboratory analyst began purchasing samples of both organic and commercial plant foods. He wanted to know why organic foods were getting so much attention, and if that attention was warranted. For over two years he studied each of his samples for trace elements. Take a look at his conclusions and decide for yourself whether raw organic plant food should take pride of place in your diet:

1. Organically grown pears had two to nearly three times more chromium, iodine, manganese, molybdenum, silicon, and zinc.
2. Organically grown corn had twenty times more calcium and manganese, and two to five times more copper, magnesium, molybdenum, selenium and zinc.
3. Organically grown wheat had twice the calcium, four times more magnesium, five times more manganese, and 13 times more selenium than the commercial wheat.
4. Organically grown potatoes had two or more times the boron, selenium, silicon, strontium, and sulphur, and 60% more zinc.

His other findings were that organic foods also had lower quantities of toxic trace elements, such as aluminium, lead, and mercury. There's usually a section in every supermarket now where you can buy organic cooked food such as organic biscuits, crisps etc. Organic food is not enough, foods must be 'raw-ganic' if you want the very best.

SPICE UP YOUR FOOD AND SPICE UP YOUR LIFE

If you want to build an unshakeable foundation, some of your meals must tickle you taste buds and have you drooling for more. From Italy to the Far East or from France to Mexico, you'll find every culture has its own preferred style and own preferred blend of herbs and spices that create distinctive textures and flavours. But don't think that ALL you meals have to be appealing to the eye and senses. A simple meal made with superior foods can be just as important as a 'Cordon Blue' delight. Begin experimenting today!

♦   Chinese: Anise, garlic, and ginger
♦   French: Bay leaves, garlic, rosemary, tarragon, and thyme
♦   Greek: Cinnamon, garlic, mint and oregano
♦   Indian: Cardamom, coriander seeds, cumin, curry, fenugreek, ginger, mustard seeds, and turmeric
♦   Italian: Basil, bay leaves, fennel seeds, garlic, marjoram, oregano, red pepper flakes, rosemary and sage
♦   Mexican: Chilli, cilantro, cinnamon, cumin, coriander, and oregano
♦   Middle eastern: Cinnamon, cumin, garlic, mint, parsley, and oregano

Herbalists know that spices can help with ailments as diverse as stomach problems, toothache and chilblains. In response to hot and spicy food, your brain produces pain-killing endorphins that promote a mini-euphoric high! More about this phenomenon later.

ARE YOU READY FOR THE CHALLENGE?

No stone is left unturned when it comes to understanding how various foods affect your magical being. Knowledge is power and this chapter is only the beginning. Start today and remember one thing. If you've spent your whole life trying to lose unwanted fat, or trying to get control of your health, or trying to break the barriers of a personal best, let the struggle come to a grinding halt! What you've done in the past may have had some degree of success, but what you are learning now will exhaust every avenue necessary, allowing you to become an unrivalled success. Be the best you've ever been. Now is the time and this is the book.

Over a short period of time, a diet rich in raw, living foods will accelerate your progress towards scintillating health. Here's why:

♦ You'll begin to radiate more energy. Andre Simoneton found that we radiate more energy if we eat foods that also give off a high level of radiance. Examples are chlorophyll rich greens, wheatgrass juice, Blue Green algae, organic vegetables/fruits and sprouted nuts, seeds, pulses and grains along with many mineral rich raw superfoods and juices.

♦ Raw foods cleanse your body of stored wastes and toxins. These wastes interfere with the proper functioning of cells and organs and are responsible for lowering your energy.

♦ Raw foods restore optimal sodium/potassium and acid/alkaline balance allowing you to increase the charge of electricity around every cell in your body. More about this later.

♦ Raw foods offer, in perfect and complementary combination, all the nutrients essential for maximum vitality at the cellular level. If you doubt the quality of the foods you buy from the supermarket, you can invest in an inexpensive superfood that will make up the deficit. See Appendix 1 – AGGRESSIVE HEALTH Superfoods and goto www.aggressivehealth.co.uk for more information.

♦ Raw foods increase the efficiency with which your cells take up oxygen. Oxygen is necessary for your cells to release energy and carry out an infinite number of critical life processes.

♦ Raw foods increase the micro-electrical potential of your cells, improving your body's use of oxygen, energising your muscles and brain.

♦ You'll begin to unlock nature's pharmacy, as you tap into the unlimited storehouse of phytochemicals (plant chemicals) present within plant foods. Phytochemicals not only prevent many diseases, but virtually guarantee unrivalled health. To maximise your phytochemical intake, focus on a variety of colourful raw foods. Did you know that scientists have found over 10,000 vital nutrients in an apple? Do you think you'll get all of them in a vitamin pill?

♦ One research group found that people who ate a lot of fibre – via raw fruits and vegetables – excreted more calories on a daily basis than those on a cooked diet of the same caloric content but without the fibre.

♦ Forget calorie counting once and for all. It is impossible to put on extra fat content by eating raw foods alone. More about this later!

♦ Raw foods prevent a build up of waste matter between the target tissue within your cells and the protective endothelial cells that are in direct contact with the bloodstream. This space, known as the interstitial space needs to be kept clear to allow optimal exchange of nutrients and hormones. More about hormones later!

♦ Did you know that the number of old cells being replaced on a day to day basis is between 300 billion and 800 billion? The difference – approximately 500 billion! That's a big difference, especially if you can influence it! And the only way to prevent such dramatic losses is to minimise cooked/processed food and replace them with raw-ganic foods.

♦ Raw plant foods are easily digested, and within only 24-36 hours pass easily through your digestive tract. Cooked/dead foods in comparison take 40-100+ hours and can clog your system.

♦ There are distinct physiological differences between animals that feed exclusively on raw foods and animals that feed on cooked foods. Shouldn't they be biologically identical if both food types have the same physiological effect?

Instinctively, I want you to realise that raw foods and superfoods are the no.1 priority for your body. Not the ONLY priority, but the No.1 priority. You may still eat cooked foods when you choose, in order to complete your ultimate fuel mix, but you'll always be motivated to reach for raw, living, vibrant foods as the foundation to your diet.

Roll up your sleeves, sharpen your knives, clear some space in your refrigerator, and let's begin. It's up to you to take action to create momentum. Begin slowly and remember, wherever you go and whatever you do, always search for foods that ultimately create biochemical harmony in your body. The choice is yours, dead food and a lifeless body, or live raw food and a vibrant body.

THE AGGRESSIVE HEALTH EVALUATION:
Do you eat a variety of colourful raw foods every day?
Have you begun creating your own favourite vegetable juices?
Do you ensure the foods you eat are delicious and mouth watering?
Do you use nutrient dense superfoods for the nutritional insurance needed for
AGGRESSIVE HEALTH?

When you begin any life-changing program, you need momentum! You need to ensure that every action you take propels you towards unlimited success. With this kind of momentum you go far and you go fast. Let the journey begin...

CHAPTER 2

DISCOVER THE HEALTH SECRETS OF THE GODS WITH ELECTRICALLY CHARGED GREENS AND ALKALISING VEGETABLE JUICES

Until man duplicates a blade of grass,
Nature can laugh at his so-called scientific knowledge.
– Thomas A. Edison

Whether you want to increase your strength and body mass, lose unwanted fat or increase your general health, begin loading your diet with green leafy vegetables. Constipated? – Eat more greens. Want more iron? – Eat more greens. Want more calcium – Eat more greens. Think about it, where does a cow get her calcium from for her milk? Mineral-rich green grass! I don't expect you to begin grazing in the nearest field, but I do expect you to begin seeing the magic inherent within green leafy vegetables. This chapter will open your eyes to their true power. Chlorophyll-rich foods and juices are the blood of life and critical building blocks in the foundation of AGGRESSIVE HEALTH.

NATURES No.1 SUPERFOOD FOR RESTORING BALANCE TO A WEAK AND TIRED BODY

Before you sneak off in the middle of the night, rob your local farmer, and load up on greens, let me introduce you to one of nature's most remarkable gifts. Imagine a super-food so potent and so densely packed with nutrition, that it could, if it had to, supply almost all your nutritional needs. Imagine a super-food teeming with essential amino acids, essential fatty acids, enzymes, glucose, vitamins, minerals, phytochemicals, along with powerful blood building/cancer fighting qualities. Imagine no more. Wheatgrass juice has the power to reconstruct your body into a temple of exuberance and youth. Drink it often, and it won't be long before the air around you is crackling with electricity!

Dr. Arthur Robinson, director of the Oregon Institute of Science and Medicine credits wheatgrass as having the most preventative and restorative properties known to mankind.

In 1978 at the Linus Pauling Institute, Dr. Robinson completed a research project in which wheatgrass and live foods were fed to mice with squamous cell carcinoma (a cancer that develops in levels of the epidermis that are closer to the body's surface. They commonly appear on sun-exposed areas of the body such as the face, ear, neck, lip and back of the hands.)

Dr. Robinson's excitement was clear, "The results were spectacular. Living foods alone (including wheatgrass) decreased the incidence and severity of cancer lesions by about 75%. This result was better than that of any other nutritional program."

CANCER: OXYGEN DEFICIENCY AT ITS WORST

1 in 3 people now die from cancer, but does it have to be this way? Even whilst the struggle continues, a German biochemist, Dr Otto Warburg, won a Nobel Prize for his research into cancer and oxygen. He discovered that cancer cells thrive in an oxygen-poor environment and concluded that cancer is nothing but the process of cell mutation caused by oxygen deprivation on the cellular level. Even though he arrived at this discovery more than fifty years ago, his theory has never been discredited.

DO YOU WANT TO INCREASE THE OXYGEN CARRYING CAPACITY OF YOUR BLOOD?

Wheatgrass juice is your answer! Do you remember the last time you cut yourself? Do you remember seeing *red oxygen rich blood?* The reason it was red is because of the pigment Haemoglobin, but haemoglobin is more that just a pigment, it brings life to every part of your body. And in the same way, chlorophyll is the *green oxygen rich pigment* that brings life to plants. Think of chlorophyll as 'green plant blood'!

In 1930, Dr Hans Fisher and a group of associates won the Nobel Prize, after making a groundbreaking discovery. Their work was based around the mysteries of the red blood cell. To their amazement they found that on a molecular level, haemoglobin in human blood is practically identical to chlorophyll (plant blood). The ONLY difference between the two pigments is that chlorophyll has a core of magnesium, whilst haemoglobin has a core of iron.

The resemblance between the two is so striking that:

- When crude chlorophyll is fed to rabbits with anaemia (low serum iron count) it restores normal red blood cell counts within approximately 15 days and is completely non toxic.
- A simple injection of crude chlorophyll increases red blood cell counts in healthy animals that already have normal haemoglobin levels.

USING THE POWER OF NATURE TO CURE ANAEMIA

Are you anaemic? As many as 30% of all women beyond the age of puberty in the United States may be anaemic. For men the rate of anaemia begins to increase by age 50. The major symptoms of anaemia are fatigue and loss of appetite and these symptoms usually coincide with deficiencies of various nutrients, such as B12, folic acid, iron, copper, potassium and protein.

In 1936, research into the power of chlorophyll went one step further. Scientists J.H. Hughs and A.L. Latner of the University of Liverpool conducted some groundbreaking experiments. In their study, reported in the Journal of Physiology in 1936, they created a number of anaemic animals by bleeding them at regular intervals. Once the animals' haemoglobin levels were slashed in half, they were divided into ten different groups.

- Five of the groups were fed various types of chlorophyll in their diet.
- The other five groups of control animals were fed no chlorophyll.

The animals that received *raw, unrefined* chlorophyll experienced a regeneration of their blood haemoglobin levels 50% above average. In less than two weeks their blood haemoglobin levels were normal! The group receiving synthetic chlorophyll made no marked improvements, highlighting that only *raw, unrefined* chlorophyll can be converted into haemoglobin. Synthetic versions created by decomposing natural chlorophyll and combining it with a copper ion proved to be incredibly stable, but CAUSED nausea and anaemia rather than curing it!

EMBRACE AGGRESSIVE HEALTH TODAY WITHOUT WASTING MONEY ON USELESS SUPPLEMENTS

When compared to many of today's expensive supplements, wheatgrass is not only far superior, but easy to grow and easy to use. Simply take a handful of wheat berries, some water, a tray filled with an inch of topsoil and a cover. Within seven days at a cost of 7p a tray, you'll have enough wheatgrass to juice. Drink it daily and you'll maximise the charge of electricity around each and every one of your ten trillion cells. Wheatgrass juice is not only a superior source of chlorophyll, but also gives you a concentrated dose of high-quality water, oxygen, enzymes, phytochemicals, carotenoids, fatty acids, trace minerals, antioxidants and amino acids. If you want to stand out from the crowd, with a glint in your eye and a magic about your aura – drink wheatgrass juice. It is alive, and brings life to your body in every way. It will help you to release an unnatural build up of excess fats and mineral deposits. It will also help you to release proteins trapped in your blood, organs and bowel. Every element within wheatgrass juice rushes to revitalise your entire being! Awesome!

YOU ARE ONLY AS YOUNG AS YOUR BLOOD

Dr Bernard Jensen, author of 'Chlorophyll Magic From Living Plant Food' has used green juices and wheatgrass juice to treat low serum iron counts and toxic conditions of the blood, with unrivalled success. He was able to double patients' red blood cell count in a matter of days, by prescribing 'chlorophyll water baths' and including green juices such as wheatgrass juice into their diet. If your blood is rich in iron, it will deliver more oxygen to your cells.

According to Dr Yoshihide Hagiwara's research, it is the fat solubility of chlorophyll that allows it to be converted directly into haemoglobin in the lymphatic system. Chlorophyll-rich foods invigorate every fibre of your being, injecting you with life and energy.

PERFORM AT YOUR BEST
IN SPITE OF DEADLY POLLUTION

WARNING: OUR FOOD, AIR AND WATER IS CONTAMINATED
Unless you have a proven system to detoxify your body on a *DAILY* basis you may be in great danger! Many pollutants are carcinogenic, responsible for the rise in cancer, whilst others are capable of altering genes or DNA, affecting future generations. If you want to increase the strength and resistance of your body so you can co-exist with them, rather than be devastated by them, pay close attention.

Wheatgrass juice acts like a detergent, purging the liver, scrubbing the intestinal tract and oxygenating blood. The elements within wheatgrass chelate and remove heavy metals from your body. Did you know that even your faecal matter is likely to have a higher heavy metal count after you've ingested wheatgrass juice, highlighting its eliminative power?

BANISH ACCELERATED AGEING
WITH WHEATGRASS ENZYMES

Did you know that at this very moment millions of enzymes are participating in thousands of never-ending chemical changes in your body? Without them you wouldn't be able to digest food, absorb nutrients, eliminate waste, repair damaged tissues or maintain a powerful immune system. Quite simply you'd be dead. Fortunately you can provide a powerful enzyme boost to your body with enzyme rich raw food, none more powerful than wheatgrass juice. Here is a list of the most important enzymes found in wheatgrass:

♦ Cytochrome oxidase - Your cells will become energised with this antioxidant required for proper cell respiration.

♦ Lipase - Your ability to digest fat will improve with the inclusion of this fat digesting enzyme.

♦ Protease - Your ability to digest and break down undigested protein remnants left in your digestive tract will improve as you increase the consumption of this protein digestant.

♦ Amylase - Your ability to digest starch will improve with the inclusion of this starch-digesting enzyme.

♦ Catalase and gluathione peroxide - You'll help prevent any unnecessary ageing with the inclusion of these two enzymes. They both reduce hydrogen peroxide to water before it can combine with another superoxide free radical to form the hydroxyl free radical, the most destructive of all free radicals.

♦ Transhydrogenase - You'll ensure a healthy heart by increasing the consumption of this enzyme since it helps in keeping the muscle tissue of the heart toned.

♦ Superoxide dimutase (SOD) - You'll discover the power of SOD shortly.

As you age, your body's natural production of these enzymes dwindles, reducing your ability to handle heavy fats, proteins, and excess calories. Imagine how bright your future will be as you include an early morning shot of wheatgrass juice into your routine. It'll cause your blood stream to dance and your heart to sing! The enzymes that are found in relatively high concentrations in normal red and white blood cells are cytochrome oxidase, peroxidase, and catalase, but in the body of a cancer patient these enzymes are of a dangerously low concentration. All cancer patients should focus on increasing their enzyme intake and there is no cheaper place to begin than with wheatgrass juice. The enzymes have been found to break down tumours and cysts. If you are interested in taking a powerful enzyme supplement to further enhance your health goto www.aggressivehealth.co.uk and begin investigating Vitälzym™.

DRUM ROLL PLEASE!
PRESENTING THE KEY ANTI-AGEING ENZYME: SOD

Dr. Barry Halliwell, a biochemist at the University of London, Dr. M. Rister, at the University of Cologne in Germany, and Dr. Irwin Fridovich, a biochemist at Duke University have all tested the power of SOD (superoxide dimutase) and each one of these three experts are excited at its potential. Firstly it helps slow down cellular ageing. It does this by neutralising the toxic effects of damaging superoxides that are naturally produced in every cell in your body. If the quantity of superoxides in the cell increases without a corresponding increase in SOD production you have a recipe for accelerated ageing.

TESTING THE ELDERLY FOR SOD

Ten senior citizens with an average age of 70 took part in an experiment where they had their blood levels of various nutrients tested before and after taking a wheat sprout supplement. Usually, senior citizens are slower to respond to such experiments, but in this case their serum levels of SOD increased by an average of 230% and by 730% in one individual. 7 out of the 10 more than doubled their blood levels of this powerful antioxidant.

FREEDOM FROM DAMAGING SUPEROXIDES

A life of exposure to radiation, pollution, drugs and chemical additives (found mostly in recreational foods), increases the number of harmful superoxides in and around your cells. This gradual accumulation of superoxides damages your fats, DNA, and overall cell structure.

Have you ever met someone who told you they were 40 years old, but looked 60? What about the opposite example – someone who looks 40 but is actually 60? The difference could be the devastating effect of superoxide free radical damage. Don't let this be you! Put the breaks on the ageing process and focus on Superoxide dimutase (SOD). SOD seeks out superoxide free radicals in your body and converts them to hydrogen peroxide. Catalase and glutathione peroxidase reduces hydrogen peroxide to water before it can combine with another superoxide free radical to form the hydroxyl free radical, the most destructive free radical of all. Does sound all too technical? Fear not! All you have to do is use this information to your advantage. If your daily habits are diminishing your body's supply of SOD, your cells can become poisonous and lose their ability to renew themselves, causing premature cellular death. Any abnormal cells in your body are likely to contain a greater number of superoxide free radicals, so it's your job to electrify your bloodstream with a daily dose of SOD rich wheatgrass juice or an equivalent superfood rich in SOD. For more information on equipment you can use to begin growing and harvesting wheatgrass or for any other powerful superfoods visit www.aggressivehealth.co.uk.

STARTING TODAY - A NEW BEGINNING!

Along with wheatgrass juice and other grass juices such as barley grass juice, eat, blend and juice as many different varieties of raw/wild organic greens as you can! Choose from herbs and big leafy green vegetables. All herbs have rejuvenating properties and some of the more common varieties, such as lettuce, celery, parsley, coriander (cilantro) etc. are very powerful foods. I juice a lot of spinach, kale, spring greens, parsley, cucumber and celery. Remember there isn't a laboratory in the world that is a complex as the one found within the photosynthetic green leaf organs of plants.

GO HUNTING FOR WILD GREENS
AND PREPARE FOR THE ULTIMATE 'HIGH'

The idea of eating and juicing more green-leafy vegetables, especially wild herbs, is to significantly alkalise your biochemistry and electrify your blood. But what does this REALLY mean? Most of the junk that lines the supermarket shelves (the coffees, cola, beer, spirits, pizza, chips, cake, sweets etc.) create an acidic environment. In an acidic environment, vital minerals are used up to neutralise the acid, oxygen levels are depleted and as a consequence energy plummets. At this point most people reach for another stimulant such as coffee or chocolate when all they need to do is begin to alkalise their body. This is where greens and vegetable juices exert their power. Use them daily and you can turn poor health into EXPLOSIVE HEALTH! If you want to feel a surge of electricity through your bloodstream and through you body, green foods are the answer.

Over time, let green vegetable juices step in to provide you with (what will feel like) rocket fuel to launch you into your day. But wait! There exists another superfood that has five times more chlorophyll than wheatgrass juice and a potent mineral content to match.

E3LIVE - NATURE'S MOST COMPLETE FOOD

Unlike fruits or vegetables that lose many of their vital nutrients during packing and transit, nature has created a food that grows thousands of miles from your door, but can be delivered to you frozen, maintaining every vital nutrient. This food is Aphanizomenon flos-aquae (AFA). It is a blue green algae grown/harvested in its natural state from the mineral rich waters of the Upper Klamath Lake in southern Oregon. It is genetically prepared for extreme alterations in temperature, especially in winter when parts of Klamath Lake freeze over. But when the weather warms up, the algae comes out of its frozen dormancy and resumes its active growth cycle. AFA algae is high in lipids and free fatty acids, which protect it from crystallising in low temperature conditions. Bee pollen works the same way, it can be frozen without losing any of its nutritional value. Marvellous!

WITH FIVE TIMES MORE CHLOROPHYLL THAN WHEATGRASS -
ENSURE YOU DON'T MISS OUT!

E3Live has the highest concentration of bio-assimilable chlorophyll than any other food. It has five times more chlorophyll than wheatgrass, twice as much as spirulina algae, and slightly more than chlorella algae. Chlorophyll is the lifeblood of AFA algae. According to biochemist Lita Lee, Ph.D.,

> "Chlorophyll appears to stimulate the regeneration of damaged liver cells, and increases circulation to all organs by dilating blood vessels. In the heart, chlorophyll aids in the transmission of nerve impulses that control

contraction. The heart rate is slowed, yet each contraction is increased in power, improving the efficiency of cardiac power."

E3Live is 100% AFA (Aphanizomenon Flos-Aquae). It is 60%+ protein, containing all the amino acids, making it 100% natural brain food. AFA algae is 97% absorbable by the body, contains every B vitamin (including B12) and every known trace mineral. AFA algae contains 10 to 50 times as many minerals as vegetables and is extremely rich in (hard to find) trace minerals, which you may be deficient in. Without trace minerals, many of your enzymic reactions can be compromised. E3Live is also abundant in enzymes, phytochemicals and essential fatty acids, especially the important Omega 3 fatty acids that you need for the formation of eicosanoids. You'll learn about these super-hormones in chapter 8.

DOCTORS ARE PRAISING THIS 'MIRACLE' FOOD

Dr Gabriel Cousins, M.D., holistic physician, psychiatrist and internationally respected author of the classic 'Conscious Eating' and 'Rainbow Green Live Food Cuisine' has incredible praise for E3Live – "There is no other blue green algae that is alive and active as E3Live. E3Live is the only really live algae we have now. The life force aspect of E3Live is probably the most important factor that singles it out. E3Live has the strongest possible effects, and represents a qualitative leap compared to any other algae coming out of Klamath Lake"

E3LIVE AND ATHLETIC PEAK PERFORMANCE

Many athletes have broken through their limits and gone on to achieve remarkable success in their chosen field by choosing E3Live as one of their preferred forms of nutrition. Do you want to join this elite group, who are smashing personal bests and becoming champions in their chosen endeavour? Here are just a few:

- Grant Hackett, Long Distance Swimmer, 2000 Olympic Gold Medal Winner in the 1500 meter freestyle.
- Ky Hurst – Australian Iron man Triathlete Champion.
- Mary Louise Zeller – 57 year old Tae Kwon Do US National Champion, Gold Medal International Champion competing against opponents 40 years younger.
- Lynne Taylor – Miss Natural Olympia 1999 – Drug-free World Champion Body-Builder – Mother of Four.
- Ryk Neethling – Olympic Swimmer and World Record Holder.

HORMONAL CONTROL AND BRAIN REGULATION –NORMALISE BLOOD SUGAR LEVELS WITH E3LIVE

E3Live is a valuable asset to anyone suffering with diabetes. The elements within it assist in the restoration of an over-worked pancreas. With its exceptional blood sugar balancing qualities, it helps eliminate the craving for alcohol and drugs whilst enhancing brain function (brain function is immediately optimised when blood sugar levels are stabilised. Chapter 11 will spill the beans on this subject.)

EXPEL PROZAC FROM THE EARTH –
USE E3LIVE TO RESTORE MENTAL HEALTH

E3Live is incredibly rich in amino acids, providing the necessary raw materials for the brain to manufacture serotonin-based neuro-transmitters. These go on to support the master glands of the entire endocrine system, creating a harmonious inner environment. You'll discover the power of neurotransmitters in chapter 14.

RESTORING BRAIN FUNCTION AND BALANCE
TO YOUR CENTRAL NERVOUS SYSTEM

The brains of drug addicts, sugar addicts and alcoholics are often functioning very poorly. They have unbalanced brain wave readings, and a lack of mood and memory control. By using E3Live along with other dietary changes, electroencephalogram (EEG) readings can be normalised, if not optimised, restoring balance to the central nervous system.

As long as someone's brain function is only 'sub-clinically' out of balance showing unbalanced EEG readings (and not dramatically out of balance like those who suffer epileptic seizures), E3Live can help to restore balance and harmony. There isn't a supplemental food as pure and natural as the AFA algae found in E3Live.

BOLSTERING UP YOUR IMMUNE SYSTEM WITH E3LIVE

A recent study showed that E3Live activates up to 40% more of the immune system's beneficial natural killer cells. These cells hunt out viruses and bacteria, even if they are deep within the body's tissues. According to Dr Gabriel Cousins, AFA algae has some anti-HIV effects, although more research needs to be done in these areas.

POWER UP YOUR VITAMIN B12 STATUS
AND MAXIMISE YOUR OXYGEN UPTAKE

AFA has the highest active vegetable source of vitamin B12, in a form that is totally usable by the body. It has 65 times more B12 than kelp and 700 times more B12 than alfalfa. Without enough vitamin B12 oxygen uptake is compromised and according to Dr. Otto Warburg, oxygen deprivation is the major cause of cancer.

The key difference between taking supplements and taking E3Live is that AFA algae is recognised by the body as food. This means it is immediately available with a greater than 90% assimilation rate. It is so powerful that NASA have been studying the algae as a possible food source for space missions, whilst Russians have used it to treat patients exposed to radiation in the Chernobyl nuclear disaster.

MAINTAINING THE CRITICAL
ACID/ALKALINE BALANCE IN YOUR BODY

Green leafy vegetables, wheatgrass and other grass juices, along with E3Live help to restore your body to a more favourable alkaline state. Too many people are suffering the perils of over acidification – BE UNIQUE and embrace the power of a balanced diet and become the king or queen of greens! Green leafy vegetables provide the necessary nutrition to prolong exceptional health and allow you to maintain an excellent calcium-phosphorus balance.

The best green leafed vegetables include:

> All wild edible greens and grasses (including wheatgrass juice), algae (blue-green, chlorella, and spirulina, these are alkaline green protein foods, they are not true leafy-vegetables, but can be used in this category). Bok choy, celery (very important, an excellent source of sodium), coriander (cilantro), crane's bill, collard, dandelion, dark green cabbage, endive, fennel (wild), kale (especially dinosaur kale), lamb's quarters (goose foot), lettuce (all types), malva, mustard (wild), parsley, spinach, spring onions (green), sunflower greens, wild radish, all green herbs.

If you find it impossible to get enough greens into your diet, you can also use a powerful green superfood supplement. There are many that are overpriced and lacking quality. For information on the latest and most health restoring green superfoods, along with E3Live contact me at www.aggressivehealth.co.uk. Take a look at Appendix 1 for more information.

ARE YOU READY FOR THE CHALLENGE?

AGGRESSIVE HEALTH begins by building a powerful foundation for success. First you make your positive addictions and then you spit out your negative ones. Throughout our journey together you'll discover which foods are best and why. You'll learn to work with them, play with them and experiment like never before until you discover what you enjoy and what works for you.

In the absence of light there's darkness, and these early principles shine the light of nutritional success down upon you. Look to the light and you won't see the shadows. Look to the light and your old negative addictions will fade away and be forgotten!

Wheatgrass juice, E3Live or any raw green juice/superfood should be the first thing you drink in the morning, and the last thing you drink at night. You'll feel it rushing through your body every time you drink it, raising the hair on the back of your neck. Here's a re-cap why:

♦ Numerous experiments on animal and human subjects have shown chlorophyll to be effective in treating anaemia (a low serum iron count).

- Green vegetables contain every amino acid necessary for a life of vitality. These amino acid chains (polypeptides), are absorbed directly into your blood, and can neutralise toxic substances like cadmium, nicotine, strontium, mercury, and polyvinyl chloride, by changing them into insoluble salts that your body can eliminate more easily.
- Green vegetables are both rapidly assimilated by your body and help stimulate cellular metabolism.
- Green vegetables are rich supplies of bioflavinoids and used to help cleanse the blood and tissues, detoxifying cells and preventing their deterioration.
- Green vegetables will cause your blood vessels to dilate, leading to an increase in overall blood flow. The delivery of nutrients to your cells will be enhanced, the elimination of waste speeded up and with an increased blood flow, oxygen delivery is enhanced.
- Choline, magnesium and potassium are three compounds found abundantly in wheatgrass. They are essential for detoxification and help the liver stay vital and healthy.
- Even offensive body odour can be neutralised if chlorophyll is consumed consistently over the course of a few weeks.
- Wheatgrass is an abundant source of enzymes, which among other things help to detoxify the pollutants that are part of every day life. They also increase your ability to digest food more fully, dissolve excesses of fat and protein, and in some cases may even break down tumours and cysts.
- Wheatgrass is a superior food source of Superoxide dimutase (SOD), the true anti-ageing enzyme.
- P4D1 and D1G1 are two glyco-proteins found in wheatgrass that have excellent anti-inflammatory actions, anti-ulcer actions and a powerful antioxidant potential. P4D1 has the ability to stimulate the production and natural repair of human reproductive sperm cells and DNA.
- Wheatgrass is abundant in vitamin B17 (laetrile) that can selectively destroy cancer cells, leaving non-cancerous ones alone.
- Wheatgrass has the power to simultaneously neutralise the toxic effect of fluorine, and convert it into an ally that helps in the maintenance of healthy bones and teeth.
- 2oz of wheatgrass juice has the equivalent vitamin and mineral content of roughly 4lbs of organic green vegetables. On an empty stomach, it is assimilated into the blood in about 20 minutes and is charged with 'chi' electrical energy. The vitality lasts throughout the day.
- Wheatgrass juice has been shown to build red blood cells quickly after ingestion. It normalises high blood pressure and stimulates healthy tissue-cell growth.
- Drs Hugh and Latner found that small doses of **pure** chlorophyll regenerate blood haemoglobin levels, but large doses appeared to be toxic to bone marrow. **Crude** chlorophyll, on the other hand was found to be non toxic even in large doses.
- Chlorophyll doesn't play much of a role in medicine because its inherent

instability prevents it from being stored. Like fresh fats and oils, fresh vegetable and fruit juice, when exposed to light and air deteriorate/oxidise very rapidly.

♦ If you have any concerns about osteoporosis, let them be banished. Chlorophyll promotes calcium absorption because it has a similar action to vitamin D in your body. When you consume wheatgrass juice, you'll also be tapping into an excellent source of vitamins A and C and the mineral magnesium, all of which help you absorb more calcium.

♦ Green vegetables/superfoods are excellent transition and detoxification foods (especially for overcoming heavy metal poisoning). The earth is covered with grass. Four of the world's top five crops come from it. Muscular 2000lb animals sustain themselves on it and science has found every nutrient in it.

♦ Having spent many years researching plant foods, Brian Clement, director of Hippocrates Health Institute in West Palm Beach, Florida, has reported that wild greens have the highest energy frequency of any food. Wild greens should be your preference, but if you can't get wild you should buy organic!

No 'one food' should be eaten exclusively, but once you've experimented with greens, you'll instinctively be drawn towards them. Not only do they deliver an abundance of nutrients and vitality, but they'll also cause you to feel sharp, alert and centred.

The choice is yours – dead food and a lifeless body – or live raw food and a vibrant body. As Dr. Bernard Jensen said, "If you're green on the inside, you're clean on the inside."

THE AGGRESSIVE HEALTH EVALUATION:
Do you eat/juice a variety of green foods on a daily basis?
Do you enjoy a regular shot of wheatgrass daily ?
Have you begun to use E3live?
Do you use a powerful chlorophyll based superfood for nutritional insurance?
Do you create a variety of green drinks that tickle your taste buds?

CHAPTER 3

TRANSFORM YOUR WINDOW SILL INTO A MASS PRODUCING ORGANIC FARM AND BEGIN HARVESTING ELECTRICALLY CHARGED SUPERFOODS TODAY

'Life force' is a term used to describe the universal energy and innate intelligence that gives life to everything living. Without it, a cut wouldn't heal. Without it, there would be no nerve vitality. Without it, your spinal fluid wouldn't possess life and power. All health, energy, happiness and longevity is directly related to the amount of life force flowing through you at any one time. Once that flow ceases – you cease!

DISCOVER HOW THE POWER OF LIFE FORCE HELPED HEAL EPILEPSY AND TWO BRAIN SEIZURES

In the 1970s, Loretta Harmony Kohn underwent medical treatment for a variety of difficulties. The most problematical were two brain seizures. Shortly after the treatment she was diagnosed with epilepsy and her driving licence revoked. Her physical condition deteriorated and as time drifted by she suffered with severe depression. In 1979, after her second epileptic seizure, she felt alone, stranded and wanted to give up on life. On the brink of suicide she read a book by the late Ann Wigmore entitled, 'Be Your Own Doctor: Let Living food Be Your Medicine'. Ann's approach was to use raw foods for healing, none more important than sprouted alfalfa seeds, wheat berry sprouts and wheatgrass juice.

INSPIRATION LED TO REGENERATION

Having been inspired by what she had read, Loretta made the decision to visit The Hippocrates Health Institute in Boston, Massachusetts, founded by Ann. She packed her belongings and moved there for one month in a last ditch effort to regain her health.

Ann informed Loretta that her seizures were due to an over toxic body. Years of nutritional/lifestyle abuse had got her into this mess, but raw plant foods were going to help her out of it! When Ann was alive she worked with hundreds of sick people, relying on 'live foods' (sprouted salads, sprouted juices, and other sprouted foods) to eject, eradicate and expel the toxic sludge from their bodies. People often arrived barely able to move or speak, and left being able to walk, run, swim and play tennis!

SIMPLE RITUALS, POWERFUL RESULTS

As part of Loretta's routine she was given juice in the morning made with 50% alfalfa and 50% wheat sprouts, a salad or sandwich abundant in alfalfa and wheat sprouts for lunch, and another sprout juice with a baked vegetarian sprout loaf or vegetable/sprout burgers for dinner. Within a few short days, excess fat began melting off her body and her energy began to replenish. For 120 days she continued these simple rituals until she felt convinced she was healed. At this point she wanted medical proof. She decided to visit a physician at Brigham and Women's Hospital in Boston and submitted herself to have an electroencephalogram (EEG). When the results came back from the laboratory, Loretta couldn't believe it! The liberating diet Ann had given her had not only allowed her to recover from her low energy and depression, but had also freed her from epileptic seizures. Loretta could begin driving again.

CREATING A MAGICAL DIET FROM MAGICAL MATERIALS

If Loretta's story inspires you, imagine what 'live' sprouted foods can do for you. Remember, in their original form, these foods have a low water content and are very concentrated. However, when you sprout them their nutritional content explodes and they transfer their life-force directly to you! Pound for pound you won't find a cheaper food on the planet. Begin experimenting TODAY.

◆ The Pulses: Adzuki beans, chickpeas, lima beans, blackeye peas, lentils, mung beans, navy beans, etc.
◆ The Seeds: Hemp, Pumpkin, sunflower, mustard, fenugreek, alfalfa, radish, buckwheat, sesame, etc.
◆ The Nuts: Brazil nuts, almonds, hazelnuts, pine nuts, pecans, pistachios, walnuts, etc.
◆ The Grains: Quinoa, rye, rice, oats, millet, wheat, barley, maize, etc.

PERFECT NUTRITION AND PERFECT HEALTH

You've seen how a tiny seed can sprout and force its way through a slab of stone! Well imagine what that kind of life-force and energy can do for your body! Each and every seed contains enough stored energy to send it on its way in life, and all the genetic information necessary to grow and develop into a plant. These intelligent little powerhouses know up from down, light from dark and moist from dry. They are the secret weapon in your AGGRESSIVE HEALTH arsenal. Eat them and thrive! Neglect them and you'll never know the true meaning of explosive health. Take a look at why they will become your No.1 nutritional super-foods:

♦ They are the fresh, easy to prepare and grow energetically until YOU decide to eat them.
♦ Pound for pound they are the cheapest food in existence, putting money back in your pocket where it belongs.
♦ They have a higher nutrient ratio than any other food.
♦ They have a life force and radiance that they pass directly onto you.
♦ As a premier raw food they are perfect for people who don't want to spend time in the kitchen but want to get busy living.
♦ They are the most enzyme rich foods you are likely to eat, powering up your digestive process simultaneously.
♦ For all your sprouting needs goto www.aggressivehealth.co.uk

SPROUTS, UNLIMITED HEALTH AND CANCER PREVENTION?

As far back as 1978 Dr. Charles Shaw and Dr. Chiu-Nan at the University of Texas Cancer Centre tested a variety of foods to determine whether they had any anti-cancer properties. The chosen foods included lentil sprouts, mung bean sprouts, wheat sprouts, as well as carrots and parsley. The foods were then tested on mice inoculated with carcinogens (cancer causing substances). Although the carrots and parsley did show an inhibitory effect on the carcinogens, the true heroes of the experiment were the sprouts. They inhibited the activity of the carcinogens, even when small dosages of the sprout extracts were used. The other major benefit was that the extract wasn't toxic even in high dosages. (Most known inhibitors of carcinogens are toxic at even moderately high levels of concentration.) With this information fresh in your mind, let me introduce you to my secret for weapon for power packed workouts and life energy that is second to none…

THE POWER OF SPROUTED BEANS

Sprouted beans are true magic. Not only do they provide an abundance of hunger-cutting protein, but they also replace the calcium that is lost through diets high in animal protein.

♦ **Eliminate Cravings Today** – Sprouted beans are so nutritionally dense and fibre rich, they will satisfy you in every way. Their bulkiness and low-calorie profile will help eliminate cravings and make them the perfect food for life-extension.

♦ **Develop An Outstanding Blood Profile** – Long-term studies carried out by Dr. James W. Anderson at the University of Kentucky showed that as little as 50grams of beans per day can reduce serum cholesterol levels and actually increase serum HDL-cholesterol levels. Forget cooking beans altogether. Start sprouting today! You'll preserve the vital nutrients that assist in their digestion and assimilation.

♦ **Stablilise Blood Sugar Levels** – The soluble fibre in sprouted beans gels in the intestines and prevents any dramatic rises in blood sugar. The importance of maintaining stable blood sugar levels cannot be over emphasised. If you want to lose unwanted flab and have a mind that is sharp and alert, it's time to get out your sprouting trays and begin.

♦ **Energise Your Brain For Peak Performance** – Beans contain high levels of the amino acid tyrosine. You'll read about tyrosine in chapter 14 – Food For Thought. It is a critical amino-acid necessary for the synthesis of the neurotransmitter dopamine. As you spark the fire of your brain's dopamine receptors, your outlook on the world will become ferocious. You'll feel more energy and vigour, cut stress and develop laser-like concentration, all whilst feeling more lively and buoyant. Dopamine will also help you exercise become more explosive in the gym and in the bedroom. With your dopamine levels high your sexual vigour will soar!

♦ **No More Unwanted Gas** – It was discovered at the U.S. Department of Agriculture near Berkeley, California that a group of complex sugars called oligo saccharides found in beans cause excessive flatulence. Fortunately though, when a bean is sprouted it secretes an enzyme called glastosidase. This enzyme breaks down the sugars and prevents the formation of excessive gas.

FORGET EXPENSIVE SUPPLEMENTS AND EMBRACE
21ST CENTURY SUPER FOOD

Imagine how much money you'd save if the main bulk of your diet cost as little as 30p per day. That's the reality when it comes to sprouting. You can load up your cupboards with a few months supply of beans and seeds and turn your window sill into a nutritional goldmine. They will grow in any season, are simple to harvest and can be eaten immediately. Growing them at home takes no time at all. You will have a new harvest every few days. Choose either low cost sprouting trays or a state of the art 'EASYGREEN™ Automatic Sprouter'. Whatever your choice, make sure you always have some sprouts either soaking or growing. Sprouted foods are the foundation to AGGRESSIVE HEALTH.

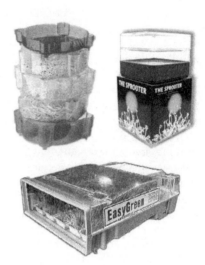

IGNITING THE FLAME OF YOUR SEXUAL FIRE
WITH SEXY SPROUTS

One interesting study performed by the Agricultural Experiment Station in Beltsville, Maryland demonstrated the ability of sprouted grains to restore fertility to cows that lost or outgrew their ability to reproduce. One study used cows that had never shown any signs of reproductive capacity. Each animal was fed five pounds of sprouted oats daily along with its usual food. Would you believe that after just sixty days all the cows were pregnant!

I don't know how you assess your sexual vigour, but since Viagra 'popped up' a few years ago, it has become one of the fastest selling drugs in history. I'll let you make your mind up about how seriously people take their sexual prowess. Let sprouts be your starting point if you need your sexual functions rejuvenated and restored.

Almonds should also be at the heart of your campaign if you are looking to boost or regain your sexual crown. They have long been considered a powerful aphrodisiac and are also key for athletes looking to maximise their anabolic cycle for gains in size and strength. More about this later.

Sprouted seeds are an important part of the diet of the long-lived Hunza people of the Himalayas. Not only do the Hunzas have one of the highest percentages of centenarians, but they are also very active up until the time they pass away, especially sexually! They also have very efficient digestive systems, which brings me onto the subject of enzyme inhibitors...

DESTROYING ENZYME INHIBITORS
COOKING -V- SPROUTING

Seeds need to be tough to survive the most adverse of conditions which is why all their nutrients are packed away in a tough woody matrix. To release the arsenal or nutrition and enzymes within you must soak them to remove the enzyme inhibitors. Think of it like this – all seeds have the potential to grow into a huge plant, but the conditions must be right for germination. Each potential sprout contains enzyme inhibitors to prevent the seed from 'awakening' at the wrong time. When you soak the seeds, the inhibitors are removed, giving you unlimited access to the massive enzyme content within. Most people cook beans and pulses to release the nutrients, but in doing so destroy the enzymes. If you destroy the enzymes, you place an unnecessary demand on your pancreas and other organs to release extra enzymes to make up the difference. Did you know that compared to any other species on earth, in proportion to body size and weight, humans have the largest overworked pancreas in existence? Without sprouts and other enzyme rich foods/supplements you increase your chances of becoming part of this statistic.

BREAK UP THE FAT IN YOUR BODY, DEVELOP A POWERFUL BRAIN AND TRANSER MORE NUTRIENTS TO YOUR CELLS – IT'S ALL POSSIBLE WITH LECITHIN

In the process of germination, one of the compounds that increase as your sprouts grow on your window sill is lecithin. When you include more lecithin in your diet you supply a critical element necessary for optimising mental performance and brain power. You'll learn more about this later. Lecithin will also help your body break up and transporting fats and fatty acids around your body and encourage the transport of nutrients through cell walls. Do you need any more reasons?

UNLEASH THE MOST ENZYME RICH FOODS INTO YOUR BODY AND SLOW DOWN THE PASSAGE OF TIME

Enzymes digest food, break down toxins, cleanse the blood, strengthen the immune system, build protein into muscle, assist in muscle contraction, eliminate carbon dioxide from the lungs, and reduce stress on the pancreas and other vital organs.

According to Dr Edward Howell, an 18 year-old body produces 30 times more amylase (carbohydrate digesting enzymes) than a 69 year old. Dr Howell suggests if you eat an enzyme poor diet, you are inviting premature ageing. In fact the more lavishly a young body gives up its enzymes, the sooner the state of enzyme poverty or old age is reached.

♦ Enzyme function is suppressed in an acidic environment. To alkalkise your body focus on chlorophyll rich foods, vegetables, sprouted foods and vegetable juices. Without active enzymes, intracellular activity begins to decline.

- Enzymes have as much of an impact on your health and well being as any other vital nutrient. Without them, vitamins, minerals, phytochemicals, proteins, fats and carbohydrates would be rendered useless! Forget supplementing with multiple mineral and vitamin supplements without first bolstering up your enzyme account. The most powerful enzyme supplement on the planet is called Vitälzym™. It eats away at scar tissue, can restore aged organs to a youthful placid state. One capsule has the power to break a 14oz steak into its basic amino acids – that's power. Visit www.aggressivehealth.co.uk for more details.
- Enzymes are your body's labour force. Without them you'd be nothing more than a pile of lifeless chemicals.
- Enzyme rich, sprouted foods help transform undigested food into its basic components. These are then absorbed and used to build cells, tissues and organs. They also form the basis of a healthy digestive system.
- When introduced directly into the bloodstream, enzymes tend to concentrate at the site of a wound, a tumour, inflammation, or immune system activity. Their ability to break down protein and fat molecules in various tissues of the body has been shown to reduce the size of blood clots and tumours, reduce inflammation, and speed tissue repair.
- Supplemental digestive enzymes such as Vitälzym™ can dramatically reduce inflammation and autoimmune activity in arthritis and other degenerative and inflammatory conditions. According to Dr Wong (www.drwong.info) – In tests conducted to find a fibrinolytic enzyme to go along with their natural cancer therapy, the University of Southern California, through the Apex Research Institute tested 70 of the proteolytic enzyme products available today for enzymatic action. Of the 70, Vitälzym™ ranked #1! For more information on Vitälzym™ visit www.aggressivehealth.co.uk.
- At body temperature, a tiny amount of pepsin (one of the gastric enzymes used to digest protein) will break down the white of an egg into small chain peptides within just a few minutes. To accomplish this feat in a laboratory would mean boiling the egg white for 24 hours in a strong acid or alkali solution. That's the power of enzymes.
- As you increase the enzyme content of your diet through sprouted foods and Vitälzym™, your bowel movements will become more regular, maybe more than twice a day. This is all possible with an enzyme rich existence.

THE POWER OF PRAYER... SOMETHING TO THINK ABOUT

A botanist by the name of Dr Robert Jerome, at the University of Mexico, found that by intentionally sending out loving thoughts to his plants, he was able to make them grow much faster. He also discovered that by sending out hateful thoughts, he was able to cause plants to wither and die in five weeks (even when receiving proper care of soil, water and sunlight). It makes you wonder doesn't it? Prayed over seeds grow faster than ones that are left to their own devices. Minister Franklin Loehr and his researchers have performed experiments with 20,000 seeds and have satisfactorily demonstrated that prayer affects germination and growth if it is done repeatedly. When you send out loving thoughts to help them grow and ingest them, you are eating 'love consciousness'. Sounds very airy-fairy – but every living thing has a consciousness. I suggest you develop a relationship with your sprouts because they are going give you more than you could ever wish for.

ALFALFA SPROUTS – THE BASIS OF QUALITY NUTRITION

Alfalfa sprouts are possibly one of the most nutritionally rich foods you'll ever eat. Not only do they have an incredible vitamin and mineral content, but they are 40% protein and contain every amino acid. For years, people have eaten alfalfa sprouts and experienced remission from a number of ailments. They provide an excellent calcium-phosphorus ratio (2:1). They supply your body with a large quantity of low-calorie liquid nourishment that is easily digested and used as fuel. In addition, the liquid helps to flush toxins out of the body and is an excellent source of trace elements such as iodine, zinc, selenium, chromium, cobalt, and silicon. Alfalfa sprouts and sprouted pumpkin seeds are especially potent sources of zinc. Zinc is necessary for all sexual functions, the healing response, protein synthesis and liver functions. Selenium is abundant in alfalfa sprouts and is now being tested for anti-cancer properties

GANGRENE CURED WITH ALFALFA SPROUT JUICE

In the late 1970s, a middle aged man suffering from gangrene in his right leg visited Ann Wigmore at her institute. Poor circulation due to acute diabetes had been the cause of this problem, but Ann seemed to have the answer. She gave him four glasses of alfalfa and wheat sprout juice to drink daily. To make this juice, simply put equal parts with a little water in a blender for three minutes. Ann also used the concoction for bathing the afflicted limb on a daily basis. Can you believe it took only two weeks for the gangrene to completely heal!

MUNG BEAN SPROUTS –
THE MAGICAL SPROUT/FRUIT LINK

After 5 days of sprouting Mung beans transform into a superfood that surpasses any fruit in existence. Mung beans sprouts have the carbohydrate content virtually identical to that found in a casaba melon. They increase in water content from 10.7% found in the seed to 88.8% in the sprout. The protein content is similar to that found in a dry fig, whilst its calorie content is similar to that of a papaya or honeydew melon. Mung sprouts have a vitamin C content similar to that found in a pineapple, vitamin A content of a lemon, thiamine content of an avocado, riboflavin content of an apple, niacin content of a banana, calcium content of damson plums, potassium level of papaya and iron percentage of a loganberry. Mung sprouts are good sources of the iron needed for red blood cell formation and the transport of oxygen from the lungs to the cells. And unlike most fruit found in todays supermarkets, Mung beans won't result in a sugar high. Mung beans are also high in B17 (laetrile). This powerful nutrient selectively destroys cancer cells, leaving non-cancerous ones alone. It was discovered by Dr. Ernst Krebs, Jr. (a highly respected biochemist and researcher) and in parts of the world where the incidence of cancer is almost non-existent, nutritional intake of vitamin B17 is about 400 times higher than here in the west. In fact, in a later chapter you'll read about the Hunzas, a population that has been cancer free for over 900 years of its existence. The Hunzas base much of their diet around sprouted foods but they also have secret weapon that has begun helping people in the west win the war against cancer – apricot kernels. Found inside an apricot stone an apricot kernel has the highest active B17 content of any food. You can also find B17 in buckwheat sprouts, macadamia, wheatgrass juice and the seeds of the common fruit.

DISCOVER HOW MUNG BEANS AND THE PENTOSE PHOSPHATE PATHWAY CAN PROTECT YOUR DNA AND MAKE YOUR ENERGY LEVELS SOAR

Because beans help stabilise blood sugar levels and decresase serum lipids they simultaneously have a positive effect on a critical energy system of the body - the pentose phosphate pathway (PPP). Not only does 30% of glucose oxidation in the liver occur via this pathway, but it is a major player in other areas such as protection against DNA damage, oxidative stress and toxin overload through the generation and utilisation of NADPH – an essential energy molecule.

Without going over board on the technical aspect, if you want to stimulate PPP activity, eat mung beans – they are rich in pentose and PPP enzymes. Can life get any better?

ARE YOU NUTS ABOUT NUTS?

Researchers recently found that women who ate nuts regularly had a 32% lower risk of having a non-fatal heart attack and were 39% less likely to die of a heart attack than those who never or rarely consumed nuts. The amount of nuts needed to provide the protection was very low – only five ounces a week. A handful of walnuts, macadamias, almonds, pecans, or hazelnuts can do more for your health than you think. Similar results from the Physician's Health Study suggest that frequent nut consumption benefit men in the same way.

BRAZIL NUTS FIGHT THE CANCER BATTLE

Brazil nuts have been found to increase cancer resistance due to their exceptionally high levels of selenium. Researchers at Roswell Park Cancer Institute showed that animals fed the tropical nut increased their resistance to tumours more significantly than a group fed a walnut-enriched diet. Even supplementation of selenium didn't prove any more powerful than eating a daily serving of brazil nuts. When it comes to the anti-cancer properties of selenium, brazil nuts lead the pack.

TAKE MACADAMIA NUTS TO HEART

Macadamia nuts have been found to improve fat metabolism efficiency according to a preliminary study conducted by researchers at the University of Hawaii in Honolulu. High levels of omega 6 fatty acids counteract the beneficial effects of omega 3 fatty acids. Macadamia oil has only 3% omega 6 fatty acids. Macadamias are also high in B17 (laetrile). B17 consumption is 400 times higher in populations that have no signs or recorded cases of cancer.

USING WALNUTS IN THE FIGHT AGAINST HEART DISEASE

In the spring of 1993 researchers at Loma Linda University Medical School (California) made some exciting discoveries. They reported that after comparing the results of two four week long dietary intervention trials in 18 men, eating moderate amounts of walnuts, without increasing total dietary fat and calories, "decreases serum cholesterol levels and favourably modifies the lipoprotein profile in healthy men."

LOAD UP YOUR DIET WITH ANTIOXIDANT FOODS

The amino acids cysteine and glutathione are powerful antioxidants. They protect against car exhaust fumes, carcinogens, infections, alcohol excess and toxic metals. They also help make one of the body's key antioxidant enzymes, and help detoxify the body. Cysteine and glutathione are particularly high in lentils, beans, nuts, seeds (especially hemp seeds), onions and garlic. They have been shown to boost the immune system and increase antioxidant power.

POWER UP YOUR ANTIOXIDANT STATUS
WITH ELLAGIC ACID

In the October 1968 Journal of Pharmaceutical Sciences (57:1730-31) you can read a study where ellagic acid from black walnuts was injected into a group of mice before they underwent electroconvulsive shock. With the presence of this substance in their blood they remained alive for longer than other rodents that were shocked but received no injections. This suggests that ellagic acid has a protective effect on the myelin sheathing (fatty protein substance) encasing each strand of nerve.

Between 1985 and 1990 researchers at the Medical College of Ohio in Toledo began investigating ellagic acid's effects on cancer growth. They found that ellagic acid competes for DNA receptors that are also used by carcinogens. Thus with more ellagic acid in your diet you give your body greater strength and a greater chance against the diseases of modern civilisation. Ellagic acid is found in blackcurrants, grapes, raspberries, strawberries, and some nuts such as brazil nuts and walnuts.

POWERFUL PISTACHIOS PACK A MIND BOOSTING PUNCH

In a study back in the 1960s, alcoholics were given the opportunity to relieve their addiction by taking part in an experiment using high doses of glutamic acid (GA). They were given 2 grams, 3 times a day for the first month, 12 grams a day for the second month and finally 15 grams for months 3 and 4. Compared to the control group taking placebos, 75% of the experimental group reported remarkable control over their drinking habits. A cup of pistachios supplies about 6 grams of GA. Glutamic acid forms a partnership with gamma-aminobutyric acid (GABA) and glutamine (GAM) causing your brain reactions to run more smoothly. GA is a stimulating neurotransmitter, whilst GABA calms the brain. GAM on the other hand performs so many different functions it's hard to classify. Out of all the amino acids, GA is the most abundant one in the brain and its main role is to help in the production of mental energy. If you're doing anything that requires intense mental concentration and an excellent memory, and you want a snack, choose a handful of raw pistachios. Another food rich in GA that you'll soon realise is a powerful key to unlocking the secrets of AGGRESSIVE HEALTH is the hemp seed.

WARNING: YOU'RE ABOUT TO LEARN ABOUT THE MOST POWERFUL FOOD IN EXISTENCE. IF THIS FOOD DOESN'T TAKE PRIDE OF PLACE IN YOUR DIET THEN YOU'LL NEVER REACH THE HOLY GRAIL OF AGGRESSIVE HEALTH! THIS FOOD ALONE CAN HEAL THE WORLD!

Curious? I hope so. So was I when I began investigating this magical food. But let me tell you something. Nothing (and I mean NOTHING – no food supplement or superfood) has had as much impact on my health and vitality as this. In my opinion, this food should be the first food you turn to if you are serious about AGGRESSIVE HEALTH. It's an exceptional food if you want to detox/lose weight and an ABSOLUTE MUST when you start to exercise frequently. In fact, if you are committed to looking like a muscular athlete rather the victim of a concentration camp, this food will become your saviour! If you want to sculpt your body and stay lean and slim, this food will help you recover faster and give you more sustained energy levels, making your workouts something you love, not something you 'put off until next week'! Lastly, if you are sick or 'dis-eased', this food can set you on your way to faster recovery as you take the first step towards a life of joy and vibrancy.

WELCOME TO THE PLANETS MOST SUPERIOR FOOD!
WELCOME TO THE WONDERFUL WORLD OF HEMP!

There are many reasons why hemp seed is critical if you want to master AGGRESSIVE HEALTH, but one of the most important reasons is protein. Some people avoid it on high carbohydrate diets. Some people rave about it on high protein/weight loss diets. The truth is simple: PROTEIN IS CRITICAL – but the secret is in selection. Animal protein can drain the body of pancreatic enzymes, but that doesn't mean you should never eat it. Awareness is the key. Remember, food has to be broken down in order to feed your cells. If you eat too much meat, eggs or dairy, digestion can sap the life-force out of you. Make sure you eat an abundance of live food with your meat, including sprouts to assist digestion. Also, invest in an enzyme supplement such as Vitälzym™ to assist your body.

The great news with sprouts is that they are pre-digested before you even take your first mouthful, meaning they can instantly supply your cells with optimal nutrition to create their maximum electrical charge. In fact if you used to be a lover of 'The Atkins Diet' – here is your chance to create REAL HEALTH – not JUST weight loss. Sprouted foods are exceptional sources of amino acids, the building blocks of protein and sitting on the throne of AGGRESSIVE HEALTH is the hemp seed! Take a look for yourself.

- If you are very active and concerned about protein, hemp is your answer. Hemp contains up to 30% highly digestible protein with the perfect ratio or amino acids. It won't cause flatulence often associated with Soy products and isn't hard to digest like meat and diary.
- The protein in hemp is about 65% Edestin and 35% Albumin. You'll find both Edestin and Albumin are highly digestible. Edestin aids digestion and is also considered the backbone of your cells DNA. Albumin is an excellent source of free radical scavengers.
- The 'high protein' Atkins diet may be effective for losing unwanted fat for the first few weeks, but in the long run the high protein consumption stresses your kidneys and causes fatty acid imbalances (because all the meat is cooked). With hemp, not only will you be getting the essential fatty acids (EFAs) and fibre often lacking on many of the high protein diets, but you also get the best source of dietary protein in existence.
- Hemp seeds provide a perfect ratio of essential fats needed to assist the detoxification process, create a powerful brain, speed up the recovery process, oxygenate your cells, digest and absorb nutrients more efficiently, promote healthy intestinal bacteria… the list goes on.
- Hemp seeds contain an array of vital nutrients including Magnesium, Phosphorus, Potassium, Sulphur and Manganese that assists the metabolism of the essential fatty acids (EFAs). Hemp is also a great source of Zinc, Calcium, Iron and Vitamin A.
- Hemp is a critical food if you want to create hormonal mastery. It's nutritional profile will help you reach your perfect weight and feel phenomenal.
- Hemp is high in dietary fibre helping your body expel waste more efficiently.

Find out what works best for you when it comes to hemp. I tend grind up the seeds with their shell once they've been soaked for 8-12 hours and don't let them sprout for too long. You can buy the seeds without the shell (vacuum packed preferably to keep Mother Nature out – in the same way the shell does). You can also use hemp oil on salads and in juices, but as always, the whole food is best choice. It is an excellent source of Vitamin E. If any one food encompasses all the principles of AGGRESSIVE HEALTH, it is the hemp seed.

SPROUTED FOODS ARE THE CRITICAL MISSING LINK
IF YOU WANT THE VERY BEST BRAIN NUTRITION

From chapter 12 onwards, you'll learn exactly what it takes to feed your brain. You'll learn about the superstar neurotransmitter acetylcholine. It is the most abundant neurotransmitter in the brain and essential to higher mental processes such as learning and memory. If you want develop a brain that soaks up information like a sponge and can focus like a laser, you want to focus on foods high in choline. Choline is a natural precursor for acetylcholine and can be found in hemp seeds. It is vital for nerve impulses from the brain through the nervous system and assists liver and gall bladder function. But that's not all! Hemp seeds are also rich in two other brain nutrients inositol and lecithin. Inositol is calming to the nervous system, promoting harmony and balance. Lecithin is a lipid found in the protective sheaths surrounding the brain and nervous system. Many people buy lecithin for its ability to break down fat, not realising it also enhances liver activity and enzyme production. Why waste your money on another supplement when you can get your lecithin from hemp.

HEMP IS BECOMING THE FOOD OF CHOICE FOR ATHLETES
EVERYWHERE

When the blood profiles of marathon runners were studied, choline levels fluctuated dramatically. Researcher Richard Wurtman discovered that after 26 miles of running, choline drops by a staggering 40%. Studies also show that swimmers are able to swim for longer, without the perils of muscle fatigue, when they include choline rich foods such as hemp seeds and other sprouted foods into their diet. The best way to incorporate all of this into your life is to begin today with the…

AGGRESSIVE HEALTH RITUAL:
THE ULTIMATE SALAD

If you want my key to success with sprouts pay attention. Treat them as your No.1 bulking agent for your diet. I very rarely let a day go by without having a sprouted salad feast. Forget the limp, lifeless little salad you see in most restaurants! We're talking about something that's going to fill you up and make you feel fantastic. You can throw in as many of your favourite salad veggies as you like, add a tasty dressing of your choice, some all powerful green leaves and you're on your way to OUTSTANDING HEALTH.

Most of my salads include either chickpea, mung bean, aduki bean or lentil sprouts. I love to blend soaked hemp seeds into a nutritionally dense mix that supplies everything from protein to essential fats and other critical nutrients. Almonds are great if you want to maximise your anabolic pathway and increase size and strength through effective training. Mung Beans are great to keep your pentose phosphate pathway optimised for energy. The list goes on. Experiment with sunflower, pumpkin and sesame seeds. You can blend them up, put them in salads add them to stew or soups (but don't cook them or you kill vital enzymes), or simply eat them as a snack. The options are endless. In today's 'protein motivated society' sprouted foods will soon become the food of choice and MUST be at the heart of your diet.

ARE YOU READY FOR THE CHALLENGE?

One of the mysteries puzzling scientists for years is how one tiny seed can develop into a fully grown plant. The answer can be found when you appreciate the mysterious force that governs all creation. This is why sprouts are one of the most superior foods on the planet. If you see sprouting as a problem there is only one solution: Go out and buy as many different varieties of nuts, seeds, pulses and grains, and make it your commitment to sprout all of them. Treat it like your ultimate experiment. Call it personal responsibility. It represents the beginning of a richer, more fulfilling life. Be the best you've ever been. Now is the time and sprouts are the all-singing, all-dancing super food that will propel you down the road towards scintillating health. Here's a re-cap:

♦ Sprouts are low on the glycemic index and help keep blood sugar balanced. This is critical for consistent energy and optimal brain function.

♦ Sprouts offer all the nutrients essential for maximum vitality. Levels of vitamins and minerals increase during the sprouting process. Some as high as 600%.

♦ Sprouted beans supply high levels of the amino acid tyrosine, a critical building block for dopamine – the neurotransmitter that affects how alert you are.

♦ Brian Clement, Director of The Hippocrates Institute recommends sunflower sprouts to all athletes, especially body builders with concerns about protein.

♦ Sprouts form part of the diet of the long-lived Hunza people of the Himalayas. Is it any wonder they have one of the highest percentages of centenarians in existence today?

♦ Sprouts increase the micro-electrical potential of cells, improving your body's use of oxygen so that both muscles and brain are energised.

♦ In the process of germination the brain boosting phosphorus compounds such as lecithin increase.

♦ Sprouted beans provide an abundance of hunger-cutting protein and replace the calcium that is lost through diets high in animal protein. They fill you up, improve your blood profile, keep blood glucose levels balanced and energise you.

♦ Alfalfa sprouts provide an excellent calcium-phosphorus ratio (2:1) and are excellent sources of trace elements such as iodine, zinc, selenium, chromium, cobalt and silicon.

♦ Mung bean sprouts are rich in pentose and PPP enzymes necessary for DNA protection and the fight against free radicals.

♦ Brazil nuts pack a healthy selenium punch offering anti-cancer properties.

Macadamia nuts have been found to improve fat metabolism. Pistachio nuts are excellent brain food, and walnuts help develop optimal blood profiles.

♦ Without the shell, hemp seeds have a 30% protein content. With the shell they are an excellent source of dietary fibre. They have the perfect ratio of amino acids to allow optimal assimilation. They provide essential fats in a ratio that is perfect for your body. They contain an array of vital nutrients including Magnesium, Phosphorus, Potassium, Sulphur, Manganese (which assists the metabolism of the essential fatty acids (EFAs) that it naturally contains). Hemp is also a great source of Zinc, Calcium, Iron and Vitamin A.

♦ Remember to pray for your sprouts and watch as your loving thoughts cause them to grow full of life and vitality.

♦ Hemp seeds are the ultimate food for unrivalled nutrition and could eradicate every case of essential fatty acid imbalance/deficiency, protein malnourishment and many mineral deficiency symptoms.

♦ Due to their inherent life force, sprouts are the most enzyme rich foods in existence. Add in a powerful enzyme supplement as well and you'll be able to have an enzyme level of a teenager. Remember, according to Dr Wong (www.drwong.info) – In tests conducted to find a fibrinolytic enzyme to go along with their natural cancer therapy, the University of Southern California, through the Apex Research Institute tested 70 of the proteolytic enzyme products available today for enzymatic action. Of the 70, Vitälzym™ ranked #1! For more information on Vitälzym™ goto www.aggressivehealth.co.uk.

THE AGGRESSIVE HEALTH EVALUATION:
Do you sprout your own pulses, legumes, seeds, nuts or grains?
Do you soak the majority of your nuts and seeds?
Do you have at least one all powerful sprout salad daily?
Is the hemp seed at the heart of your health regime?
Do you take a regular dose of Vitälzym™ to ensure you maintain the enzyme levels of a teenager?

CHAPTER 4

TO WIN THE RAGING WAR AGAINST OBESITY AND CREATE OUTSTANDING HEALTH DEVELOP A LOVE AFFAIR WITH FAT

Three simple letters, F, A and T. Put them together and you have one of the most emotionally charged words in existence.

HIGH FAT, LOW FAT OR NO FAT - WHAT'S THE STORY?

Have you been conditioned to think that *all* fat is bad? Would you be surprised to find that some fats are considered poisonous, whilst others are as essential as air and water? Ultimately, if your body is out of balance and you are suffering ill health, you may need a series of tests to determine what course of action is best for you and which fats to focus on to restore balance. If you're interested in complete biological terrain testing that includes these tests contact me at www.aggressivehealth.co.uk. If you are in good health, the simple inclusion of a few basic foods will be a massive step in the right direction, helping you to master this piece of the AGGRESSIVE HEALTH puzzle.

HOW A SIMPLE LESSON IN HISTORY WILL CHANGE YOUR RELATIONSHIP TO FAT FOREVER

In Europe, before the Second World War, oil pressing was a home and cottage industry. Every large estate and small town usually had an oil mill and many villages had an oil beater. The oil beater would put flax or other seeds into a funnel, place a steel wedge on top of the seeds, and then pound the wedge with a sledge hammer – crushing the seeds and pressing the oil into a barrel. Once or twice a week the oil beater would put the barrel of oil onto his wagon and ride through the village selling it. People stored the fresh pressed oil in a ceramic container in a cool dark place. Storage was critical because of its short shelf life. It was treated like milk, eggs and bread, spoiling quickly if not consumed.

In the 1920s the oil trade became big business and almost over night people discovered how to press oils in huge quantities and preserve them for greater profit. But there was an enormous price to pay.

Imagine warehouses full of oil that had been heated to such high temperatures that all the vital nutrients were destroyed. Imagine bottles of chemically refined oil, pale in colour and bland in taste. Imagine bottles of oil lacking the essential fatty acids (EFAs) that your body needs at all costs to create and maintain health.

As usual, money, greed and big business took over and the oil business boomed. The result was oils that had more stability and a longer shelf life, but at the same time, the power to totally destroy your body.

WHY ALL THE FUSS ABOUT FAT?

Since the oil trade became big business, the majority of fat eaten in Western civilisation has been cooked, processed or both. Cooked fat kills! Whenever fat is cooked, trans-fatty acids are produced, and they represent one of the most destructive elements of any cooked food diet.

On November 20th 1997, The New England Journal of Medicine reported the results of a 14 year study of more than 80,000 nurses. During this time 939 heart attacks were documented and among the women who consumed the largest amounts of trans fatty acids, the chance of suffering a heart attack was a staggering 53% higher than those who limited their intake.

THE LAW HAS BANNED TRANS-FATTY ACIDS IN BABY FOODS – BUT NOT IN YOURS!

Did you know that it is illegal to put trans fatty acids into baby foods? But somehow, 'the powers that be' didn't think that if it is dangerous for babies it might be dangerous for you. Figure that one out! Here are 13 reasons why trans fatty acids from cooked/processed fat can kill.

♦ They are a major source of damaging free radicals which cause your body to age at an accelerated rate.
♦ They are difficult to digest.
♦ They cause the mitochondria (energy centre of your cells) to swell and malfunction, compromising energy production.
♦ They interfere with cell respiration and the function of your immune system
♦ They decrease testosterone production and increase abnormal sperm.

♦   They interfere with milk production and encourage low birth weights.
♦   They interfere with blood insulin function which can result in blood sugar imbalances and increase fat storage.
♦   They interfere with the liver enzymes necessary for detoxification. This system, the cytochrome P450 system is essential for eliminating chemicals, hormones, drugs and metabolic waste from the body. It's also necessary for eliminating excess estrogen, ensuring optimal testosterone balance.
♦   They change the fluidity of cell membranes, making them harder and slowing down their reactions, lowering cell vitality and making cell membranes leakier.
♦   They make platelets stickier because natural dispersing properties are lost when they are created.
♦   They increase the ratio of LDL (bad) cholesterol to HDL (good) cholesterol, increasing your chance of heart disease.
♦   Whenever you eat fat, it is incorporated directly into the walls of your cells. When trans-fatty acids are incorporated into the cell wall, the cell begins to lose control over which substances pass through the cell membrane into the cell, opening the doorway to salt, carcinogens, damaging free radicals, and chemicals from unnatural food sources. As they gradually accumulate within a cell, the cell becomes susceptible to ultra-violet radiation and cancer. (Research shows that cooks who spend time wok or pan-frying have a higher incidence of lung cancer.)
♦   They also raise the level of Lp(a), the strongest known risk factor for cardiovascular disease. Lp (a) carries a protein called apo(a) which is used for tissue repair. Along with fibrinogen/fibrin it can thicken arteries.

BEWARE – THEY ARE EVERYWHERE!

Trans-fatty acids (hydrogenated or partially hydrogenated oils) are widespread in your foods. You can find them in breads, cakes, cookies, crackers, digestive biscuits, breakfast cereals, instant soups, chocolate bars, desserts, fruit cakes, crisps, convenience and junk foods, peanuts and peanut butter. Even in the croutons used to make the so-called 'healthy' caesar salad. If the law prohibits trans-fatty acids from being used in baby foods, can there really be any purpose for them in your body?

ITS TIME TO BEGIN YOUR LOVE AFFAIR WITH FAT – THE FAT THAT BUILDS EXPLOSIVE HEALTH

How would you like to know which foods you need to consume on a regular basis to virtually guarantee superior health? How would like to begin using fat today to gain the edge in your quest for radiant health?

        If you've spent a lifetime eating health destroying fats in one form or another, I'm about to share with you cutting edge information that could save your life. As with most aspects of health, misinformation can lead to imbalance and the only way to ensure your health is balanced is through specific testing (I go into this in more detail in chapter 17). For now, when it comes to choosing fats for

AGGRESSIVE HEALTH there are a few key players: Whole foods such as sprouted/soaked nuts/seeds, avocados, flax oil, hemp oil, coconut oil/butter, and extra virgin olive oil.

YOUR BODY DOESN'T MANUFACTURE ESSENTIAL FATS SO THEY MUST COME FROM YOUR DIET

Plain and simple. If you haven't been eating omega 3 fatty acids, you will be deficient in them. Separate yourself from this crowd today. In fact symptoms of omega 3 deficiency are so common and varied it would take another book to list them all! Fortunately you can take a giant step towards superior health by including one food and its oil into your diet. This food is so powerful that it has been used for centuries to help people regain their energy and health and restore flagging omega 3 deficiencies. The food is flax.

GRIND YOUR OWN FLAX SEEDS, ELIMINATE ALL OMEGA 3 DEFICIENCIES AND REDISCOVER EXUBERANT HEALTH

If you want to immediately take charge of your health and reverse any fatty acid deficiencies, grab your hand blender and a few tablespoons of flax seed, grind them up and you're good to go! When you grind up the seeds into a seed meal, breaking up the tough protective coating, you unleash an arsenal of nutrition ready to serve your health in every way. Not only is flax meal cheaper than buying the oil, but you get the freshest oil possible. Limit your intake of flax seeds to 6 tablespoons per day. This will give you the equivalent of 2 tablespoons of fresh oil. I'll explain why shortly.

A STOREHOUSE OF LIFE ENHANCING NUTRIENTS

Ground up flax seeds can be found to have 35% oil content (containing lecithin), 26% protein, 14% fibre, 12% mucilage, 4% minerals and 9% water. Other compounds that you'll find in the flax meal are lignans. Lignans have powerful anti-viral, anti-fungal, anti-bacterial, and anti-cancer properties. Another important benefit according to Udo Erasmus, author of Fats That Heal – Fats That Kill is that lignans contain anti-estrogenic properties which have a powerful effect on ensuring testosterone production doesn't drop to unhealthy low levels, making flax a key superfood for the athletes. Now, imagine unleashing this arsenal of nutrition upon your cells. Flax meal has 100 times more lignans than the next best source – wheat bran. That's nutritional power.

USE THE FAT IN FLAX TO RESTORE OMEGA 3 DEFICIENCY ONLY

The key to using fats for AGGRESSIVE HEALTH is balance. Now pay attention at this point. Too many people over consume omega 6 fatty acids and neglect omega 3s. They often begin to suffer the perils of omega 3 deficiency and regain health by restoring essential fat balance. For general health, your diet should contain a 1:3 ratio of omega 3s to omega 6s. In your brain the ratio of omega 3s to omega 6s should be 1:1. In your fat tissue it is about 1:5 and in most other tissues it is about 1:4. Flax oil is so heavily weighted on the omega 3 side it is capable of turning around imbalances very quickly.

WARNING:

You only need about 3 litres of flax oil, consumed over a few months to restore a flagging omega 3 deficiency. But be warned. According to Udo Erasmus, it only takes between 10 months and 2 years of exclusive flax oil consumption to develop omega 6 deficiencies – tipping the scales in the other direction! He tells the story of how prolonged use of flax oil caused his skin to become thin and 'papery'. He goes on to say that eventually it dried out and cracked easily. Don't let this scare you. People suffering from degenerative diseases (obesity, cancer, cardiovascular disease, diabetes, and liver degeneration) usually have very low levels of essential fats in their tissues and flax is best choice of oils for restoring levels to normal. If you're not suffering ill health, regular use of ground flax seeds will be your best option.

If you are an athlete who is interested in maximising your growth potential you may be wish to keep your omega-6 to omega-3 ratio as high as 5:1. For more information go to www.aggressivehealth.co.uk and invest in the book, Maximum Muscle, Minimum Fat by Ori Hofmekler.

30% OF THE POPULATION EXPERIENCE CONSTIPATION – ELIMINATE IT WITH FLAX MEAL

Imagine having access to a food that would virtually eliminate any chances of constipation EVER again. The mucilage within flax seeds is a superior laxative that soothes and protects your stomach and intestinal lining. All you need to be aware of is that with flax meals' affinity to absorb water, you must drink at least 5 times as much water as flax. Why? Flax swells up to 20 times its dry weight making your bulky stool something to be proud of!

Another great advantage of flax mucilage is that it is excellent at buffering excess acidity in the body helping to maintain harmonious pH levels, a critical component of AGGRESSIVE HEALTH. Flax mucilage also helps you maintain 'rock steady' blood sugar levels by slowing down the rate at which sugar is absorbed by your intestinal tract and is also an excellent food for your friendly intestinal bacteria.

ONE FOOD ALONE WILL SUPPLY YOU AN ABUNDANCE OF SUPERIOR NUTRITION

Now, if you thought flax was good - Imagine a plant that grows as tall as its does deep. Imagine a plant with roots that penetrate 10 feet into the ground, drawing out vital minerals from the earth. Imagine a plant that needs no fertiliser or pesticides and that can turn carbon dioxide into oxygen and fibre faster than any other plant (including grasses and trees), making it perfect for reversing the 'greenhouse' effect.

Imagine a plant that is so resilient, it attracts no bugs or pests. Finally, imagine a plant that concentrates so much nutrition in each of its seeds, it can be considered an almost perfect food. Imagine no more. The hemp plant and its seed could single handily save the human race. You discovered the power of hemp in the last chapter, but this food is so powerful you're going to learn more! If one food was to be crowned king and had to sit on the throne of AGGRESSIVE HEALTH, it would be the hemp seed.

TOTAL NUTRITION FOR AGGRESSIVE HEALTH

Hemp oil pressed from the seed contains the perfect balance of essential fatty acids (EFAs). A 3:1 ratio of omega 6 fats to omega 3. Unlike flax which is heavily weighted on the omega 3 side, hemp is in perfect balance. Don't fear flax for its unbalanced fatty acid content – simply use it wisely. Awareness is everything. Flax is perfect for restoring a fatty acid deficiency and hemp is perfect for maintaining balance.

CREATE SUPERHORMONES WITH GLA

The other great benefit of hemp oil is that it is one of the only foods on the planet to contain GLA (gamma linoleic acid). GLA can be made by your body, but this takes an optimal environment as you'll discover in chapter 8. For now remember this – when you consume hemp seeds and their oil you get direct access to this critical fatty acid. Hemp seeds contain about 2% GLA and as you'll discover in chapter 8, GLA is critical for the formation of the super hormones 'eicosanoids'.

ELIMINATE THE NEED FOR EXPENSIVE FISH OILS

If you want to save money and eliminate the need for buying expensive fish oils, the hemp seed may be for you. As you may know, the two fats most talked about in fish oil are eicosapentaenoic acid (EPA) and docosahexaenoic acid (DHA). Fortunately for you, another advantage of the hemp seed is that it contains 2.5% stearidonic acid (SDA), which your body can use to produce EPA. So there you have it. Not only do you get essential fats, but you also get protein, fibre, minerals, vitamins, chlorophyll. The hemp seed is king.

THE PROTEIN AND FAT COMBINATION PAR EXCELLANCE.

As far back as 1888 a researcher, Lebedow discovered that when starving dogs were fed either protein or fat they die even faster than if they are left to starve, but if they were fed a combination of good protein (rich in sulphur containing amino acids methionine and cysteine) along with EFA rich oils they quickly recovered. Although most animal proteins (dairy, beef, chicken fish, shellfish, and egg) are seen as a good source of these amino acids, the cooking process alters the protein, making them difficult to digest for some people. Hemp seeds however are abundant in the sulphur containing amino acids, are easy to digest **AND** contain a perfect balance of essential fats. Awesome.

RESPOND TO YOUR BODYS CRY FOR MINERALS

If you want to ensure your mineral intake is optimal take note. The hemp plant reaches 10 feet below the earth's surface drawing out vital minerals that can powerfully impact your health. Whether your need is for more phosphorus, potassium, sodium, magnesium, sulfur, calcium, iron, or zinc, the hemp seed delivers. Many people who eat an abundance of fruit may suffer from a lack of phosphorus. In the medical reference Calcium Homeostasis, Gregory Mundy, MD, states that serum phosphorus can fall by 33% within two hours after eating a carbohydrate rich meal. Reduce sugar TODAY and redirect your focus. This is the beginning of nutritional mastery.

EMBRACE THE GREAT BALANCING ACT:
SATURATED AND UNSATURATED FATS

Another myth surrounding fat is that ALL saturated fat is bad. What you very rarely hear is that your cells use long-chain saturated fats to build cell membranes. With too many unsaturated fats and not enough saturated fat you begin to lose vital balance at the cellular level. The aggregating action of saturated fats balances the dispersing action of the unsaturated fats found in hemp and flax. One oil stands head and shoulders above the rest for its saturated fat content. Are you ready for another key player in the AGGRESSIVE HEALTH line up?

IMMEDIATELY REDUCE YOUR CALORIE INTAKE TODAY BY
CHOOSING COCONUT OIL

Did you know there exists a fat that is lower in calories than all other fats? Did you also know that this fat can stimulate your metabolism, help you lose fat, protect you against 'superbugs' by boosting your immunity and also feed your cells quickly and efficiently, giving you access to immediate energy? The fat I'm talking about is coconut oil. Most fats contain 9 calories per gram, but coconut oil with its high content of MCFA (medium chain fatty acids) contains only 6.8 calories per gram. Can you imagine how delighted most dieters are when they hear this?

IF CALORIE RESTRICTION DOESN'T IMPRESS YOU
DISCOVER THE TWO SECRETS OF ENERGY METABOLISM THAT
MAKE COCONUT OIL A MUST FOR FUELING THE NATION

When you eat coconut oil, the MCFA are broken down almost immediately by enzymes in your saliva and gastric juices. Once broken down, MCFA are absorbed directly from your intestines into your portal vein and sent straight to your liver where they are, for the most part, burned as fuel much like a carbohydrate. But it doesn't stop there! Inside each of your cells is the energy producing factory of the cell called the mitochondria. Mitochondria are encased in two membranous sacs which normally require special enzymes to transport nutrients through the double membrane, slowing energy production and taxing enzyme reserves. Not with MCFA found in coconut oil. They easily permeate both membranes without the need of enzymes, providing your cells with an immediate source of energy.

A FOOD OF CHOICE FOR THE SMALL AND SICK

Even premature babies and sick infants with underdeveloped organs benefit from coconut oil. Studies show that they absorb MCFA with ease, whereas other fats can often be found passing through their systems undigested. Coconut oil has the highest MCFA content of any food at 63%, making it critical for AGGRESSIVE HEALTH. MCFAs rev up your metabolism and increase your fat burning potential. MCFAs allow you to absorb more minerals, vitamins and amino acids. MCFAs are one of the reasons why breast milk is THE food of choice for new born babies.

WHY BREAST FEEDING CREATES STRONGER, HEALTHIER, HAPPIER BABIES

If you could feed your baby a food that doesn't tax their digestive system, supply unrivalled nutrition and protect against viruses such as HIV and herpes, bacteria such a chlamydia and H. pyloris, fungi such as Candida and protozoa such as giardia, would you dismiss it? Of course not! That's the promise of MCFAs found abundantly in breast milk.

When pregnant and lactating pigs were fed diets containing either long-chain fatty acids from vegetable oil or medium-chain fatty acids from coconut oil there was a dramatic difference in both survival and growth rates. The piglets whose mothers received the MCFA grew faster and healthier and had a survival rate of 68% compared to 32% and it's no different for humans. For example, coconut oil was added to the formula of 46 very low-birth weight babies. Just as expected, the group consuming the coconut oil grew quicker and became larger without storing any extra fat. Simply put, the coconut oil was easily digested, where as the vegetable oils were seen to be passing through their digestive tracts undigested.

COCONUT OIL AND THE PROTECTION AGAINST VIRUSES, BACTERIA AND INFECTIONS

In a world where supergerms are on the increase, how can you guard against them? Simple, a small daily dose of coconut oil. When it is eaten your body transforms its unique fatty acids into powerful antimicrobial agents that have the power to over throw some of the most insidious disease causing micro organisms. If you think this is just more hype about another fatty acid, I assure you – it's not. If you were breast fed, lauric acid, found abundantly in your mothers breast milk, would have been your first line of defence against disease. Your body would have converted the lauric acid to a fatty acid derivative (monolaurin), which would have protected you from viral, bacterial or protozoal infections.

Whether you're dealing with viruses, bacteria, yeast, fungal infections or any other pathogenic micro organisms, begin using coconut oil – without it you may not be getting enough lauric acid into your diet. Even sufferers of chronic fatigue are now using coconut oil to ward off herpes, Epstein-Barr virus, Candida, giardia and a whole host of other infectious organisms. Lauric acid is now being used to treat the symptoms associated with AIDS.

LEARN FROM THE FARMERS WHO TRIED TO FATTEN THEIR CATTLE, BUT ENDED UP WITH A FIELD FULL OF LEAN, MEAN, HEALTHY COWS!

Rather than dig out sophisticated studies, ask a farmer about the power of coconut oil. Farmers will do anything to fatten up their livestock! As you can imagine, the fatter the animals the fatter the profits! But when farmers decided to use coconut oil because of its saturated fat content they were horrified at the results. The animals actually lost weight! It wasn't long before they put them back on their usual diet of high polyunsaturated oil from corn and soybeans causing them to pack on the pounds for market. Ray Peat, Ph.D, an endocrinologist specialising in the study of hormones highlights the dangers of unsaturated oils. He explains that unsaturated oils can block thyroid hormone secretion and movement in the circulation, thus inhibiting its overall action in the body. If your thyroid hormones are deficient, your metabolism will become depressed and weight gain is the result.

WARNING: Polyunsaturated oils encourage weight gain more than any other fat!

REV UP YOUR METABOLISM WITH COCONUT OIL AND SHIFT INTO A CALORIE BURNING GEAR

Why did the farmers end up with lean, mean, healthy cows after feeding them coconut oil? If you want a perfect analogy describing the difference between MCFA found in coconut oils and LCFA (long chain fatty acids) found in polyunsaturated fats listen to Dr Julian Whitaker.

"LCFAs are like heavy wet logs that you put on a small campfire. Keep adding the logs and soon you have more logs than fire. MCFAs are like rolled up newspaper soaked in gasoline. They not only burn brightly, but will burn up the wet logs as well."

In one study MCFA given over a six-day period increased diet-induced fat-burning by 50%! In another study, researchers compared single meals of 400 calories composed entirely of MCFA (medium chain fatty acids) and of LCFA (long chain fatty acids). The fat burning effect of MCFA over six hours was three times greater than that of LCFA. The simple fact is that when you replace cooked fats and oils with coconut oil you immediately benefit from the effects MCFAs. Refined vegetable oil promotes weight gain by supplying more nutritionally void calories, and by harming the thyroid

– lowering metabolic rate. Coconut oil does the exact opposite and because it is primarily a saturated fat, the heat of cooking does not create a free radical soup like it does with other vegetable oils. If you are going to use oil to cook with, choose coconut oil/butter. It is the most stable of any known oil/butter (up to 170 degrees Fahrenheit)

THE YIN AND YANG OF FAT METABOLISM
IF A LITTLE IS GOOD...

An excess of any food can cause problems and it's no different with fat. For example, as good as coconut oil is, if you consume too much you'll interfere with the chemical conversion of essential fatty acids into eicosanoids. But at the same time, if you do include it in your diet it improves the utilisation of the essential fatty acids and protects them from oxidation. Dr Doug Graham author of Food 'n' Sport and Grain damage recommends less than 10% of calories to come from fat. Udo Erasmus, author of Fats That Heal Fat That Kill recommends 15% or less. Other authorites go as high as 30%. What they don't tell you is that if your beta-oxidation pathway is strong you'll be able to easily use fats for energy. If it is weak and your metabolism is stuck in the tricarboxylic acid pathway (carbohydrate burning) you may have trouble dealing with a high fat load. What's important here is for you to realise that you have your own unique fuel mix. For some people, high protein/high fat/low carb works really well. For others, high carbohydrate/low fat/low protein is key for optimal health. For me, it's a balance – but that doesn't mean it's a balance for you. For more information on these essential energy pathways and how biological terrain testing can highlight imbalances at the core homeostatic level, contact me at www.aggressivehealth.co.uk. Ultimately I want you to find your correct fuel mix. In order to do so experiment with different combinations (high/low protein, high/low fat, high/low carbohydrate) because this will give you insight into how you operate at your very best. The best advice for now is to experiment with the good fats. Flax will help regain balance, hemp will help you maintain balance and your use of coconut oil and extra virgin olive oil along with sprouted foods will help complete the picture.

THE PHYTOCHEMICAL REVOLUTION:
MINOR INGREDIENTS FROM EXTRA VIRGIN OLIVE OILS

Extra virgin olive oil is such a key food for AGGRESSIVE HEALTH is because of the minor ingredients (phytochemicals) it contains? Although they only make up about 2% of the oil these phytochemicals are nature's pharmacy and must remain in foods if they are to create outstanding health.

- ◆ Minor ingredients found in extra virgin olive oil:
- ◆ Help lower cholesterol, and block cholesterol absorption from foods.
- ◆ Improve cardiovascular function.
- ◆ Improve digestion, and stimulate pancreatic enzyme production.

+ Improve liver and gall bladder function, and increase bile flow.
+ Act as anti-oxidants and stabilise essential fatty acids against oxidation (rancidity).
+ Act as anti-inflammatory agents.
+ Protect visual functions, and improve brain function.

Extra virgin olive oil contains a mono unsaturated fat called oleic acid, which will help you maintain youthful, supple arteries allowing you to maintain exceptional health.

THE MAGIC OF THE AVOCADO

Avocados are marvellous! Not only will they help you eliminate any cravings for cooked/processed fats, but they will leave you feeling full and satisfied.

Avocados are a rich source of a monounsaturated fat called oleic acid. "We've found that these monounsaturated fats improve fat levels in the body and help control diabetes," says Abhimanyu Garg, M.D., associate professor of internal medicine and clinical nutrition at the University of Texas' South-western Medical Centre at Dallas.

In a study from Mexico, researchers compared the effects of two low-fat diets. The diets were the same except that one included avocados and the other didn't. Amazingly, by including this powerful food, LDL cholesterol was lowered, HDL cholesterol was raised and triglycerides were lowered. You couldn't get a more favourable cholesterol response. Avocados are also excellent at helping re-establish hormonal balance within the system:

+ They also contain a seven-carbon sugar that depresses insulin production, making them an excellent choice for people with hypoglycaemia.
+ One of the most important functions of fat is to slow the rate and speed of which sugars enter the digestive tract – blunting insulin response.

Join the elite group of AGGRESSIVE HEALTH enthusiasts who know how important avocados are and enjoy clear smooth skin, stable energy levels and exceptional health. Avocados are also rich in fibre, potassium and folate – all critical for AGGRESSIVE HEALTH. But there's more:

+ One avocado contains 10 grams of fibre. That's more than a bran muffin and is 40% of your daily need.
+ "You can never get too much potassium," says David B. Young, Ph.D., professor of physiology and biophysics at the University of Mississippi Medical Centre in Jackson. Avocados pack a huge potassium punch – about 1100mg, a third of your daily requirement. Studies indicate that people who eat diets high in potassium rich foods have a significantly lower risk of high blood pressure, heart attack and stroke.

♦ One avocado will also provide a third of your folate requirements, a nutrient that helps prevent life threatening birth defects of the brain and spine. All you potential mothers out there, take note! Folate is essential for keeping nerves functioning properly.

♦ Avocados, like all raw foods, are full of enzymes assisting your body in a multitude of ways.

♦ Use raw fats to your advantage, it stimulates the release of the hormone cholecystokinin (CCK) helping to promote a feeling of fullness, allowing you to feel fuller for longer.

ONE FINAL TIP WHICH MAY EXPLAIN WHY HIGH FAT DIETS CAN CAUSE HEART DISEASE

Dr Kilmen, M.D. Professor of Pathology at Harvard Medical School states that the original injury in heart disease is caused by a series of events initiated by a deficiency of vitamin B6, and an increase in the toxic substance, homocysteine. Homocysteine is a breakdown product of the amino acid, methionine, but when vitamin B6 is present, homocysteine is unable to do its destructive work. Vitamin B6, acting as a co-enzyme, facilitates an enzyme reaction, which quickly converts homocysteine to cystathionine, which is non toxic and is safely used by the body in other pathways. But what has this got to do with a high fat diet? Simple. B6 gets used up at an acclerated rate when you ingest a lot of fat. The answer: Learn to love foods high in B6 content. Now, a few select foods have a highly desirable B6/methionine ratio:

1. Bananas with 10:1
2. Carrots with a ratio of 15:1
3. Onions with a ratio of 10:1
4. **Bee Pollen with a ratio of 400:1. FOUR HUNDRED TO ONE!**

Now since vitamin B6 gets used up rapidly on a high fat diet you can see the link between too much fat and heart disease. For more information about bee pollen visit www.aggressivehealth.co.uk.

SELECTING THE FINEST FATS

Here is a selection of the best fats. Choose whole foods for fat first and oils second. Add these to your shopping list:

Hemp seed and its oil, coconut butter, flax seed and its oil, olives and their oil (stone pressed extra-virgin if possible) akee (a relative of the durian fruit found growing in West Africa and the West Indies), borage seed oil, durians, grape seeds, nuts of all types, raw nut butters (almond butter is excellent), pumpkin seeds and their oil (cold pressed), sesame seeds, sunflower seeds, Tahini (sesame butter), unhulled Tahini (an alkaline fat, high in calcium), young coconuts (available at Asian markets).

ARE YOU READY FOR THE CHALLENGE?

Although fats have been seen as the enemy for many years, essential fatty acids are your closest friends. Respect them, use them to your advantage and reap the rewards.

- EFAs absorb sunlight, increasing their oxygen reacting ability a 1000 times, making them very chemically active.
- EFAs hold oxygen in the cell membranes where they prevent foreign organisms such as viruses and bacteria entering by creating a barrier. Such organisms cannot thrive in the presence of oxygen.
- EFAs are the precursors of a gang of hormone-like substances known as eicosanoids.
- EFAs help carry toxins and other substances to the surface of your skin, intestinal tract, kidneys, or lungs where these substances are discarded. The slight negative charge carried by raw plant fats allows them to do this. They disperse concentrations of substances, causing them to spread out in a very thin layer over surfaces. This charge also prevents each molecule from aggregating as they repel one another.
- EFAs are the precursors of the highly active, very highly unsaturated fatty acids required for brain cells, synapses, retina, adrenal glands, and testes to function properly.
- EFAs improve performance by improving calmness under pressure and improving your ability to concentrate. They also help you sleep better and decrease your sleep requirement.
- EFAs improve performance because they improve the capacity of your liver and kidneys for detoxification. They also enhance the ability of glands such as the thyroid.
- EFAs improve performance by improving gut integrity, allowing you to digest and absorb nutrients more efficiently. They help prevent energy-robbing allergic reactions secondary to poor digestion. They also help you maintain a healthy intestinal flora.
- In your immune system, EFAs protect your genetic material (DNA) from damage. Omega 3 essential fatty acids have anti-oxidant-like functions in the oil soluble system of your body (similar to the anti-oxidant functions of vitamin C in the water-soluble system). Their anti-oxidant ability protects you from the damaging effects of free radicals. Your immune cells use raw plant fats to make oxygen 'bullets' to kill infectious foreign invaders preventing them from eating your tissues.
- EFAs protect you from the toxic influences of oil-soluble pollutants such as pesticides, PCBs and chlorinated hydrocarbons. These oil-soluble poisons exit your body with the oil.
- EFAs help treat fungus infections like athlete's foot and yeast over growth (candida). They've also been known to inhibit tumour growth.
- EFAs elevate mood, lift depression and help prevent cravings of all kinds.

- EFAs help your kidneys dump excess water, decreasing unnecessary bloating. Without them, your kidneys cannot do their job properly and you'll retain water in your tissues.
- EFAs lower the glycemic index of sweet and starchy foods, preventing wild blood sugar fluctuations.
- EFAs improve your immune cells' ability to produce hydrogen peroxide (made by oxidising essential fatty acids) that they use to kill unwanted bugs.
- EFAs help control yeast overgrowths (like Candida) that can be found in your intestinal tract.
- EFAs make skin soft, smooth and velvety, and are excellent internal, edible cosmetics. The best way to oil the skin is from within. You'll tan better, burn less, get relief from eczema, acne, psoriasis, and other skin conditions.
- Sperm formation requires essential fatty acids. In the female reproductive cycle, they help prevent pre-menstrual syndrome.
- EFAs contain an abundance of antioxidants that deactivate free radicals by giving them electrons. The spare electrons in fats help sweep toxins along to the liver. In a healthy body, when there are spare electrons, ageing is slowed.
- EFAs can buffer excess acid as well as excess alkalinity in your body.
- Essential fatty acids lower fibrinogen/fibrin levels. Vitamin C and other antioxidants can help lower Lp(a) and apo(a) that can thicken arteries. Your initial priority is in eliminating the cause – trans fatty acids. If you are interested in a vitamin C/antioxidant supplemental superfood that I rate as the best in the world go to www.aggressivehealth.co.uk.
- Donald Rudin, MD, showed that when juvenile delinquents were given omega 3 rich oils, they became more responsive to counselling. The human brain is made from food, and requires essential fatty acids to function. It's up to us as parents to take responsibility and feed our children raw plant fats. Lead by example.

FEROCIOUS ENERGY, PERFORMANCE AND STAYING POWER WITH RAW PLANT FATS

- If you are serious about exercise and fitness, you'll be interested to know that heavily processed fats change the outer layer (membrane) of your muscle, preventing the flow of nutrients and glucose to muscle cells, compromising performance. Eliminate them!
- When athletes optimise their fat intake, their performance both in strength and in endurance increases dramatically. High fat meals can help promote steroid production as long as calorie supply is sufficient.
- EFAs improve performance by making red blood cell membranes more flexible, allowing them to slide through your capillaries more easily, which in turn improves the delivery of nutrients and oxygen to your cells, tissues, organs, glands and muscles.
- EFAs attract oxygen like a magnet! EFAs are involved with the transfer of oxygen from the air in the lungs – through the alveolar membrane – through the

capillary wall – into the blood plasma – across the membranes of the red blood cells – to the haemoglobin – to all cells in the body. They make oxygen available to the tissues, by activating oxygen molecules.

♦ EFAs help you recover from fatigue quicker, because recovery requires oxygen, and essential fatty acids increase the body's ability to metabolise oxygen.

♦ EFAs help you to lose unwanted body fat by increasing the rate at which you burn calories. They make you feel more energetic and therefore more physically active. Refusal to exercise is usually due to lack of energy. EFAs provide that energy, where as cooked fats make you feel lazy and lethargic and slow your metabolic rate. EFAs have anti-inflammatory properties. They help minimise joint, tendon and ligament strain.

♦ EFAs decrease recovery time of fatigued muscles after exercise, by facilitating the conversion of lactic acid to water and carbon dioxide. If you workout with weights you'll perform better, grow faster and recover quicker. (Combine EFAs with green leafy vegetables after a workout for excellent results.)

♦ EFAs are anti-catabolic. They are part of protein metabolism, and prevent muscle breakdown. Without EFAs, protein can become toxic (a warning for those who eat lots of protein to build muscles and avoid fats because they have been misinformed by those with a rampant fat phobia).

♦ EFAs are required for testosterone production and insulin function, both of which are important for muscular development. Body builders on low fat diets fail to gain the development they strive for, because testosterone is required for muscle development.

In 1900, deaths from cardiovascular disease accounted for only 15% of all deaths from all causes. But today, 100 years later, with an increase of over 350%, it kills over 50% of the entire population.

In 1900, cancer killed 1 person in every 30. Today it kills over 1 in 3 of the entire population. So much for medical advances! If you were to chart the increases in disease from other forms of fatty degeneration such as diabetes, multiple sclerosis, kidney degeneration and liver degeneration you'd find similar increases. Tissue and blood levels of people with diseases of fatty degeneration (Cardiovascular disease, cancer, diabetes, arthritis, obesity, mental dysfunction) are low in essential fatty acids. When essential fatty acids are added to the diets of these people, the symptoms surrounding the diseases begin to fade. When fat is cooked, diseases and deaths prevail. Be warned! Your body instinctively craves fat. It's up to you to supply the right kinds at the right time. If you want a complete biological terrain analysis along with live blood microscopy to assess your current health status contact me at www.aggressivehealth.co.uk. More about these tests later.

THE AGGRESSIVE HEALTH EVALUATION
Do you happily eat a small variety of flax seed, hemp seed, coconut oil, olive oil, avocados and other sprouted/soaked nuts and seeds?
Have you eliminated processed/cooked fat from your diet?

The world can be a harsh place. Toxicity is everywhere and nutritionally void food is becoming common place. If you don't do everything you can to eliminate this waste and keep your body clean, toxicity can drain the life right out of you.

CHAPTER 5

IS YOUR BODY A FILTER FOR WASTE, POLLUTION AND TOXICITY? LEARN HOW TO STOP THE ROT

Health is as infectious as disease, given the right conditions for its spread –
Dr George Scott-Williamson, 1943

The current perception of detoxification needs a face-lift. People tend to think they have to be on a detoxification diet for detoxification to occur. Wrong! Whenever waste matter passes out of your body via your skin, bowels, urine, breath etc. you are ridding your body of waste. This is the natural process of detoxification and it is happening every minute of every day, by embracing it, you'll begin to eliminate waste faster and set the stage for exuberant health. Every natural process in your body is designed to preserve life. If you don't assist the detoxification process on a regular basis, you'll never eliminate the obstructions that can eventually lead to your demise.

BEGIN RESTRUCTURING YOUR BODY TODAY!

Today you have the opportunity to make a very important decision. Over the course of the next two years, 98% of the atoms in your body will be completely replaced. Over the course of the next seven years, 100% of your body will be replaced. What does this mean? With a powerful vision and the love of creation, you can literally rebuild a new you. You are constantly recreating yourself out of the food you eat, the air you breathe and the water you drink.

If you make the decision to embrace detoxification and completely clear your body of ALL unwanted waste, it'll be one of the most rewarding journeys you'll ever take. Ultimately you'll have the joy of knowing that every cell and atom in your body is crackling with energy and built from something alive and vibrant. Whether you're in your teens or about to reach 100, it's never too late to regenerate.

THE TUBES OF DETOXIFICATION

The best way to think of detoxification, intoxication and digestion is to imagine that your body consists of three layers of 'tubes'.

1. The first tube is your digestive system or alimentary canal. It runs from your mouth to your anus and consists of the mouth, oesophagus, stomach, intestines, and colon. Each of these organs help to break down and assimilate foods. As you'll soon discover, when this tube is obstructed by a substance called mucoid plaque it can lead to a whole host of problems.
2. The second tube is your circulatory system and it draws in whatever is present in the first tube. If you've just ingested hemp seeds for example, the chlorophyll, enzymes, amino acids, vitamins, minerals, phytochemicals and trace elements will enter your bloodstream ready to create amazing health. If you've eaten a meal of cooked meat and pasteurised milk, your bloodstream will draw in those elements and your blood will thicken and slow down. This second tube consists of arteries, veins, capillaries, and the heart.
3. The third tube is the lymphatic system. It's the lymph fluid that bathes every cell, organ, muscle and tissue drawing nutrients (and waste) from the bloodstream before delivering them to the cells. If the bloodstream is full of powerful nutrients, the cells will get a good feed. If the bloodstream is full of the waste, the cells will be poorly nourished. The lymphatic system also returns the waste products of cell metabolism back to the blood and back to the intestines. Did you know that you have four times as much lymph in your body as you do blood? The lymphatics also hold 80% of your body's antioxidant capacity, necessary for the fight against free radicals. The liver is also filled with lymphatics, highlighting the importance of keeping this tube flowing freely and unobstructed. When you create a free flowing bloodstream, the lymph fluid can mobilise any waste that may have built up around the cells and eliminate it.

Now that you are aware of the three tubes of detoxification, you need to know what can be done to bring each 'tube' back to perfect functioning. Let's begin with the Tube 1 - Your digestive system or alimentary canal

A PICTURE OF IMPERFECT HEALTH
EMERGES FROM INSIDE

Take a look at the following pictures.

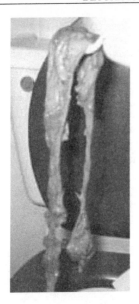 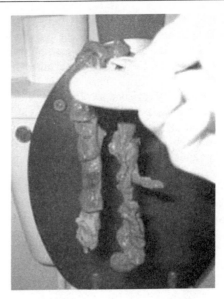

If you knew that deep within your body, coating your alimentary canal (from your tongue to your anus) there was a thick, rubbery, slimy mucus layer that was preventing you from getting the MAXIMUM nutrition from food – would you want to get it out? What if this foul smelling layer was harbouring parasites, preventing nutrient absorption and basically robbing you of life – would you be motivated to rid your body of this hazardous material?

SO WHAT IS THIS THICK RUBBERY MUCUS AND WHY IS IT SO DANGEROUS TO OPTIMAL HEALTH?

If you've spent a lifetime eating an acidifying diet, full of meat, dairy, sugar, bread, wheat, fried food, fizzy drink etc. with very little nutrient rich food, your body will have responded by creating an internal shield to help prevent the devastating effect of the excess acidity. This shield consists of mucin, a glycoprotein mucus secreted by your intestinal glands. It lines the intestines in an effort to protect you from acids and other irritants. If this situation persists, layers of mucus build up until they form mucoid plaque. This plaque is so insidious it prevents normal digestion and assimilation NO MATTER HOW GOOD YOUR DIET IS! It harbours toxicity, causes your bowels to lose efficiency and destroys the balance of healthy bacteria in your gut, opening the door to bowel disease, the forerunner to almost ALL diseases of modern civilisation.

TAKING A STRANGLE HOLD ON YOUR HEALTH

Mucin, mucoid, glycoprotein or mucoprotein – call it what you will, is strangling the health out of millions of people, and maybe you are one of them. You may not notice it now, but once you expel it from your body, the mere experience of not having it will be so powerful; you'll want to shout it from the rooftops.

In his book Tissue cleansing through bowel management, Dr Bernard Jensen D.C., N.D., Ph.D. shares a powerful example of how insidious mucoid plaque can be,

"One autopsy revealed a colon to be 9 inches in diameter with a passage through it no larger than a pencil. The rest was caked up layer upon layer of encrusted faecal material. This accumulation can have the consistency of truck-tire rubber. It's that hard and black. Another autopsy revealed a stagnant colon to weigh in at an incredible 40 pounds. Imagine carrying around all that morbid accumulated waste."

If you are highly motivated to lose weight, and 'your key to happiness' is seeing a low reading on the scales, focus on eliminating the mucoid plaque that may be weighing you down. A healthy colon should only weigh between 4 and 6 pounds –not 40!

ONLY WHEN YOU EXPEL THIS THICK RUBBERY, FOUL SMELLING MUCUS FROM YOUR BODY CAN YOU EXPERIENCE THE JOY OF AGGRESSIVE HEALTH

Do you know what happens to mucoid plaque if it isn't dealt with? It gets thicker, harder and more toxic. Before long it becomes the home for a whole host of pathogenic micro organisms and parasites. How can any attempt be made to regain health if this filth isn't removed?

AGGRESSIVE HEALTH CANNOT BE ACHIEVED UNLESS YOU RID YOUR BODY OF MUCOID PLAQUE

Whether you're reading this because you feel sick and are worried about your future or if you consider yourself in good health – until you rid your body of mucoid plaque your attempts to accelerate down the path to explosive health may be compromised. Don't get me wrong, you can still make incredible progress, but talking from personal experience, the difference before and after doing the cleanse is like night and day. Every disease known to man can be traced to a foul putrefying internal state. Clean tube No.1 and you march towards AGGRESSIVE HEALTH with CERTAINTY!

RIDDING YOURSELF OF MUCOID PLAQUE ONCE AND FOR ALL

THE BIG QUESTION: How do you eliminate mucoid plaque? ANSWER: By embracing a 3-4 week cleanse program designed specifically to soften the plaque and expel it from your body. Even after years of eating a high raw diet I still managed to expel length after length of foul smelling, rubbery mucoid during this cleanse. Take a look at those pictures again. I took these pictures 2½ weeks into the cleanse once the mucoid plaque started to exit my body. Let me tell you – it had an odour like burn't rubber mixed with the smell of an old peoples home. Get it out!

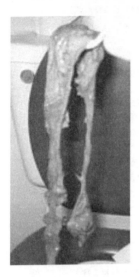
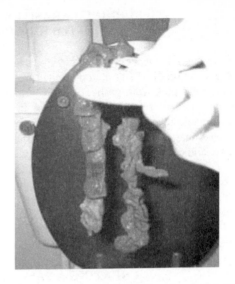

After seeing this it begs the question. How can ANY diet be truly successful if mucoid plaque remains stuck to the alimentary canal preventing the maximum absorption of nutrients? Many experts have suggested that nothing is able to get this rid of this foul smelling waste other than a highly sophisticated program designed to soften the plaque and expel it. For more information goto www.aggressivehealth.co.uk. One of the keys to AGGRESSIVE HEALTH is being systematic in your approach. When you clean the first tube via a herbal cleanse and eliminate mucoid plaque you set the stage for perpetual health.

CREATE A HARMONIOUS ENVIRONMENT
WHERE PARASITES DON'T WANT TO LIVE

There is a lot of talk about parasites in today's society, but without mucoid plaque to 'get their teeth into' they can't even get a foot hold in a strong powerful body. Imagine layers of sticky, slimy faeces attaching itself to your intestinal tract, building up into a tough, rubbery foul smelling substance. In the same way that mosquitoes love a stagnant pond environment, parasites love a stagnant mucoid covered environment to live and feed on. Again, it's not a parasite problem as much as it is a problem with the internal terrain and internal pollution. Parasites protect themselves by burying inside or under the layers of filth and remain there until the mucoid plaque is eliminated. Once it has, you can then focus on restoring optimal bowel pH and create a healthy environment for the good bacteria. Simple. Anyone who disagrees hasn't had the experience of this 'stuff' being eliminated.

BURNING PARASITES OUT OF YOUR BODY
WITH RIPE HOT PEPPERS

Commercial meat is loaded with parasitic worms. Parasites feed on toxicity, especially cooked starch and animal protein. A great ritual to keep them at bay is to take your pick from garlic, onion, ripe hot peppers, ginger, radishes, etc. and ensure you eat them regularly or use them in your vegetable juices. Ripe hot foods are invaluable to health. Not only do they burn parasites out of your intestines but they also stimulate the intestines. It's important to know that parasites can prevent weight gain and cause emaciation.

Hot peppers are excellent foods to eat if you live in the city. Every city has its fair share of people who are either ill or very toxic. If you live in the city, you are likely to come into contact with these people on a moment-to-moment basis. Hot peppers are antibiotic, wiping out harmful bacteria and boosting your immune system. If hot peppers are too strong, try garlic, onions or ginger as an alternative. Use them in your vegetable juices for an all powerful AGGRESSIVE HEALTH cocktail.

CREATING A PASSAGE TO BE PROUD OF!

Now that you're committed to experiencing explosive health, book an appointment with a colon hydrotherapist. Colonic hydrotherapy is a gentle internal bath using warm, purified water that can help to eliminate stored faecal matter, gas, mucus and toxic substances from the colon. Once the colon is clean and more efficient, detoxification and elimination will be enhanced dramatically. Combine colonics with a herbal cleanse and in only a few weeks you'll feel like you've been given a new lease of life. This is more than just hype. This is one of the most important aspects of AGGRESSIVE HEALTH.

Did you know that the transit time of food through your body should be less than 24 hours? On average in the UK it is now 60 hours for men and 70 for women. The United Kingdom is the most constipated nation in the world and has the highest incidence of bowel cancer with over 20,000 new cases every year.

Unless you are sick, I don't believe it is a good idea to completely clean your colon with a series of colonics until you're regularly incorporating juicing, sprouting and a high raw diet. Once your diet is built on this powerful foundation, colonic irrigation will be another tool in your AGGRESSIVE HEALTH arsenal!

"I WOULD TRAVEL 1000 MILES FOR SOME COLONICS BEFORE I
WOULD ALLOW MYSELF TO BE TAKEN TO HOSPITAL"
DR NORMAN WALKER, AUTHOR OF COLON HEALTH

Dr. Bassler repored that by reducing intestinal toxaemia, he had 100% success eliminating cardiac arrhythmia.
C.W. Hawley, M.D., treated many cases of eyestrain and disease with success by relieving intestinal toxaemia.
In 1892, a Dr. Herter (M.D.) linked intestinal putrification to epilepsy in 31 patients.

If you suffer from any of the following afflictions, book a series of colonics today. It'll be the best money you've ever spent.

Constipation, fatigue, poor eyesight, hearing loss, asthma, prostate trouble, colds, allergies, nagging back ache, respiratory disorders, excessive gas, abdominal pain, colitis, thyroid deficiency, diabetes, hayfever, tonsillitis, sore throat, chest problems, glandular problems, heart problems, liver difficulties, gall bladder problems, over-exhausted pancreas and breast lumps.

WHEN YOUR COLON IS COMPLETELY CLEAN
YOUR HEALTH WILL BE REVITALISED

Imagine working as a colon hydrotherapist and seeing 100 patients with hay fever walk through your door. Imagine giving them all a series of colonics and finding that every last patient was 'cured' from their symptoms! You may think it strange to blame the symptoms of hay fever, a runny nose and sore throat on the condition of the colon, but nearly everyone who has experienced colonic irrigation has benefited from complete remission. Dr Norman walker states in his book 'Colon Health' that every X-ray taken of a hay fever sufferer shows blockages in exactly the same area of the colon.

> *William Lintz, M.D., successfully treated 472 patients suffering from allergies by cleansing the bowel.*
> *Allan Eustis, M.D., Professor at Tulane University of Medicine in 1912, cured 121 cases of bronchial asthma by intestinal cleansing.*
> *D. Rochestoer, M.D., University of Buffalo School of Medicine in 1906, made the statement that after 23 years of observation, he concluded that toxaemia of gastrointestinal tract origin is the underlying cause of asthma.*

Even those who have been advised to go under the knife of the surgeon for breast removal (due to lumps being found in the breast tissue) have found that after a series of colonic irrigations, the lumps completely disappeared in a matter of days!

WARNING: JUST AS DIARRHOEA CAUSES RAPID ELECTROLYTE DEPLETION, SO DO COLONICS. IDEALLY YOU'D FINISH A COLONIC WITH A WHEATGRASS ENEMA. IF THIS ISN'T POSSIBLE FOCUS ON VEGETABLE JUICES AND SUPERFOODS TO RESTORE ELECTROLTYE BALANCE.

Taking care of the first tube of detoxification often maximises the efficiency of both tube 2 – the bloodstream and tube 3 – the lymphatic system. But for maximum results let's dig a little deeper.

TUBE 2 – THE BLOODSTREAM
ALLOWING THE RIVER OF LIFE TO FLOW

As Dr William Wong so eloquently puts it, "The bloodstream is the river of life, but is also the river of trash." Cleansing your bloodstream and bringing it back to an optimal state is critical for AGGRESSIVE HEALTH.

Here are two pictures. One of them is of healthy blood and one is taken from the excellent book 'How You Rot And Rust' which can be ordered from www.biomedx.com. It is from a patient diagnosed with inoperable cancer and given 30 days to live by her doctor. The picture shows deterioration on the slide after 30mins. Which picture would you want for your blood?

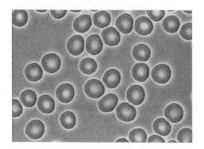 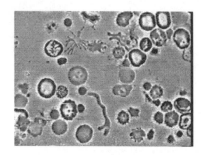

As you can see, the bloodstream is a powerful mirror image of your current state of health. In the healthy blood, red cells are of a similar size and shape, reside freely in their own space and gently bounce off each other. The goal of AGGRESSIVE HEALTH is to get your blood looking like this. Remember the simple formula – when your blood looks great, you feel great! In the other picture the blood stream looks like a war zone. If you are interested in live blood analysis contact me at www.aggressivehealth.co.uk where we discuss these principles in more depth.

Note: A website exists called www.quackwatch.org that highlights live blood analysis as 'another gimmick to sell you something'. As with all disciplines, there will be helpful practitioners and unhelpful ones that will indeed, just try to sell you something rather than educate you. I use live blood analysis to compliment biological terrain testing. Often times what you see in the live blood confirms findings found in the biological terrain. Ultimately, if your blood looks anything other than perfect, there is room for improvement through education and effective action. In the UK you can visit www.lifephorce.com and access 'The UK Live Blood Network' for a list of practitioners.

COOKED WASTE CLOGS THE BLOODSTREAM

To illustrate the power of food on the bloodstream, watch the video by Dr. Michael Klaper, entitled 'A Diet For All Reasons'. Dr. Klaper shows you the effects of a typical cooked meat and pasteurised milk diet. After only a few hours of ingesting this waste, the blood becomes very thick and heavy! Did you know that there are more heart attacks in the United States on Thanksgiving Day than any other day of the year? Is there a connection here?

SURGEONS KNOW THIS – WHY DON'T YOU?

Did you know that surgeons refuse to operate on a patient unless they've fasted on water for at least 8 hours? They know from first hand experience the dangers involved when the bloodstream isn't flowing freely enough. Cooked foods insulate and dampen your body's electrical nervous system. Senses become dulled and life becomes grey rather than colourful. Enough. What can you do about this situation today?

STEPS TO PERFECT HEALTH THROUGH
FOCUSING ON THE BLOOD

Many of the principles discussed so far, namely a high raw diet, plenty of chlorophyll rich foods (wheatgrass juice, E3Live, green superfoods and juiced greens), a high volume of sprouted foods (pulses, seeds, nuts and grains), along with healthy fats can make all the difference to the look of your blood and the way you feel. One critical reason why all of these principles work so well is their direct effect on supplying alkalising minerals to the body.

WHY pH AFFECTS EVERY ASPECT OF AGGRESSIVE HEALTH

Did you know that every minute of every day your body is striving to maintain the pH of your blood in a very narrow range around 7.3? Any shift either side of this and there can be devastating consequences. Although your body has a number of powerful mechanisms to keep blood pH in this range, the over indulgence in processed/junk foods can often use up these resources leaving you in a vulnerable position. pH is so important that if you don't do all you can to ensure balance you can create an environment that can have the following effects.

1. Oxygen delivery to your cells declines fostering an anaerobic environment.
2. As an anaerobic environment develops, microorganisms in your blood begin to evolve into forms that rob you of your health. In excess they literally strangle the life force right out of you. It's these kinds of organisms that cause your body to rot when you die. This is a natural process in an oxygen deficient environment, but sadly, many people begin to create a 'deathly' environment in their youth and feel dead long before they pass away.
3. Enzymes are like keys that need to fit specific locks in the body. When pH is off, the keys don't fit the locks as well and consequently the thousands of life processes that require enzymatic activity begin to suffer – therefore life suffers. As you already know sprouted foods not only supply you with an abundance of alkalising nutrients but are also very enzyme rich – a one-two punch in your favour. The same is true of wheatgrass juice and other green

superfood supplements and the systemic enzyme formula Vitälzym. For more information visit www.aggressivehealth.co.uk.

4. Hormones – The function of insulin is under pH control. An alkalkine urine pH can point to strong insulin response. An acidic urine pH can point to a weak insulin response. For more info on biological terrain testing contact www.aggressivehealth.co.uk.

5. Serum phosphorus levels are critical to the pH buffer system that helps maintains pH balance. A regular supply of green leafy vegetables, almonds, eggs, pumpkin seeds will help raise levels. Phosphorus levels can fall as much as 33% within two hours of a sugary meal. For more information read Calcium Homeostasis by Gregory Mundy, MD.

6. Mineral assimilation is controlled by pH. On the lower end of the atomic scale minerals can be assimilated in a wider pH range, but those higher up the scale require a narrower pH range.

Sodium and magnesium have a wide pH assimilation range
Calcium and potassium have a narrower range
Magnesium and iron narrower still
Zinc and Copper narrower
Iodine narrow

The functioning of your thyroid is optimised by the mineral iodine. As you can see iodine needs near perfect pH for assimilation. If you are overweight and have blamed your 'under functioning thyroid', maybe you need to focus on balancing your pH with the principles of AGGRESSIVE HEALTH. Malfunctioning thyroids have been connected to cold intolerance, depression, fatigue, sleepiness, muscle weakness, brittle finger nails and hair, elevated cholesterol, dry skin arthritis and ultimately heart attacks, diabetes, cancer. Are you taking pH control and the principles of AGGRESSIVE HEALTH seriously enough? Biological Terrain Analysis leads the way when it comes to addressing imbalance that may be preventing optimal health. Visit www.aggressivehealth.co.uk for more information.

HOW YOUR BLOODSTREAM'S
AFFECTED BY DETOXIFICATION

If it were as simple as cleaning the blood overnight and forgetting about years of nutritional abuse, more people would find themselves on the path to AGGRESSIVE HEALTH. In the same way nutrients end up reaching your cells via tube 1, 2 and 3 (your digestive system, bloodstream and lymphatic system), waste leaves varying sites of your body in the reverse order (lymph, blood, organs of elimination). This is easy to understand if you remember the concept of diffusion from chemistry class. The principle of diffusion states that molecules move from an area of greater concentration to an area of lesser concentration. Detoxification begins when the blood is thinner than the lymph fluid, allowing trapped toxicity in the lymph to diffuse back into the blood to be eliminated. When you begin to eat in alignment with the principles of AGGRESSIVE HEALTH, your bloodstream will flow more efficiently and any toxic undigested molecules trapped in your lymph fluid will begin to enter your bloodstream. The importance of thinning the blood naturally cannot be overstated. The cleaner you keep your blood, the quicker the lymphatic system will be able to release stored toxins. Eventually, there will be no more toxins left in the lymphatic system leaving only room for AGGRESSIVE HEALTH.

SYSTEMIC ENZYME THERAPY CAN KEEP THE BLOOD CLEAN DURING THE MOST THOROUGH DETOX

As long as you aren't taking any prescription drugs, especially blood thinners, an enzyme formula such as Vitalzym will go along way to keep your bloodstream clean in the event of rapid detoxification. During this time obstructions such as cooked fat, cooked protein and other toxins pass easily into the lymph during detoxification, making the blood very thick, sometimes even causing blood pressure to rise, whilst overworking the liver and other organs of elimination.

Live Blood Analysis
Using Vitalzym for 60 Days

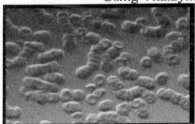 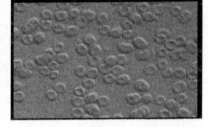

Before

Stacked red blood cells – Rouleau – often reflects poor protein digestion, the pancreas may be off, poor assimilation. Eating too much animal protein, toxic blood from stress. and generally acute phase of protein elevation in the blood. Signs: Fatigue, stress on heart, cold hands/feet – poor circulation. This person has high cholesterol, high triglycerides, and high C reaction protein levels, which indicates high levels of inflammation. This patient has also been made aware of the infestation of parasites and has severe allergies.

After

The red blood cells are no longer stacked, allowing for better circulation to the hands and feet through the small blood vessels and has resulted in much higher energy levels. RBC's are now re-oxygenating the body tissue and the stress level has been reduced considerably. The excess protein has been removed by the proteolytic enzymes and has made a major impact on cholesterol, triglycerides, and GI balance. The C reactive protein levels have reduced to normal levels and so has the pain and inflammation.

WITH THE USE OF VITÄLZYM YOU CAN HELP ELIMINATE ALL DETOXIFICATION SYMPTOMS

Remember it takes years for your tissues to become clogged by toxicity, and in the same way, can take time to dissolve, dislodge and eliminate these materials. Be patient. As long as you employ as many of the principles of AGGRESSIVE HEALTH simultaneously you can make a remarkable difference very quickly in the way you look and more importantly feel. I put my mother on a unique program to help her restore health after she'd been diagnosed with a potentially life threatening disease. Within 3 days she felt incredible and for the whole 4 weeks experienced no detoxification symptoms. I can attribute my mother's success to many factors but I believe Vitälzym™ played a powerful role in keeping her feeling good during this stressful time.

TUBE 3 – THE LYMPHATIC SYSTEM
DELIVERING NUTRIENTS, ELIMINATING WASTE

The importance of your lymphatic system should NEVER be understated. On a moment by moment basis, it rids your body of toxins, dead cells, cancer cells, nitrogenous wastes, trapped protein, fatty globules, pathogenic bacteria, infectious viruses, foreign substances and heavy metals. If it is congested, you need to take immediate action today to stimulate its flow. Failure to do so could result in your cells stewing in their own waste, starved of nutrients.

THE MOST EFFECTIVE WAY TO
STIMULATE LYMPHATIC FLOW – REBOUNDING

As you know, you have four times as much lymph fluid as you do blood, but you don't have a pump (like the heart) to keep the lymph fluid flowing. So what can you do to stimulate your own lymph flow? Rebounding. That is, buy a mini trampoline and bounce!

> "The lymphatic flow becomes very active during rebounding but sluggish under resting conditions," states Arthur C. Guyton, M.D., chairman of the department of Physiology and Biophysics at the University of Mississippi School of Medicine. "During rebounding, the rate of lymph flow can increase as much as 15 times because of the increased activity."

Your lymphatic system is filled with many valves allowing lymph to flow in one direction away from gravity. The rhythmical bouncing causes all of the one-way valves to open and close simultaneously increasing lymph flow. The lymph ducts expand during rebounding and the increased lymph flow flushes more toxins through your lymphatic system. Now you have no excuses! For as little as £20, you can increase your lymphatic flow by 1500%!

LYMPHOLOGISTS DISCOVERA RAPID CAUSE OF DEATH!

After months of investigation and research, Dr. C Samuel West, chemist and lymphologist, concluded that: "If blood proteins cannot be removed from the spaces around the cells by the lymphatic system, they can cause death within just a few hours."
This is where rebounding exerts its power. The gravitation force your body will experience during rebounding allows trapped blood proteins to be removed increasing your chances of experiencing flow.

RESTORING REGULAR BOWEL MOVEMENT CAN BE ACHIEVED THROUGH A DAILY BOUNCE

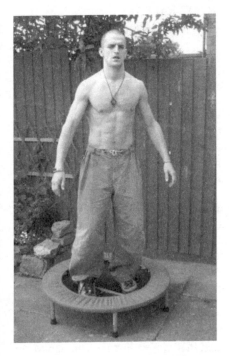

When you begin rebounding, don't be surprised to find yourself making a more regular visit to the toilet, even if you're chronically constipated. The regular bounce causes the nervous system to transmit messages to the part of your brain responsible for regulating your intestines, thus restoring optimal bowel activity.

SPACE REASEARCH DISCOVERS MIRACULOUS EXERCISE

Researchers at N.A.S.A. found that rebounding was 68% more efficient than treadmills or other forms of exercise. One N.A.S.A study called rebounding a *"miracle exercise"*. N.A.S.A. also found rebounding to be the most effective exercise for helpful astronauts rebuild bone and muscle mass lost in the non-stimulating weightlessness of space.

TARGET YOUR SKIN AND ENHANCE LYMPHATIC FLOW EVEN FURTHER

The largest organ of elimination is your skin. It is responsible for 1/4 of your body's daily elimination of waste, with one pound of waste being discharged through it EVERY day. If the pores of your skin become choked with dead cells, so does its ability to eliminate, but fear not! One of the most effective methods for keeping this vital organ functioning perfectly is dry skin brushing. Not only does it help maintain excellent skin tone, but it improves your digestion, stimulates lymphatic flow and strengthens your immune system.

TWO MINUTES PER DAY IS ALL YOU NEED

Simply buy a natural bristle brush with a long wooden handle and brush your entire body. Start with the soles of your feet (the nerve endings here affect your entire body) and brush towards your heart. Do circular counter-clockwise strokes on your belly and remember to avoid your face and nipples. The best time to do this is in the morning before your daily bath or shower, when your skin is completely dry. Also, never share your brush with anyone. Wash it every couple of weeks.

PREPARING FOR SHORT-TERM PAIN
TO ACHIEVE LONG-TERM GAIN

As you unburden your lymph of undigested proteins, toxins and unwanted chemicals, you may experience any number of short-term symptoms of detoxification. Take a look at these symptoms and prepare yourself – It could be you!

> Fevers, diarrhoea, desires for poor foods, tastes of old medicines, mucus discharges, bad breath, coughs, cold symptoms, drowsiness, momentary aches, nausea, unclear thinking, weight loss, intestinal discomfort, gas, headaches, light-headedness, rashes, cloudy urine, swelling of the feet, dryness and itching of the skin and scalp.

To eliminate all this unwanted waste from your body, your body will make use of all the eliminative organs, including your bowels, mouth, sinuses, skin, and kidneys. A great indicator is your urine. If it is clear, your blood is clean (at that moment). If it is dark or cloudy then your body is releasing toxins and you may be dehydrated.

You may also experience emotional detoxification, where emotions such as anxiety, depression, and other imbalances expel themselves from your body. Many authorities believe stored emotions can reside within mucoid plaque. Why? Because on the release of that foul smelling substance people often lose the negativity they've been holding onto for years. I'll let you make your own mind up at this point. If you experience any of these symptoms, feel delighted that you've had the courage to see the process through to the end. I send you my congratulations.

REJUVENATE WITH SAUNA DETOXIFICATION

A gentleman in America spent the best part of his working life surrounded by diesel fuel and exhaust fumes. He experienced constant migraine headaches, varying sickness, had achy joints and was so allergic to most modern buildings and appliances that he was considering moving to the desert! Fortunately a close friend told him about a sauna detoxification centre and the gentleman checked in.

When the gentleman began the program, the detoxification process was so powerful, that the other people in the sauna were forced to leave. Eventually the centre built a special exhaust vent to expel the fumes out of the building! That's how powerful the detoxification process can be!

CRITICAL POINT:

If you suffer from constipation on an ongoing basis, or a lack of sleep, it may be that you have an anabolic/catabolic imbalance. When you wake in the morning your body switches from an anabolic state into a catabolic state. In this catabolic state you spend your energy/charge during the day. When you retire for the evening your body switches from a catabolic state to an anabolic state to rebuild/recharge your system. Constipation can often be linked to anabolic imbalance, where a person loses the ability to switch from an anabolic state to a catabolic state. This switch is critical. All the colonics in the world will never create the results you desire unless you address this imbalance. For more information on biological terrain analysis contact www.aggressivehealth.co.uk.

SPARKLING FROM THE INSIDE OUT

Once you've eliminated the toxins from your body, the future automatically becomes bright and inspiring. Here's what you've got to look forward to:

♦ Increased endurance and energy, faster reflexes and increased sexual vigour.
♦ A more peaceful rejuvenating sleep.
♦ Greater concentration, improved memory and mental focus, clearer more logical thinking and increased creativity.
♦ Fresher breath, decreased body odour, a better sense of smell and hearing, and improved eyesight.
♦ Elimination of pollen and animal allergies and the ability to breathe deeper.
♦ Increased resistance to hot and cold weather.
♦ Quick and strong growth of hair and fingernails.
♦ Controlled temper, decreased stress, and increased confidence.
♦ The ability to fast with no adverse side effects.
♦ Increased individualism, a superior attitude towards life, nature, and the order of things, and a closer relationship with natural forces.

ARE YOU READY FOR THE CHALLENGE?

Increasing the amount of raw food you eat in your diet is an excellent starting point. Systematically cleansing the three tubes of detoxification is a whole new level of responsibility. Here's a re-cap:

- Detoxification is something that is going on in your body all the time. If you embrace this natural process and assist it, you'll eliminate waste faster, remove obstructions from your body and allow exuberant health to emerge
- Over the next two years, 98% of the atoms in your body will be completely replaced! Over the next seven years, 100% of your body will be replaced! Detoxify and eliminate the waste, setting the foundation for the ultimate re-build.
- Imagine that your body consists of three layers of 'tubes', your digestive system, your circulatory system and your lymphatic system. Detoxification begins as soon as the blood is thinner than the lymph fluid, allowing trapped toxicity in the lymph to diffuse back into the blood to be eliminated.
- The cleaner your your blood, the quicker the lymphatic system will be able to release stored toxins, leaving room for exceptional health.
- Layers of mucoid plaque can prevent optimal digestion and assimilation, eliminate it. Goto www.aggressivehealth.co.uk for details. A healthy colon should only weigh between 4 and 6 pounds. A stagnant colon can sometimes weigh up to 40 pounds!
- A typical cooked meat and pasteurised milk diet leaves the blood thick and heavy.There are more heart attacks in the United States on Thanksgiving Day than any other day of the year.
- Surgeons won't operate on a patient unless they've fasted on water for at least 8 hours because of the dangers involved when the bloodstream isn't flowing freely enough.
- Garlic and onions thin the blood naturally. Systemic enzymes such as Vitälzym™ have a dramatic effect on blood cleansing.
- Rebounding can stimulate lymphatic flow by as much as 1500% and has been proven by N.A.S.A. to be the most effective exercise for rebuilding bone and muscle mass after the non-stimulating weightlessness of space.
- Skin brushing stimulates lymphatic flow and is a very simple daily routine.
- Saunas are great if you want to speed up the detoxification process.
- Choose wheatgrass juice and E3Live. The chlorophyll and the alkaline compounds in green leafy vegetables/AFA algae can combine with heavy metals, allowing for their rapid elimination.
- Ripe hot foods burn parasites out of your intestines. Parasites can prevent weight gain and cause emaciation. Use garlic, onion, ripe hot peppers, ginger etc.
- Whole hempseeds are a remarkable laxative. This is due to its high fiber and soothing qualities causing them to stimulate bowel action rather than being an irritant to the intestines.
- Scientists from the University of Vienna proved that raw food nutrition is the best method for eliminating the sticky marsh that surrounds cells, optimising nutrient and hormone transportation and restoring optimal sodium/potassium balance inside and outside of cells.
- The healthy transit time of food through your body should be less than 24 hours. On average in the UK it is now between 60 and 70 hours.

- When you fast you are on natures operating table. Regular juices fasts, 1 day per week will add up to 52 days of juice fasting per year. This is a powerful recommendation employed by Brian Clement, director of Hippocrates Institute in Florida and will maximise your detox potential.
- The UK has the highest incidence of bowel cancer in the world with 20,000 new cases every year.
- Alexis Carrel of the Rockefeller Institute and two-time recipient of the Nobel Prize, kept a chicken heart alive for 29 years until someone failed to cleanse away its excretion!

Be strong! Stick to your guns and prepare to embrace illuminating health with open arms. Use what you've learned and bulldoze through any negative impulses or unnatural desires and engrave positive nutritional habits into your mind. As you embrace detoxification on a daily basis, you'll lose weight as diseased cells, fat excretions, dead water, and other poisons rush into the bloodstream to be purged from the system. Over a period of time, your body will change in front of your eyes, from a solid, rigid, weakened condition, to a free, elastic, fluid, and energetic condition. The unnatural part of you will waste away, leaving a new and vibrant you.

The cell is immortal. It is merely the fluid in which it floats that degenerates –
Dr Alexis Carrel, French born American surgeon and biologist and winner of the
1912 Nobel Prize.

THE AGGRESSIVE HEALTH EVALUTIOIN
Have you begun cleansing the three tubes of detoxification?
Have you embraced a 4 week herbal cleanse program and colonic hydrotherapy
to eliminate mucoid plaque?
Is your diet built on a foundation of raw living foods?
Are you rebounding and dry skin brushing?

If you want an abundance of health and longevity in your life you must stay active. Your body was designed for movement, not stagnation! All the best foods in the world mean nothing if you don't remain active, agile and physically strong.

CHAPTER 6

APPLY THE SECRETS OF ELITE ENDURANCE ATHLETES AND ACCELERATE DETOXIFICATION BY 800%

AGGRESSIVE HEALTH doesn't pull any punches. You're going to learn the most effective way to approach exercise and movement health to ensure a lifetime of play, freedom and fluidity throughout your body and joints. It's impossible to present everything in the chapters that follow, but you'll learn enough to get a taste of things to come. You can find out more by visiting www.aggressivehealth.co.uk. Start with the basics and build from there - Just take a look at the following studies.

♦ A Harvard University study, documented in the New England Journal of Medicine, followed almost 17,000 men to determine the correlation between exercise and longevity. It showed that men who walked more than nine miles per week (enough to burn off 900 calories) had a risk of death 21% lower than that of men who walked less than three miles weekly.

♦ Dr Ralph Paffenbarger of the University of California at Berkeley conducted a second long-term study of 10,000 Harvard graduates. It clearly showed that men aged between 45 and 84 who take up moderately vigorous forms of exercise (tennis, swimming, jogging, or brisk walking) reduce their overall death rates by as much as 29% and have a 41% lower risk of coronary artery disease.

♦ An eight-year study conducted by the Stanford University School of Medicine, Palo Alto, California, looked at the health habits of 10,269 Harvard University alumni over an eight-year period. The study showed that moderately active men, who took part in such sports as jogging, swimming, and running, had a 23% lower risk of dying from any cause than men who never exercised.

♦ Another study, sponsored by the Institute for Aerobics Research in Dallas, followed more than 10,000 men and 3,000 women for an average of more than eight years. They found that exercising participants in the study had lower reported rates of colon cancer, coronary heart disease, hypertension, and stroke.

♦ In a study conducted at the University of Utah Medical School, researchers found that regular participation in such activities as walking, bowling, raking leaves and ballroom dancing were enough to reduce the risk of heart attack by 30%. Another study at the University of Wisconsin Medical School showed that when heart attack patients took part in special exercise programmes, they cut their death rate from coronary artery disease by 25% – about the same rate achieved by the use of drugs, but without any toxic side effects!

♦ The benefits of exercise are so far-reaching that they even extend to organs that you wouldn't usually associate with physical fitness, such as the eyes. Exercise significantly reduces pressure against the eyeball, which causes glaucoma and frequently leads to blindness. Exercise even optimises the eyesight of people with no vision problems. A study of regular exercisers with 20/20 vision revealed that they had visual skills far superior to those sedentary people who also had 20/20 vision.

♦ But that's not all. Exercise is also a great appetite stabiliser. People with sedentary lifestyles tend to have poor appetite control and eat more than their body requires. Physical activity appears to be essential to balance appetite in line with body needs.

Need I say more! You are designed to move, remain agile and fully active until your final moments on earth! The important question is:

WHAT KIND, HOW MUCH, HOW OFTEN, AND HOW HARD?

I don't know whether you've ever 'stepped inside a gym' or work out every day. Maybe you consider yourself somewhere in between. One thing is for sure, there are no excuses. Movement is as critical as any nutrient! You are about to learn about the bare minimum, the base line standard, the level that you will always strive to stay above, whatever challenges life throws at you. If you are an athlete, the first part of this chapter isn't for you, but you might know of someone who could benefit from the following prescription. For everyone else, ask yourself the following question: What is the minimum amount of exercise necessary before reaching a point of no returns, with regard to longevity?

IF THIS ISN'T EASY ENOUGH,
YOU ARE READING THE WRONG BOOK!

The following table was compiled through research taken from Harvard graduates. Treat this as your minimum daily requirement and success is yours.

Activity	Male (time in minutes)	Female (time in minutes)
Rowing	24	32
Bicycling	26	35
Swimming	26	35
Stationary bike	30	40
Jogging slowly	30	40
Rebounding	30	40
Walking briskly	35	47
Walking slowly	69	94

So what do these figures equate to in terms of calories? Answer: An approximate calorie expenditure of 2000 calories per week/just under 300 calories a day. But let's forget calories! If you're female, two 20 minute sessions on your rebounder every day will reduce your risk of breast cancer by a staggering 70%. Amazing!

WHY WILL AEROBIC EXERCISE CHANGE YOUR LIFE?

The term 'aerobic' means, literally, 'with oxygen,' and refers to of moderate exercise you can sustain over long periods of time, rather than short intense bursts. As you gradually demand more from your aerobic system you condition your heart, lungs, blood vessels, and aerobic muscles. If you want to tap into your fat burning potential, aerobic exercise will increase your sensitivity to the hormone insulin, the importance of which will become apparent in the next chapter when you learn how to kick-start your fat metabolism.

CHOOSE AEROBIC TRAINING AS A CRITICAL TOOL
IN YOUR INSULIN CONTROLLING ARSENAL

By the end of AGGRESSIVE HEALTH, you'll have a clear understanding of how and why you need to control the hormone insulin if you ever want to optimise your health. Insulin is critical to health, but it is also your body's primary 'fat storage' hormone. If over stimulated, it can rob you of your health.

Researchers at UCLA demonstrated that forty-five minutes of aerobic exercise has the same effect in lowering blood sugar levels as a single maximum injection of insulin. When you exercise, your muscles engage in continuous rhythmical contractions that draw sugar into the muscle. As sugar is utilised by the muscles, your body doesn't have to make as much insulin. Researchers at Duke University have found that by lowering blood-insulin levels, you engage the receptors on fat cells to release fat to be used for energy. Even after you've finished exercising, insulin in your body continues to operate more effectively for the next twenty-four hours. Gradually, through consistent conditioning, you'll also speed up the rate at which enzymes in your muscle cells utilise oxygen.

PRINCIPLES OF AGGRESSIVE HEALTH PROPEL ATHLETES TO A WHOLE NEW LEVEL!

In the 1930s Professor Karl Eimer, director of the Medical Clinic at the University of Vienna, devised an excellent experiment to test the power of a high raw diet on several top athletes in his country. He put them on a high-intensity physical training program for two weeks without making any alterations to their diet, then, without any transition, he placed them on a diet of 100% raw foods. Every single athlete experienced faster reflexes, more flexibility, and improved stamina.

Remember a diet rich in raw living foods will:
♦ Stimulate muscle cells to absorb nutrients and excrete waste more efficiently.
♦ Flush away the toxic residue that can develop between cells if too much refined 'junk' food has been eaten.
♦ Increase the exchange of oxygen, wastes, and nutrients at a cellular level leading to total cell efficiency.
♦ Give the muscle cells the ideal conditions to thrive and generate energy.
♦ According to Dr. Arthur Robinson, co-founder of the Linus Pauling Institute, wheatgrass juice causes your blood vessels to dilate, leading to an increase in overall blood flow, enhancing athletic performance.
♦ Many athletes have shattered personal bests with the inclusion of chlorophyll rich foods and E3Live in their diet. Use it!

OXYGEN: THE FAT LOSS KEY

Although a well-maintained hormonal system will ensure you burn fat primarily (as you'll learn in the next two chapters), oxygen is the key for releasing it. The greater your supply of oxygen to all parts of your body, and the greater your ability to make use of it, the higher your metabolic rate, and the more success you will have in burning unwanted fat. Whenever you're inactive for extended periods of time your system doesn't eliminate toxicity as efficiently.

Brian Clement, director of the Hippocrates Institute states that over time, aerobic exercise can increase your ability to eliminate toxins by as much as 800%. A lack of activity also leads to poor control over blood insulin levels, leading to less appetite control.

THE ONLY WAY TO LOWER YOUR BODY'S SET POINT
AND INCREASE YOUR METABOLIC RATE

If you've ever starved yourself in an effort to lose weight, you've probably experienced the 'set point' phenomenon. Let me explain. Your body has an internal mechanism that regulates the amount of body fat you store. After a few days of reduced calorie intake, your body adjusts by lowering its basal metabolic rate (BMR), to ensure a more efficient use of the calories. This automatic biological response (the set-point phenomenon) makes it progressively more difficult to lose weight whilst dieting. How do you reset your body's set point? The answer: Exercise regularly. To date, this is the only known way to lower your set point, raise your metabolic rate, and "program" your body to store less fat than it did before. When you improve your body's use of oxygen through regular exercise, you increase your overall metabolic rate. Studies with athletes show that even 15 hours after strenuous exercise the metabolic rate is distinctly elevated, sometimes as much as 25% above normal.

Diabetics must begin to use aerobic exercise to their advantage. The rise in metabolic rate associated with this type of exercise enhances absorption of glucose into cells. For this reason it is critical for both Type I and Type II diabetes.

CHOOSE YOUR FUEL WISELY

Wouldn't you love to know that with every running stride, or every pull of the rowing machine, or with every pedal of the bike, you are stripping your body of unwanted fat? The secret is in the intensity of the exercise. Take a marathon runner for example. To complete a typical marathon, a runner will use approximately 2000 calories of energy. Question: Where does this energy come from? The two primary sources are as follows:

1. 2000 calories represents the maximum amount of carbohydrate a runner can store within their muscles and liver. This is obviously an *ineffective* source of fuel.

2. Let's now look at stored body fat as a source of fuel. A typical 150-pound marathon runner with 10% body fat, would carry 15 pounds of total fat. 3 pounds of that total fat is not accessible for energy because it's in places like the brain, and surrounding vital organs, leaving about 12 pounds of fat for possible energy use. Do you have any idea how many calories are in a pound of fat? ...3500! So with a few more calculations it is easy to see that this 150-pound runner has a potential of 42000 calories of energy tucked away as fat. Follow the principles of AGGRESSIVE HEALTH and you'll immediately tap into this source of unlimited energy.

When it comes to maximising human potential in the realm of health and fitness, look no further than...

STU MITTLEMAN: WORLD RECORD HOLDER
FOR RUNNING 1000 MILES IN 11 DAYS AND 19 HOURS

Stu Mittleman made it his mission to break a world record! For eleven straight days, he ran 21 hours a day and slept a mere 3 hours a night as he focused entirely on his goal. Stu demonstrated the unlimited physical potential that resides within us all. He broke the 1000-mile record by running for eleven days and nineteen hours, at an average of 84 miles per day. His demonstration was simple. Anything is possible if we make the right demands upon ourselves INCREMENTALLY.

THE POWER OF ROLE MODELS

Whenever you study any area of life, always look for someone who is producing results, so you can emulate them. If you speak to anyone who witnessed the amazing 1000-mile record, they said Stu looked better at the end than he did at the beginning. He experienced no injuries, not even a blister! The distinction that he made which you'll also make is that health and fitness are not the same.

♦ Fitness is the physical ability to perform athletic activity.

♦ Health, however, is defined as the state where all the systems of the body – nervous, muscular, skeletal, circulatory, digestive, lymphatic, hormonal, etc. – are working in harmony.

Most people think that fitness implies health, but the truth is that they don't necessarily go hand in hand. It's ideal to have both health and fitness. The optimum balance of health and fitness is achieved by training your metabolism. Remember Stu was running 84 miles a day for 11 days. Marathon runners don't even reach 30 miles!

BUILDING THE FOUNDATION OF SUCCESS

Do you want to follow in Stu's footsteps? Probably not! But do you want to apply the same principles he applied so you too can achieve amazing results? If the answer is yes, you need to realise that all exercise programs require that you begin by building an aerobic base – a period of time during which time your exercise program is based around aerobic activity.

Properly developing your aerobic system will not only make you a better athlete, but it will also burn off any extra unwanted fat you may be carrying, improve your immune system, give you more energy, and keep you relatively injury-free.

DEHYDRATION – THE WORRYING HEALTH HAZARD

In 1982, Alberto Salazar won the Boston Marathon, but his celebrations were cut short when upon finishing he was immediately rushed to the emergency room at

Boston Hospital where he received six litres of intravenous solution to replenish lost water and salt. Dehydration had caused him to overheat.

At an iron man race lasting between 9 and 15 hours, 64 athletes were monitored for dehydration. The study showed 27% were hyponatremic (salt deficient) and 17% of them needed medical attention. Do you remember how important the electrolyte mineral sodium is? It is necessary for maintaining normal osmotic pressure and for the transport of nutrients and waste to and from cells. It also facilitates communication between cells and enables ATP generation, which is vital for energy production. The importance of sodium for athletes cannot be overstated. Remember that during stress and exercise electrolytes are used up at an alarming rate.

Whenever you train, end your workout with a celery-based juice. Celery/apple juice will taste best, but for the masters of AGGRESSIVE HEALTH celery based, vegetable juice with chlorophyll rich leaves and a drop of hemp oil will make all the difference.

USE CHOLINE RICH FOODS TO PREVENT THE PHYSIOLOGICAL HAZARDS OF ENDURANCE EVENTS

When the blood profiles of marathon runners were studied, choline levels fluctuated dramatically. Researcher Richard Wurtman discovered that after 26 miles of running, choline drops by a staggering 40%. Studies also show that swimmers are able to swim for longer (without the perils of muscle fatigue) when choline is introduced into their diet. Where do you get it from? Hemp seeds, hemp oil and another great source which is very cheap: Lecithin. Use it in your vegetable juice regularly if you're not using hemp.

A LITTLE OF SOMETHING GOOD GOES ALONG WAY – THE POWER OF MEDIUM CHAIN FATTY ACIDS (MCFAS)

Loading your diet with fat is NOT a good idea, but selecting the right kinds of fats and using them where necessary is critical, especially if you are doing a lot of endurance training. If you love your endurance events consider the power of MCFAs. In a six week study done with mice, investigators wanted to see if the daily inclusion of MCFAs would affect their endurance. The mice were placed in a 'river simulation swimming chamber' and swam until exhausted. The total swimming time was measured, and those fed MCFAs quickly began to out-perform the control group, continuing to improve throughout the six weeks.

Many sports drinks and energy bars now contain MCFAs, along with excess sugar and additives. Go to the source! As you begin to use a little coconut butter daily you may see some dramatic effects in your training capacity. Studies show that one single dose before of during competition had no measurable effect.

WATER: THE MASTER SOLUTION FOR AGGRESSIVE HEALTH

Your body is composed of approximately 67% water. Blood is 83% water, muscles 75%, brain 75%, heart 75%, bones 22%, lungs 86%, kidneys 83%, and eyes 95%. A drop of as little as 2% will cause dehydration, tiredness and fatigue. A 10% drop can cause significant health problems. Be warned!

ARE YOU READY FOR THE CHALLENGE?
THE ADVANCED AEROBIC PRESCRIPTION

Jumping on your rebounder will be enough for a great aerobic workout, but if you have a passion for fine-tuning, the advanced aerobic prescription will help you use fat as your primary fuel. If you begin exercising too hard the process that involves the transportation of fat from adipose tissue to your muscles is often compromised. Some people live for endurance events – I don't, but here's the drill.

1.   BUY A HEART RATE MONITOR TODAY!
2.   Work out your maximum heart rate.
     220 minus your age = maximum heart rate......................Never exceed this.
3.   Using your maximum heart rate work out your warm up and cool down rate.

Aerobic Warm up and Cool-down
Max Heart rate x 60% = warm up (high end)...........................
Max Heart rate x 55% = warm up (low end)........................

If you warm up for 15 minutes at this low intensity you mobilise any free fatty acids stored within your body. Fat will then get used as your primary fuel instead of stored carbohydrate. In this period of time, you give your body the time to gradually distribute blood to the areas that need it, rather than immediately shunting it away from vital organs. And that is all it takes. By controlling insulin and glucagon levels and preventing low blood sugar levels, you'll find yourself working out and feeling great. More about this in the next chapter.

4.   Once you've completed your warm-up, exercise within your aerobic training zone for between 20 and 45 minutes. Use the following formula to work out your heart rate range.

Optimal Aerobic Training Zone
180 minus your age = ...
This is your maximum aerobic heart rate during training before your body switches to anaerobic metabolism.
Take this figure and subtract 10 points, then keep your heart rate between these two figures.
Write the two figures here................. - .... This will be your optimal aerobic training zone.

Other points to remember are as follows:

- If you are recovering from a major illness or are on medication subtract an additional 10 points
- If you have not exercised before, have an injury, are gearing down in your training, or if you often get colds or flu, or have allergies subtract 5 points.
- If you have been exercising for up to two years without any real problems, and have not had colds or flu more than once or twice a year, keep your score the same.
- If you have been exercising for more than two years without any problems, while making progress in competition without injury, add 5 points.

5. Finally, remember to cool down for 15 minutes after your main exercise routine. By cooling down, you'll prevent blood from pooling in your working muscles. When people stop exercising suddenly, it's difficult for the blood to be returned for cleansing, re-oxygenation and redistribution. Joint Mobility training such as Warrior Wellness is recommended before and after any exercise routine to mobilise the joints and for 'active recovery'. For more information about Circular Strength Training™ visit www.clubbellwarrior.com.

TIME: A PERSONAL PREFERENCE

Whatever time of day you choose to exercise is up to you. You may only be able to fit exercise into a certain part of your day and have to stick to it. If you have the flexibility to try different routines then this will give you the chance to find out what works for you. The best all round day begins with joint mobility exercises designed to free up the joints and recover complete range of movement. If you train in the morning and exercise on an empty stomach you'll more efficiently access your fat stores and burn more fat. This EXPLOSION of energy will linger throughout the day. You'll automatically avoid food and caffeine to wake you up. If you choose to train in the afternoon, you'll be rewarding your body and mind with a natural endorphin high. You'll learn about the power of Clubbells®, kettlebells and other forms of resistance training in Chapter 11. For now, here's a little teaser, highlighting how seriously some people take their training.

TESTOSTERONE:
HORMONE OF STRENGTH, POWER AND DESIRE

The production of testosterone is under circadian rhythm control. It peaks in the morning, and then falls during the day. The highest levels occur between 2am and 4am and stay elevated until about 9am, making the morning a better time to train with resistance. Bill Pearl (four times Mr Universe Bodybuilding champion and the only man to defeat Arnold Schwarzenegger for the Mr Universe title) always did his training at 3am in order to utilise the maximum release of testosterone. By 3pm, testosterone levels will have dropped by some 40% compared to the morning. It's also worth noting that Bill Pearl is a strict vegetarian.

THE AGGRESSIVE HEALTH EVALUATION:
Do you engage in aerobic exercise to build unshakeable health?
Are you regularly using your rebounder for aerobic power?
Are you following the advanced aerobic prescription?

PART TWO

YOU'VE MASTERED THE BASICS NOW PREPARE TO DIAL INTO THE HIGHEST STANDARDS OF AGGRESSIVE HEALTH

CHAPTER 7

TRIGGER THE BIOLOGICAL SWITCHES THAT KICKSTART YOUR FAT METABOLISM AND STRIP YOUR BODY OF UNWANTED FAT

Many people want to lose weight and many people are on diets, but how many people do you see fail in their quest for a slim body time after time? If you want the struggle to come to a grinding halt you must learn how to control…

THE HORMONE PHILHARMONIC

The hormones of your body are like the musicians of an orchestra playing a beautiful symphony. When the orchestra is playing in tune, the symphony sounds wonderful. If, however one of the musicians plays too loudly, or is out of sync with the others, the symphony can sound horrific. In your body, if one hormone is overstimulated it can cause devastating effects and suppress the action of other hormones. In today's society with millions being spent on marketing nutritionally suicidal foods – YOU ARE THE TARGET. Most of these foods are packed full of sugar and saturated fat and over-stimulate the hormone insulin. The result – an out of control obesity crisis.

INSULIN: CRITICAL TO HEALTH
YET POTENTIALLY LIFE THREATENING

As you read AGGRESSIVE HEALTH, you'll see that insulin gets a hard time. The truth is – if insulin didn't get released from your pancreas to control the level of sugar in your bloodstream, your health would deteriorate rapidly and you'd die! If your central nervous system detects a rising in blood sugar levels, it is considered life threatening and signals are sent to the various sites in the body to release the hormones necessary to restore those levels. When your blood sugar level is normal, it falls into a range of between 60mg/dl to 120mg/dl (mg/dl = milligrams of glucose in 100 millilitres of blood). If it was to rise as high as 800mg/dl, you could end up in a coma and die. Insulin's effectiveness is governed by pH balance, highlighting the importance of a balanced biological terrain. It prevents blood sugar levels from rising too high – but at the same time…

INSULIN IS 30 TIMES MORE EFFECTIVE AT SHUNTING EXTRA CALORIES INTO *FAT* THAN INTO *MUSCLE*

30 times! That alone should make you pay very close attention to this chapter. Your goal is simple: Learn what it takes to direct the flow of fat away from your fat tissue and towards your muscles to be burnt for energy. To do this, and trigger the switch that taps into your fat burning metabolism all you need to do is stimulate the hormone glucagon and minimise insulin stimulation. Imagine insulin and glucagon sitting on opposite ends of a seesaw. When insulin is dominant fat storage prevails, when glucagon is dominant fat melts off your body like ice cream on a summer's day.

> Insulin stimulation makes you fat and keeps you fat.
> Glucagon stimulation makes you thin and keeps you thin.

BEST-SELLING 'LOW CARB DIETS'
FAIL TO TELL THE WHOLE STORY

The Atkins diet is an example of a book that focuses exclusively on nutrition for hormonal control to stimulate weight loss. You may thrive on a high fat/high protein diet, because it is the correct fuel mix for your body at this time. However, unless raw living foods are your priority (even if only in small amounts) you'll never reach your true potential. What 'The Atkins diet' doesn't tell you is that unless you eliminate the sticky marsh that surrounds your cells, hormone communication, nutrient transfer and fat burning will never be optimal. His meat/cheese/cooked fat dominant 'advice' along with the new 'Atkins' range of processed nutritional bars only add to this sludge.

LIVING FOODS ARE THE ANSWERS TO YOUR PRAYERS

Fortunately, scientists from the University of Vienna were able to show how you can systematically eliminate the sticky marsh that surrounds your cells optimising hormonal communication and therefore maximising fat burning. The answer: a diet high in raw food nutrition. Enough said. Let me introduce you to the term 'Lipolysis', because it is a magical method for triggering the biological switches that kickstart your fat metabolism…

WHY IS THERE SO MUCH MAGIC IN LIPOLYSIS?

The term lipolysis refers to the chemistry of burning fat, where fat gets broken down into glycerol and free-fatty acids. The fatty acids then break down into ketone bodies (which can be used as fuel) and a shorter fatty acid. Apart from being a storage site for poisonous wastes and toxins, your fat is nothing but stored energy. The key to storing this energy is the hormone insulin. If you want to pile on the pounds, insulin is your most valuable asset, it safely tucks fat away in the places you hate to see it, around your belly, on your hips and at the tops of your legs etc., and it also prevents the burning of fat – That is why it is critical to eliminate foods that *over*-stimulate it.

When you kickstart your fat burning metabolism you immediately enter this fat-dissolving state by putting minimal stress on your pancreas to release insulin. Remember, if your body can easily become a fat storage machine, it can also become a fat burning machine. If people can gain weight easily, science and common sense says there should be a method for stripping the body of fat as easily.

LIPOLYSIS IS YOUR ANSWER TO BURNING FAT
BUT WHAT ABOUT CALORIES?

If you've spent your life trying to lose weight, you've probably spent a lifetime worrying about calories. Let me tell you, calories should be the least of your concerns. Traditional calorie thinking says,

"A calorie is a calorie and that is all that matters. A gram of fat has more than twice the calories of a gram of carbohydrate, so you can eat twice as much carbohydrate as fat and you'll lose weight"

Wrong! The key to understanding fat loss, is understanding the effect food has on controlling your hormones. To think hormonally would be to think that a calorie of fat has a different hormonal effect than a calorie of carbohydrate, and a calorie of protein has a different effect still. Let me present you with some information about a classic study done over forty years ago.

TAKE CONTROL OF PROTEIN, FAT AND CARB RATIOS
AND PREPARE FOR SOME SERIOUS WEIGHT LOSS

In the early part of the 1950s, Professor Alan Kekwick, Director of the Institute of Clinical Research and Experimental Medicine at London's prestigious Middlesex Hospital, and Dr Gaston L.S. Pawan, Senior Research Biochemist of the hospital's medical unit embarked on a fascinating journey into the world of macro-nutrient ratios.

Their wonderful journey began when they became intrigued with various studies that suggested that weight loss was controlled by varying the macro-nutrient content of the diet (i.e. changing fat, protein and carbohydrate ratios). Their fascination was sparked by the clinical studies of Dr. Alfred W Pennington on employees of the Dupont

Corporation along with German and Scandinavian papers showing success with diet plans that had very restricted carbohydrate quantities.

They decided to conduct their own experiments on a group of obese subjects to test the results for themselves:

♦ Those on a 90% protein intake lost weight.

♦ Those on a 90% fat intake lost weight.

♦ But when subjects were given a diet of which 90% of the calories came from carbohydrates, they didn't lose a pound.

The tests performed by Kekwick and Pawan were simple, but they were both so overwhelmed by the results, they devoted nearly 20 years to researching why calories seemed to be of no importance in dieting!

SEPARATE YOURSELF FROM THE MASSES
AND WAVE GOODBYE TO FAILURE!

In their preliminary studies Kekwick and Pawan found that a diet of 1000 calories per day was only successful when most of the calories came from fat and protein, yet a carbohydrate diet consisting of 1000 calories per day produced very little weight loss. This proved that it's not the calories alone that make the difference but the foods that make up those calories. Can you see why there are such diverse results within weight loss groups? Everyone can adhere to a low calorie diet, but individual food choices will always be different. If the process of weight loss was simply a matter of controlling calorie intake, then regardless of which foods the calories came from, everyone would experience similar results.

MELT FAT OFF OF YOUR BODY
AND ELIMINATE UNUSED CALORIES

Kekwick and Pawan found that even on a balanced 2000-calorie diet, subjects experienced no fat loss. Yet when their diet was mainly fat, these same obese subjects could lose unwanted body fat even when consuming 2600 calories. Being uniquely thorough, Kekwick and Pawan did water balance studies proving that the weight being lost was mostly fat.

BRING ON THE MICE AND THE METABOLIC CHAMBER!

Next, they embarked on a study of mice in a metabolic chamber. They measured the loss of carbon in their excretions and were able to show that on the high fat diet, mice excreted considerable quantities of unused calories in the form of ketone bodies. At the end of the study period, they analysed the fat content of the animals' bodies and found significant decreases in percentage body fat.

THE MAGIC AND MYSTERY OF
THE FAT MOBILISATION SUBSTANCE

During their wonderful adventure, Kekwick and Pawan discovered and extracted a substance from the urine of the low-carbohydrate dieters. When this substance was injected into non-dieting animals and humans it caused them to experience rapid weight loss, a massive decrease in the percentage of carcass fat, an increase in ketone and free fatty-acid levels and an increase in the excretion of unused calories from 10% to 36%!

The substance they stumbled over was a fat mobilisation substance, which they soon labelled 'lipid mobilisers' along with others that they found. These lipid mobilisers are your primary weapon for kick-starting fat loss as they enable you to excrete unused calories that may have been stored in your body on the low fat-high carbohydrate diet. If you need any more evidence...

HIBERNATING ANIMALS PROVE
THERE IS ONLY ONE WAY: NATURES WAY

In the absence of carbohydrate, your body sends out a signal to release a generous influx of lipid mobilisers. If you look into nature, the burning of stored fat in the absence of dietary carbohydrate is what sustains hibernating animals. The intelligence and wisdom of your body provides a variety of natural messenger substances to ensure that fat mobilisation is efficient and quick. This is the state any obese person should be striving for and represents the road to success! The immediate feedback is great; i.e. the pounds drop off at an amazing rate and energy levels soar.

IT'S NOT ABOUT CALORIES
IT'S ABOUT HORMONAL CONTROL

I'll repeat. IT'S NOT ABOUT CALORIES! IT'S ABOUT HORMONAL CONTROL! If you've spent your whole life focusing exclusively on calories – STOP! Once you've eliminated the dreaded mucoid plaque from your body and keep your body clean with a high raw diet, your hormonal response to food should be near the top of your list of priorities. For some of you this won't be easy to digest because you've been following the low calorie mindset for so many years. There is nothing wrong with lowering calorie intake, so long as your diet is built on a foundation of superior nutrient dense raw foods.

SO MANY STUDIES, SO MANY RESULTS

Frederick Benoit and his associates at the Oakland Naval Hospital decided to compare two methods of losing weight with seven men weighing between 230 and 290 pounds. The methods are as follows:

1. A 1000-calorie diet, with 10 gram carbohydrate and high fat.
2. Fasting
♦   The first method saw the men lose 14.5 pounds, and out of this 14 pounds was body fat.
♦   On the 10 day fast, the men lost 21 pounds on average, but most of that was lean body weight. Only 7.5 pounds was body fat.

Benoit's other exciting discovery was that on these lipolysis-stimulating diets, dieters maintained adequate potassium levels, whilst those who fasted lost severe amounts of potassium. About a decade later, many dieters lost their lives on very low calorie diets similar to fasting. Many individuals hypothesised that the deaths were due to potassium losses, leading to heart arrhythmia.

If you want efficient fat metabolism then you need to take potassium seriously. It is utilised by the thyroid to make a soapy emulsifying agent used in bile for fat metabolism. But it's not enough to just load your diet with potassium; you need to ensure you have proper levels of nitrogen in your body. How do you do this – make sure you eat a regular source of protein. If you have any concerns, biological terrain analysis will be able to uncover any imbalances that may need to be addressed. Visit www.aggressivehealth.co.uk for more details.

Potassium loss is associated to sodium loss. Both critical electrolyte minerals form part of a balancing act and need to be kept in a particular ratio. If your sodium levels drop, so will potassium levels to maintain the balance. The answer: regular consumption of electrolyte rich vegetable juice with celery and chlorophyll rich greens as the main ingredients. As your sodium levels adjust, so do your potassium levels.

MAXIMISE YOUR FAT BURNING POTENTIAL

Charlotte Young, professor of Clinical Nutrition at Cornell University published an interesting study. She chose overweight young men as her subjects, and put them on various diets. Each of the three diets was based around carbohydrate restriction and consisted of 1800 calories. The results were recorded for nine weeks.

♦   Diet 1 contained 104 grams of carbohydrate and the subjects lost 2.73 pounds per week, of which 2 pounds was body fat.
♦   Diet 2 contained 60 grams of carbohydrate and subjects lost 3 pounds per week, of which 2.5 pounds was body fat.
♦   Diet 3 contained 30 grams of carbohydrate and the subjects lost 3.73 pounds per week, all of which was body fat. This group was producing ketosis and FMS.

By dropping 74 grams of insulin inducing carbohydrate and replacing it with 300 calories of glucagon stimulating protein based food, these young men lost an extra 1.7 pounds of body fat each and every week.

INSULIN: A SAVIOUR AND SILENT KILLER
THE EFFECT OF FOOD COMBINATIONS
ON INSULIN AND GLUCAGON

Through scientific investigation, subjects had their blood taken and analysed after many different food combinations to determine how much impact the food had on the two hormones of energy metabolism; insulin and glucagon. The results are as follows.

FOOD COMBINATION	INSULIN	GLUCAGON
Carbohydrate	+++++	No change
Protein	++	++
Fat	No change	No change
Carbohydrate and Fat	++++	No change
Protein and Fat	++	++
High Protein and Low Carbohydrate	++	+
High Carbohydrate and Low Protein	+++++++++	+

IF YOU WANT TO STAY FAT – UNLEASH THE BIGGEST HORMONAL NIGHTMARE OF ALL

Studies have shown that if rats are fed a diet with a macronutrient ratio equal to 40% cooked fat and 40% sugar, fat storage levels increased more than any other combination of foods. We are talking about some seriously hefty rats! If you are overweight, but don't think you eat that much, take a look at the macronutrient ratios of your diet. Are you eating small amounts of recreational food throughout the day? Even a few biscuits or the occasional chocolate bar/cake will keep your insulin levels elevated, and promote fat storage.

ARE YOU READY TO MAKE SOME CHANGES?

So there you have it, from the point of view of hormonal control, all you need is quality protein, quality fat and 'minimal-insulin stimulating' carbohydrate. Let's get to work.

YOUR ULTIMATE SOURCE OF PROTEIN –
THE RETURN OF THE HEMP SEED

Along with the flax seeds, hemp seeds can supply you with an abundance of protein. But the reason hemp sits of the throne of AGGRESSIVE HEALTH is because it is the planets most abundant source of edestin (65%). Edestin is a globular protein that is welcomed by your body with open arms. It is immediately transformed into the stuff of life – enzymes, antibodies, hormones, haemoglobin and fibrogen. No other source on earth has the essential amino acids in such an easily digestible form as hemp. The only question is, are you flexible enough to make delicious meals from hemp?

Now, when protein enters your body your body will break it down in an attempt to make globulins. If the proper quantities of globulins are not available, your performance begins to suffer and your immune system compromised.

If you want your bloodstream teeming with these critical building blocks of life, choose foods high in globular proteins – choose hemp. Just as serum globulin is found in your blood, edestin is plant globulin that is easily assimilated and utilised by your body. It is perfect for you and perfect for maintaining a powerful immune system.

FINDING THE RIGHT PROTEIN TO FUEL YOUR FIRE

Always remember the golden rule: YOU ARE UNIQUE. Just as some car engines are designed to run on petrol and others diesel, your body as its own ideal fuel mix to run efficiently. Protein is critical for health and in the same why I suggested you experiment with fats in chapter 4, I suggest you experiment with protein. One source may work well for you, but be a 'bullet to the head' for another person. You may find that diet loaded with purine-rich proteins (organ meats, wild game, anchovies, caviar, sardines, mussels, herring etc.) gets your motor running. You may find that vegetarian sources alone, sprouted beans, vegetables, salad veggies, nuts and seeds etc fire you up more than anything else. You may find that lighter protein sources such as chicken, turkey and eggs are part of your perfect fuel mix.

EXTRA INSURANCE FOR OPTIMAL DIGESTION

Whatever direction you choose to take, ensure you invest in a powerful protein digesting enzyme formula such as Vitälzym™. Too much protein can be very difficult for your body to digest without a little extra assistance. One capsule of Vitälzym™ has the power to break down a 14oz steak into its individual amino acids. Remember, when protein digestion is incomplete; it sets the stage for unwanted bacteria that can form toxic compounds.

pH IMBALANCES HALT FAT LOSS IN ITS TRACKS

'The Atkins Diet' will teach you to focus on meat as your primary source of protein. It says that when you're hungry you can eat steak, eggs, fish or certain cheeses and lose more body fat than ever before! This may come as exciting news to you, but if they don't make up your ideal fuel mix, you can be in trouble. In the wrong body, too much protein can stress alkaline reserves and invite metabolic imbalances associated with high acidity. In an acidic environment your body will gradually begin to secrete more insulin to reduce the acidity. Insulin loses its power in an acidic environment, making this a no-win situation. The excess insulin prevents further fat loss because your body is more interested in maintaining stable pH than it is burning fat! It is here where the typical 'Atkins excitement' begins to fade rapidly as people reach an unsatisfactory plateau. For more information on how your overall pH levels may be affecting your health contact www.aggressivehealth.co.uk.

WAR PROVIDES VALUABLE INSIGHTS INTO THE PERILS OF COOKED FOODS AND MEAT

Considerable evidence has been collected by research scientists all over the world showing that when animal protein is reduced, so is the incidence and growth of cancer. During the Gotterdammerung (the two world wars) under severe food rationing in Austria, Germany, Russia, Britain, and Poland, cancer deaths declined dramatically.

When the Germans occupied Norway during the Second World War, the Norwegian government was forced to sharply reduce the availability of dead animals to its citizens. The death rate from cancer and circulatory diseases plummeted. After the war, the Norwegians returned to their former diet and the death rates rose again as before. Among wild animals in nature, cancer is unknown. However, after subjecting captive monkeys to degenerated foods for extended periods of time, cancer begins to appear.

The over consumption of animal protein can drain your body of pancreatic enzymes. When levels are low, there is an increased risk of cancer. For more information read 'Cancer: Why We're Still Dying to Know the Truth' - www.credence.org.

Bolstering your intake of proteolytic (protein digesting) enzymes is critical if you continue eating animal protein. Remember, one capsule of Vitälzym is able to reduce a 14oz steak into its individual amino acids. That's power.

AVOID 'VEGETARIANISM' LIKE THE PLAGUE

Have you ever opted for vegetarianism, eliminated meat and then found your self addicted to pasta, bread, rice and baked potatoes? Many vegetarians don't even eat vegetables, but spend all day nibbling high carbohydrate foods that ultimately keep insulin levels high and fat burning low. None more horrific than refined flour.

ELIMINATE THE POWERFUL BONE DESTROYER

In his book "Nutrition and Physical Degeneration" by Weston Price, D.D.S. he tells the stories of his travels around the world. He found that when native people started eating refined flour products, it destroyed their bones in one generation. No matter what the race of natives, the results were consistent. Refined flour products transformed broad skulls, wide dental arches and beautiful bodies into deformed narrow skulls (like many if not most Western civilisations), narrow dental arches, and misshapen bodies. Do you eat a lot of white flour products? Not only do they spike insulin, but that bowl of pasta or loaf of bread are completely destructive to your bones. Any food that contains refined flour is a bone poison.

DESTROYING SEXUALITY WITH BREAD

Bread is the first food you should eliminate from your diet if you want to build any kind of health, strength or vitality. Bread contains an enormous amount of oestrogen (a female hormone) that upsets the natural balance of sexual hormones in men. The more bread you eat, the more likely your sexuality will suffer! Do you want male breast development or sexual dysfunction? I think not! Stack the odds in your favour by avoiding it. Sprouted-grain breads are an excellent choice if you find your ultimate fuel mix leans towards a higher carbohydrate diet. Sprouting increases nutrient content and destroys the enzyme inhibitors found in grains. This type of bread is also higher in protein.

AVOID MUCOUS FORMING DAIRY PRODUCTS

Cheese is another favourite food for vegetarians but is high in saturated fat. Saturated fat promotes a higher glucose load in the blood and interferes with the membranes of your cells. The result: Insulin sensors malfunction and your body pumps out more insulin to stabilise blood sugar levels. Cheese is also very mucus forming and supplies minimal nutrition.

PRIORITISE YOUR FOCUS AND ACHIEVE MAXIMAL HORMONAL CONTROL

A better strategy for long-term health is to prioritise your focus. Rather than just eliminating refined carbs from your diet and increasing protein and fat, focus your attention on the following:

1. First discover how excellent you feel once you've eliminated mucoid plaque from your body. When your body is TOTALLY cleansed, you sharpen your hormonal sensitivity dramatically.
2. Focus on becoming the 'King or Queen' of sprouting. With a mixture of sprouted foods in your diet you'll be supplying a healthy mix of enzyme rich live foods, rich in amino acids (hemp seeds, mung beans, lentils, aduki beans, alfalfa sprouts, almond etc.). FOR PROTEIN, THINK SPROUTED BEANS, along with flax meal (ground flax seeds) before you turn to animal protein.
3. Take advantage of regular 'juice fasting' throughout the day (using a variety of mineral rich vegetables/greens). 'Die Hard' AGGRESSIVE HEALTH enthusiasts concentrate on green chlorophyll rich foods and celery as the base to most of their juices. When you do this, you supply critical alkalising minerals necessary for optimal pH balance, minimising the stress on your digestive organs. Remember, digestion is the most energy sapping process in the body. Juice fasting with green vegetables will stabilise your blood sugar levels and over time increase the sensitivity of the insulin receptors on your cells. Fruit juice will create wild blood sugar fluctuations.

4. Make regular use of a wheatgrass juice, AFA Algea and other 'chlorophyll rich superfoods' to supply an abundance of amino acids (and other powerful nutrients), increasing the nutritional potency of your diet.

5. Discover which sources of protein allow you to function at your very best. Experimentation is the key. Use Vitälzym™ to help with the digestion of any animal protein you eat and to restore any enzyme deficiencies that may have developed over years of 'suicidal nutritional abuse'.

6. By selecting the most nutritious, powerful foods in existence you'll feel less hunger, will automatically eat less and overtime your stomach will shrink, your intestines will tighten, and you'll increase your body's overall efficiency.

7. Add a little hemp oil to stimulate your metabolism, an avocado to put a dampener on insulin production. Also, Dr Raymond Peat has shown that a little coconut oil is an excellent food to add to your diet as it stimulates thyroid function boosting your metabolism.

A NEW PIECE TO THE FASCINATING PUZZLE

Although it's critical to eliminate refined carbohydrates and refined sugar, there are some vegetables and fruits, which can also cause problems within the body if not monitored carefully. These specific fruits and vegetables are obviously healthier than their cooked food counterparts but can still jeopardise your progress. Ironically they are the plant foods many people are addicted to because of their high sugar content. Let me introduce you to hybrid food...

USING HYBRID FOODS TO YOUR ADVANTAGE

In a world where the mass production of fruits and vegetables has become a number one priority, crops have been cultivated and crossbred for a more appealing taste and longer durability. Over time they have grown genetically weaker regardless of their sweet flavours and durability. The protective human environments have forced the crops and fruit trees to adapt so much that they've lost their 'genetic energy' and are unable to survive in the wild.

WHAT'S THE BIG DEAL WITH HYBRIDISED FOODS?

Natural sugars from hybridised foods also upset the delicate hormonal balancing act within your body. The reason behind this is that the liver doesn't recognise these sugars and they pass directly into the bloodstream causing the familiar sugar 'high' associated with sweets, and recreational 'junk' food. For example, I used to be addicted to carrot juice! Now remember, although carrot/apple or carrot/beet/celery juice has been used to cure people of some of the most debilitating illnesses (read Jay Kordich's story in his book entitled, The Juiceman), once the healing has taken place, hybridised foods should be minimised.

In the place of carrot juice, use celery and greens. Cucumber is also great to neutralise the bitterness of vegetables and lemons can be used for a real refreshing lift.

Hybridised foods, eaten in excess, can cause the same problems associated with the high carbohydrate, low fat diet, namely – increased acidity, increased insulin production, weight gain and possibly hyperinsulinemia. The first signs are extreme tiredness and fatigue! Be warned!

Hybrid foods are also low in trace nutrients, failing to satisfy the demands of your body. You may *feel* full, but you body isn't *nutritionally* full. Too much sugar in the blood strips away the alkaline minerals from your bones and tissues in an effort to neutralise the acidifying effects of too much sugar.

WHERE TO PLACE YOUR ATTENTION

Here's a guideline to help you minimise hybrid food:

♦ Minimise all seedless fruits or fruits with non-viable seeds; they are genetically altered and weak. These include seedless apples, bananas, several date varieties (especially medjools), kiwis, seedless pineapples, seedless citrus fruits, seedless grapes (raisins), seedless persimmons, and seedless watermelons. They are all loaded with hybrid sugar and will upset the delicate endocrine balancing act if eaten in excess.

♦ Most people, who don't like fruit, like bananas. Bananas are excessively hybridised foods and as well as having a ridiculously high sugar content, also have unbalanced mineral ratios. Too much hybridised sweet fruit can lead to mineral deficiencies, minimise their use.

♦ Limit the overeating/juicing of hybrid vegetables: beets, carrots, corn, and potatoes.

♦ The same rule applies for hybrid nuts and seeds: cashews, oats, rice, and wheat.

♦ As you develop more of a love for fruits and vegetables, don't discard hybrid foods indefinitely, just be aware of their potential to upset your health if eaten in excess. Awareness is the key to your freedom.

ESCAPE THE TRAP AND LOSE A POUND OF BODY FAT
EVERY OTHER DAY!

If you are overweight and have been for some time, you've probably felt trapped. High insulin levels have kept you trapped, but by triggering the biological switches that kick-start your fat metabolism, not only do you maximise nutrient uptake with minimal food but you can lose up to a pound of body fat every other day! Think about it, if some people can put on 14 pounds of unwanted fat in a few short weeks, then the body must have a mechanism to shed body fat that quickly as well – it makes sense. And by harnessing the wisdom within this chapter you have at your finger tips a major weapon. Combine it with the other principles of AGGRESSIVE HEALTH and you can win the war against obesity with ease. In order to melt fat from your body once and for all, you need to remember a few important lessons.

- If it's got sugar in it, it will stimulate insulin production. Eliminate all processed packaged foods including, sweets, chocolate, crisps, cake, pastas, processed breads, crackers and fizzy drinks. When you limit these foods you limit insulin production and increase your chances of maintaining correct pH.
- Saturated fat and sugar form the basis of the junk foods that occupy the supermarket shelves. They cause your insulin receptors to malfunction and keep you fat. Eliminate them
- The equation is simple. Learn it, remember it and share it with others. Excess glucose/cooked fat = Excessive Insulin Secretion = Excess Fat Storage.
- If you think total elimination of carbohydrate is the answer, think again. Carbs are the main source of energy for your brain. An insufficient supply can lead to sugar cravings and compulsive binging. Focus on the best, sprouted foods, vegetables and a few select fruits. Remember, when your foundation is strong you body will better handle anything else you put into it. Don't let your diet control you, use your food selection to put you in control to create health, energy and happiness.
- Lastly, everyone has a different need for protein. Yours may be high, low or somewhere in between. Whatever it is, you need it! Experiment with high protein/low protein and judge by results. Ultimately you're searching for an ideal fuel mix that makes you feel fantastic. If you decide to eat meat (like some authorities promote), eat fresh sources of fish, fowl, eggs and red meat, but ensure you eat them on a solid foundation of veggies, sprouts, vegetable juices and other superfoods. Also, for extra insurance, ensure you take a powerful proteolytic (protein digesting) enzyme formula such as Vitälzym™, to help with protein digestion.

The ultimate question: Do you want to be permanently slim or temporarily slim? Do you want to have permanently high energy levels or temporary levels of energy? Temporary measures bring about temporary results.

PERMANENT MEASURES LEAD TO
PERMANENT RESULTS

In the UK alone, over £25million is spent on weight loss products every year and the figure is rising. What do you think the success rate is? Are you ready for this remarkably high figure? 5%. That's right, I'll even type it out – five percent. How would you describe a 95% failure rate? I'd describe it as an absolute rip-off. Very few approaches to nutrition take into consideration the biochemical factors that cause obesity in the first place. If these diets really did work, would there be an unending chain of new ones? If diets worked, wouldn't the rate of obesity in this country be decreasing instead of increasing? Dieting has been labelled a national epidemic. It is even harder to treat than the vast majority of cancers because many so-called health practitioners are using the wrong approach, time after time!

A VICTORY IS A VICTORY WHEREVER YOU SCORE FROM ON THE PLAYING FIELD

Millions of people have lost weight and kept it off through a variety of methods. Some people didn't change their diets, but began exercising. Exercise helps control insulin levels. Other people did nothing but give up chocolate and sweets, again eliminating the foods that cause excessive insulin production. High carbohydrate diets will work for some people, but with all food, the secret is in selection. You are probably beginning to see that there isn't a magic bullet ultimately, but there is an ultimate goal. That is to keep insulin under control by eliminating cooked fat and highly processed sugar rich foods and to figure out your ideal fuel mix (the ratio of protein/carbohydrate/fat) that makes you feel fantastic.

FOCUS ON THE BASICS OF AGGRESSIVE HEALTH

The basics of AGGRESSIVE HEALTH state that cooked food has a tremendously destabilising effect on blood sugar levels. When you eat cooked food you can expect blood sugar level fluctuations ten times greater than when you eat live or enzyme rich foods. Enzyme rich raw food causes a much steadier metabolic rate and greater emotional stability. Raw/living foods should be your priority, no matter what 'eating plan' you follow and what you ideal fuel mix is comprised of.

ARE YOU READY FOR THE CHALLENGE?

Regulate your insulin levels and you might as well begin the celebrations! Many people unconsciously make the association: Eating more = Getting fatter... so therefore... Eating Nothing = Maximum weight loss. WRONG! If you've ever starved yourself in an effort to lose weight, realise that all you've done is blunt your own insulin response! Yes, you probably did appear to lose weight, but at the expense of starving your body of every vital nutrient needed to survive, including vital minerals necessary to maintain a balanced pH. Not eating may appear successful to begin with because a drop in blood/insulin levels usually precedes fat loss, but once you start eating again, unchanged habits (the cause of the problem) resurface causing the classic 'yo-yo dieting' syndrome. Lipolysis reverses this trend. Simply focus on vegetable juice, veggies, greens and sprouted foods already discussed, add in your ideal source of protein to stimulate glucagons and back this up with some good quality fat to blunt the insulin response and you'll be on the fast track to success:

♦ If you are incredibly obese or simply a few stones overweight, it is likely that insulin is constantly occupying your bloodstream morning, noon and night. Excess insulin is the reason why you have put weight on and kept it on. Eliminate the cause – cooked fat and refined carbohydrates.

♦ Sleep is a time when fatty acids and ketones are *usually* converted into fuel, but this can't take place in the presence of excess insulin!

- Insulin is a storage and locking hormone. When you kick-start your fat burning metabolism you'll stimulate glucagon and be in the fat-dissolving state.
- This fat-dissolving state known as lipolysis is the opposite pathway to gaining fat.
- Fat Mobilisation Substance (FMS) and other lipid mobilisers are critical for kick-starting your journey. They enable you to effortlessly pass out unused calories from your body that may have been stored on your body on the low fat, high carbohydrate diet.
- Feeding cooked potatoes to hogs produces rapid weight gain to ensure a higher market price.
- When the entry rates of carbohydrates were studied, scientists were surprised with their findings. It was thought that simple sugars enter the bloodstream quickly, whilst complex carbohydrates slowly, but studies completely disproved this. It was found that fructose (fruit sugar) enters the bloodstream more slowly than supposedly 'complex' carbohydrates such as pasta.
- Two other studies from the same research group in Italy indicate that excessive pasta consumption is linked to increases in colon cancer and stomach cancer. On the other hand, every major study has indicated that people who increase their consumption of fruits and vegetables reduce their risk of cancer and heart disease dramatically.
- There are two types of fibre, soluble and insoluble fibre. Soluble fibre includes such things as pectin, which is found in apples. Insoluble fibre includes such things as cellulose and bran found in breakfast cereals. Soluble fibre slows the entry rate of carbohydrates into your blood stream but insoluble fibre has virtually no effect.
- Early research conducted at the University of Toronto found that table sugar enters the bloodstream more slowly than the highly recommended breakfast cereals, such as corn flakes. You may have once thought breakfast cereal was healthy but for all intensive purposes it is nothing but pure glucose linked by chemical bonds. Once these bonds are easily broken in your stomach the glucose rushes into your bloodstream at a faster rate than the carbohydrate from table sugar. Think about the effect a daily dose of cereal has on your system.
- If you want to get maximum control over your insulin levels use sprouted foods. They have the advantage of causing less insulin secretion than any other food and supply an abundance of life giving enzymes, minerals, vitamins and phytochemicals as well as being the the most electrically charged food on the planet.
- If you look into the scientific world of metabolism, you'll find the phenomenon of ketone formation documented as your major alternative fuel system. Dr George Cahill, a professor from Harvard who has respect for being a leader in the research of metabolic pathways explains how brain tissue utilises ketones more easily than glucose, being 'preferred fuel' in his opinion.
- Flax and Coconut butter increase metabolic rate. Use them to enhance fat burning.

- Cold showers can also be used to stimulate metabolism.
- Use wheatgrass juice and E3Live daily! It supplies such a cocktail of goodness you'll be on the fast track to unassailable health!
- High insulin/body fat levels increase the quantity of an enzyme that converts testosterone to oestradiol, compromising your sex drive.
- Studies have confirmed that low levels of testosterone in males correlate with an increased risk of heart disease. By lowering your insulin levels and losing body fat you indirectly decrease the quantity of the enzyme responsible for converting testosterone to oestradiol, thus maintaining optimal testosterone levels. The message: Higher insulin – lower testosterone – less sex drive! I'll let you decide how important this is!
- Protein is critical for kickstarting your fat metabolism. Hemp is the best vegetarian source along with sprouted beans, lentils etc. Finding the right protein source to make up your ideal fuel mix is your responsibility. You may prefer high protein or low protein – learn through experience. By doing so you'll gain the personal wisdom necessary for long term success. Vitalzym will assist in the break down of protein to amino acids if you decide that a high protein diet is for you.
- If you restrict carbohydrate intake to the extreme, prepare to suffer. Carbohydrates are vital for energising your brain and a lack of supply may cause you to feel anxious, dizzy, lethargic or depressed. When you don't supply enough carbohydrate, you may develop sugar cravings, which can develop into compulsive binging.

A Final Thought: Obesity is a growing national epidemic and by losing extra fat content, you immediately jump out of a group of people who are in danger of diabetes, heart disease, stroke etc. whilst immediately jumping into an elite group of people who are living the principles of AGGRESSIVE HEALTH. Come and join us!

THE AGGRESSIVE HEALTH EVALUATION:
Do you want to maximise your fat burning potential?
Have you mastered the principles of hormonal control?
Do you appreciate the role of insulin in weight gain?

If you want to know why food is more powerful than any prescription drug and how to harness this power to control every aspect of your health, pay attention. What you are about to read will revolutionise your eating habits and change the eating habits of the world.

CHAPTER 8

DISCOVER HOW TO BECOME THE MASTER OF YOUR OWN HORMONAL DESTINY BY CONTROLLING EICOSANOIDS - THE SUPER HORMONES

You are about to move swiftly into a different realm. A realm where cutting edge science takes over, a realm where fine-tuning is the key, and a realm that puts you in complete control of your health.

You may find this chapter very technical to begin with, so don't get too absorbed in the science of what you're about to read, simply learn what it takes to control eicosanoids (pronounced eye-ka-sarnoids) and watch in awe as your entire being transforms in front of your very eyes.

All you need to know is what eicosanoids are, how they are produced, why they are critical to AGGRESSIVE HEALTH, and what you can do to influence their production.

The information that follows represents the latest findings in human physiology. But hold on a minute! If what you're about to read is so ground-breaking, why haven't you heard about these super-hormones before. In fact...

IF SOME DOCTORS DON'T KNOW ABOUT EICOSANOIDS WHY SHOULD YOU?

If you've never heard of eicosanoids, don't be too concerned. Most physicians or exercise physiologists have never heard of them either. This ignorance is in spite of the fact that the 1982 Nobel Prize in Medicine was awarded to a couple of research scientists for understanding their importance in human physiology. Eicosanoids represent some of the most powerful and crucial substances in the body. They control the cardiovascular system, the immune system, and the systems that determine how much fat you store. In fact they control virtually all of your bodily functions. Yet as powerful as they are, eicosanoids are totally controlled by diet, exercise, rest and stress.

If you asked a doctor to explain the role of eicosanoids in your body, what do you think they'd say? Do you think they'd be able to tell you that almost every prescription drug directly affects eicosanoid production in your body? Do you think they'd be able to explain why a dynamic balance of eicosanoids virtually guarantees health? Do you think they'd be able to tell you that the reason aspirin is so powerful and effective is because of its eicosanoid modulating capabilities? The reality is simple – most doctors have never heard of eicosanoids. They represent the most powerful force present within your body, and the good news is that this force is controllable. Now is your chance to…

UNCOVER THE MYSTERIES OF THE EICOSANOIDS

Why is there so much ignorance concerning the importance of eicosanoids? The answer is their complexity:

1. There are currently more than 100 known eicosanoids and more are being discovered all the time.
2. Their lifetime in the body is measured in seconds.
3. They function as 'cell to cell regulators' that rarely appear in the bloodstream.
4. They work at vanishingly low concentrations.

These facts have limited the understanding of eicosanoid biochemistry to the highest levels of medical research. This data simply has not yet filtered down to exercise physiologists, physicians or athletes.

ESSENTIAL FATTY ACIDS –
THE BUILDING BLOCKS OF POWER

Eicosanoids are derived from a unique group of polyunsaturated essential fatty acids containing 20 carbon atoms (Greek *eikosi*, twenty). Think of eicosanoids as a team of at least 100 powerful hormone-like substances responsible for the control of virtually every physiological response in your body. Like most hormones, balance is the key, but unlike most hormones eicosanoids are produced inside the cells, act inside the cells, and vanish in a fraction of a second, making them more difficult to study than endocrine hormones such as insulin and glucagon.

Once an eicosanoid is excreted by a cell, its primary objective is to test the immediate environment outside the boundaries of the cell and then report back to the cell. This information is critical and allows the cell to take appropriate biological action in response to any external alterations. By continually being sent out to assess the immediate surroundings around a cell, an eicosanoid can interact with the cell receptor on the cell surface, modifying the biological response of the cell. This complex activity has only recently been discovered, but…

EICOSANOIDS HAVE BEEN AROUND FOREVER!

Even though eicosanoids have been around for more than 500 million years, the first ones were only discovered in 1936 having been isolated from the prostate gland and named prostaglandins.

At this early stage, eicosanoids were considered another endocrine hormone using the bloodsteam to get to its target cell, but this wasn't the case, leaving scientists unable to pinpoint their role in the body. It took 40 years for any breakthrough to be made, but in the 1970s with the development of exceptionally sophisticated instrumentation, scientists were able to identify more than 100 different eicosanoids and began to identify their roles.

THE MASTER CONTROL SYSTEM

By controlling leukotrienes (another subclass of eicosanoids) you can control, among other things, bronchial constriction and allergies. By controlling and balancing prostacyclins and thromboxanes, you can control heart disease. If you modify your nutritional habits and control the production of lipoxins and hydroxylated fatty acids you'll be able to control inflammation and also regulate the immune system.

So there you have it, as each year passes, more and more eicosanoids are uncovered and categorised accordingly. Prostaglandins are the most familiar eicosanoids, but represent only a small group of this very large and powerful family. If you look at the list below you'll see what I mean. Epi-isoprostanoids were only discovered a few years before the new millennium. When controlled, they have powerful anti-cancer effects similar to those found in aspirin. Here's the list.

- Prostaglandins
- Thromboxanes
- Leukotrienes
- Lipoxins
- Hydroxylated fatty acids
- Isoprostanoids
- Epi-isoprostanoids
- Isoleukotrienes

WHY ARE YOU LEARNING ALL OF THIS?

If you can control eicosanoids, you can control the finest regulators of cellular function in existence. Imagine being able to have complete biological control over the regulation of many diverse functions, such as:

- blood pressure.
- blood clotting.
- the inflammation response.
- the immune system.
- uterine contractions during birth.
- sexual potency in men.
- the pain and fever response.
- the sleep/wake cycle.
- the release of gastric acid (potent new anti-ulcer drugs currently being investigated are eicosanoid modulators).
- the constriction and dilation of airways in the lungs and blood vessels in the tissues, and many others.

YOU'RE RESPONSIBLE FOR
THE GREATEST BALANCING ACT OF ALL

Eicosanoids are the most powerful hormones in existence and must be dynamically balanced to ensure optimal health and longevity. Imbalances of any kind, left untreated, can cause major physiological problems. This chapter will allow you to fine-tune what you've already discovered and modify your nutritional habits even more to gain control and direct the balance of these super-hormones. Take a look for yourself at the powerful roles of eicosanoids and prepare to take the reins.

| EICOSANOID END PRODUCTS FALL INTO TWO BASIC GROUPS ||
GOOD EICOSANOIDS	BAD EICOSANOIDS
Inhibit platelet aggregation	Promote platelet aggregation
Act as vasodilators	Act as vasoconstrictors
Decrease cellular proliferation	Increase cellular proliferation
Stimulate immune response	Depress immune response
Decrease inflammation	Increase inflammation
Decrease pain transmission	Increase pain transmission
Dilate airways	Constrict airways
Increase endurance	Decrease endurance
Increase oxygen flow	Decrease oxygen flow

EICOSANOIDS – THE ACCELERATOR AND BRAKE OF OPTIMAL
HEALTH

Good and bad eicosanoids are like the brake and accelerator pedals in a car. In order to pass your driving test you must master the control of both. If you put your pedal to the metal and accelerate too hard, and produce an excess of good eicosanoids, you may travel down the road to exhilarating health faster, but without the brake (bad eicosanoids) you'll lose control of the car! The bad eicosanoids can be held responsible for almost every major illness that has existed within society to date, but nevertheless, like the brake pedal in a car 'bad eicosanoids' are still necessary to get you where you want to go, even though it appears they hold you back. The reason they are labelled 'bad' is because in today's society, it's easy to engage in habits that cause their runaway production and as you know it's no good trying to drive down the road to scintillating health with your foot on the brake!

Your ultimate goal is to create a dynamic balance between 'good' and 'bad' eicosanoids and when you do, your journey towards exceptional health will be fast but steady. In fact, don't be surprised to find any unwanted rashes clearing up, allergies disappearing, joints regaining mobility, headaches vanishing, nails strengthening and asthma clearing up – This is AGGRESSIVE HEALTH.

THE BENEFITS OF MAINTAINING A DYNAMIC BALANCE

Let's take a look at platelet aggregation. Platelet aggregation is the term used when platelets join together to form clumps. Good eicosanoids inhibit platelets from clumping (aggregating) and bad eicosanoids promote excessive clumping. If this clumping happens at the wrong time, a person can develop a blood clot that may lead to a heart attack or stroke. But what about if you cut yourself? If platelets lose their ability to clump together, you could bleed to death from a paper cut!

Another example is blood pressure. Over production of bad eicosanoids can cause high blood pressure by constricting the arteries (i.e. vasoconstriction), but the overproduction of good eicosanoids can cause low blood pressure (i.e. vasodilation), which can lead to shock. Very few people consistently produce too many good eicosanoids! The common diseases of civilisation are the result of the production of too many bad ones. In fact, as I've said before, the bad ones aren't 'bad', but are easy to produce in a society with so many poor eating habits.

Take a look at the relationship between various illnesses and eicosanoids:

♦ Heart attack victims are making more 'bad' eicosanoids (that promote platelet aggregation and vasoconstriction) and not enough 'good' ones (that prevent platelet aggregation and promote vasodilation)
♦ High blood pressure victims are making more 'bad' eicosanoids (vasoconstrictors) and not enough 'good' ones (vasodilators).
♦ Arthritis sufferers are making more bad eicosanoids (pro-inflammatory) and fewer 'good' ones (anti-inflammatory)
♦ Cancer victims are making more 'bad' eicosanoids (immune depressing) and too few 'good' ones (immune stimulating).
♦ Sufferers of Type 2 diabetes, are making more 'bad' eicosanoids (that stimulate insulin secretion) and fewer 'good' ones (that inhibit insulin secretion).

BAD EICOSANOIDS HAVE THE POWER TO
EXPOSE GENETIC PRE-DISPOSITIONS

If a group of individuals spent a lifetime producing too many bad eicosanoids, do you think they'd all show the same symptoms? Definitely not! Some may have heart disease, others cancer, whilst others may be crippled by arthritis or have diabetes. Many of these chronic diseases have a strong genetic linkage. The potential for their expression lies buried in your genes, and bad eicosanoids can expose these threats if over produced! The message is clear: In a world where 21st century breakthrough principles of health need to spread like wild fire to ensure people get control of their health again, disease can be looked upon as nothing but the body making more bad eicosanoids than good. The quality of your health is the quality of the balance between good eicosanoids and bad. In fact, the worst diet approach is one that was promoted in the later stages of the 20th Century…

THE EVILS ASSOCIATED WITH
A HIGH CARBOHYDRATE DIET

Up until recently, society has encouraged a very high carbohydrate diet. I used to. Years ago when I first started teaching people about nutrition, I found myself getting more and more fatigued as I forced down another bowl of pasta. I had little physical energy and my blood pressure was so high, I should have referred myself to a physician. I was playing the eicosanoid game poorly, leading to a decline in my health. Without knowing it, I was disrespecting the super-hormones that have evolved over the last 500 million years to maintain my blood sugar levels and ensure optimal health. I've learned the hard way. You don't have to! You can change your biochemistry in an instant as long as you eat in accordance with what you are about to learn. So what have you learned so far?

A Quick Re-cap:

♦ The 1982 Nobel Prize in Medicine was awared to two research scientists for understanding the importance of eicosanoids in human physiology.
♦ Eicosanoids control virtually every function of your body including the cardiovascular system and immune system.
♦ Almost every prescription drug directly affects eicosanoids.
♦ Eicosanoids are derived from polyunsaturated essential fatty acids.
♦ Both 'good' and 'bad' eicosanoids must be kept in balance.
♦ A high pasta/bread/rice carbohydrate diet will thwart eicosanoid balance.

Now is the time for you to discover the secret formula for…

BUILDING EICOSANOIDS FROM SCRATCH

With the importance of eicosanoids very clear in your mind, the question is how can you control their production? Just like any construction project, you need raw materials to begin your project. It's up to you to use these raw materials to build solid foundations. Let me take you on a journey through the production of eicosanoids. Use this knowledge for the rest of your life and you'll experience the kind of legendary health that will separate you from the masses! Your immediate priority is fat! You must ensure you get enough fat in your diet – but not just any old fat – raw plant fats that provide essential fatty acids!

WITHOUT ESSENTIAL FATTY ACIDS YOU'LL NEVER PRODUCE EICOSANOIDS

For this section, I'm not going to beat around the bush. Essential fatty acids from raw plant fats are the basic raw materials needed for the eventual production of eicosanoids. Essential fatty acids can't be manufactured in the body, so therefore have to be present in the food that you eat. If you remember one thing, remember this: no essential fatty acids – no eicosanoids.

The eight essential fatty acids fall into two categories – omega 6 and omega 3 fatty acids. The eicosanoids that come from omega 3 fatty acids are relatively neutral. The eicosanoids that come from omega 6 fatty acids form the building blocks for both good and bad eicosanoids.

STAGE 1 - EAT ENOUGH LINOLEIC ACID TO BEGIN THE PRODUCTION OF EICOSANOIDS

Linoleic acid is where you begin. Basically it's an essential fatty acid, an omega 6 fatty acid to be precise. You need to ensure you include plenty of it in your diet, so the question is: Where do you find it? Raw plant fats. With plenty of linoleic acid present in your diet, the next stage is transporting it into your cells somehow. Ironically this is a job for the so-called 'bad' low-density lipoproteins (LDLs).

LOW DENSITY LIPOPROTEINS AREN'T SO BAD AFTER ALL

Whether you are familiar with 'the old cholesterol-madness mentality' or not, LDLs used to have a very bad reputation. If you have a high LDL to HDL ratio you increase your chance of heart disease, but having no LDLs is also just as life threatening. If you had no LDLs you wouldn't be able to make any eicosanoids, which ultimately is a no-win situation. (See chapter 9 for more information about cholesterol.)

With enough linoleic acid, and a vehicle to transport it into the eicosanoid pipeline, the next stage is getting what's available into the production pathway so it can be converted to another fatty acid called gamma linolenic acid (GLA). This conversion is controlled by an enzyme, which acts like a gatekeeper, called delta 6 desaturase. You are about to learn how to control this enzyme, because if you don't, you'll never master control of the eicosanoid production pipeline. Imagine linoleic acid to be the 'goods', LDLs to be the delivery truck and delta 6 desaturase the guard that either lets you deliver your goods and convert them into GLA or turns you away! Let's look at it in detail.

THE ENZYME STANDING AT THE GATE:
DELTA 6 DESATURASE

If delta 6 desaturase is active, you're in luck! You'll be able to deliver your goods without any problems. If delta 6 desaturase is not active then you'll be turned away from the gate, the entry of linoleic acid will be denied and eicosanoid production will suffer. Your job is to do everything possible to ensure delta 6 desaturase is active. Here's how:

VARIABLES THAT GOVERN THE ACTIVITY OF
DELTA 6 DESATURASE

SPEEDS UP DELTA 6 DESATURASE	*SLOWS DOWN* DELTA 6 DESATURASE
1.Dietary Protein	1.High carbohydrate diet/sugar
	2.Trans fatty acids
	3.Alpha linoleic acid
	4.Stress
	5.Disease
	6.Ageing
	7.Zinc deficiency

DIETARY PROTEIN
Protein is critical and often overlooked. It speeds up the activity of delta 6 desaturase and provides the raw material needed for a powerful body and a biochemically balanced brain. Sprouted foods (mung beans, hemp seeds, lentils, almonds etc.), along with green chlorophyll rich foods and green superfoods will supply you with critical amino acids, but you may need more than this.

Through experimentation, you'll discover your body's demands as you figure out your ideal fuel mixture. If your body demands animal protein, don't feel guilty – your biochemistry is more important than what you've been led to believe by 'so-called' authorities. People who succeed on low protein diets will promote low protein diets. People who succeed on high protein diets will promote high protein diets. It makes sense. Remember, protein provides the amino acid tryptophan. From tryptophan, your body makes serotonin and it's serotonin that keeps you feeling balanced, calm, and productive. We'll chew over this subject more in chapter 14. Back to the chase. One last point – If you choose mostly animal protein, begin to increase your intake of metabolic enzymes, such as vitalyzm. Excess animal protein puts a drain on enzyme reserves.

Although protein is critical to speed up delta 6 desaturase, minimising the factors that slow delta 6 desaturase down is just as important. Here we go.

HIGH CARBOHYDRATE DIET

Various studies conclusively show that high carbohydrate, low protein diets inhibit the activity of delta 6 desaturase. The problem is also compounded due to the insulin producing effect of a high carbohydrate diet. This has an effect on another enzyme called delta 5 desaturase. More about that later. Alcohol is worth a mention here because its use is so widespread. It is high in sugar and interferes with the delta 6-desaturase enzyme. High sugar diets also prevent fat from being released from your own personal fat stores in your body, essentially keeping you fat! Sugar also interferes with the work of the essential fatty acids. Sugar and alcohol are also non-ionic substances that can interfere with the ionic mobility and lower zeta potential. For more information go to the article section at www.aggressivehealth.co.uk.

TRANS FATTY ACIDS

Foods that contain trans-fatty acids, especially fried foods, are dangerous to your health. They slow down the activity of delta 6 desaturase and thus inhibit the formation of good eicosanoids. Firstly they change the permeability of cell membranes, allowing unwelcome molecules in, and letting some molecules escape which would usually remain in the cell. This protective barrier is vital in keeping your cells alive and healthy. Eliminate all cooked fat and replace it with raw plant fats immediately!

Trans-fatty acids make up 37% of partially hydrogenated vegetable oils and if ingested can rapidly increase blood cholesterol level by 15% and triglyceride levels by 47%. In experiments, trans-fatty acids have been shown to have the power to increase the size of atherosclerotic plaques in the aortas of pigs. Hydrogenated oils are used in baked goods, confections such as ice cream, chocolate and sweets, and snacks such as crisps where the hydrogenated oil helps to give the product crispness. A crisp would have no crunch without the hydrogenated (hardened) oil. Eliminate them and replace them with raw plant fats!

When you look at the facts, death from cancer has increased from 1 in 30 in 1900, to over 1 in 4 in 2000. The increase parallels the increased consumption of hydrogenated vegetable oils and trans-fatty acids. Any fat that is cooked or altered is not welcome in the body.

MARGARINE MAYBE CHOLESTEROL-FREE
BUT IT INCREASES CHOLESTEROL!

Margarine may be free of cholesterol, but it increases cholesterol levels because it is a potent source of trans-fatty acids. One study showed that women who ate four or more teaspoons of margarine per day had a 66% greater chance of contracting cardiovascular disease than women who ate about one teaspoon per month. Also, women who eat trans-fatty acids found in margarine and shortening have a much higher chance of contracting breast cancer, the number one cancer killer in women. When men eat this form of fat, they greatly increase their risk of prostate cancer. Good eicosanoids reduce the manufacture of cholesterol in the liver. Raw plant fats are the only answer!

THE IMPORTANCE OF UNDERSTANDING OILS

For oils to remain fresh and deliver vital nutrients and essential fats to the body, they must be pressed and packaged in the dark, in the absence of oxygen and heat. Having been through this kind of stringent process they must then be stored in opaque containers, excluding air and oxygen. This kind of packaging allows oils to retain their goodness for years. Alternatively, nature packages these oils in nuts and seeds, in a way that keeps light, air and heat out. Seeds can protect oils for several years without spoiling. When you sprout seeds you unleash their nutrition in a way that is more easily absorbed by your body.

THE DANGERS OF HOT FAT

Many polyunsaturated fats undergo a trans-alteration during the high temperatures required for sautéing and frying, changing the molecular structure of their constituent fatty acids. Once these changes have occurred, your body finds no use for them because they can't be assimilated. Once a fat has been cooked at high temperatures, it becomes poisonous and carcinogenic (cancer causing).

Studies at the University of Helsinki, performed by Dr Rakel Kurkela showed how cooked fats can drastically reduce levels of health. He split his animal subjects into two groups:

♦   Group 1 was fed with raw, unheated safflower oil, rich in unsaturated fatty acids.
♦   Group 2 was fed with the same oil that had been heated in a frying pan.

Every other part of the diet was kept similar throughout the experiment and the results were so clear it's almost frightening. Group 1 thrived and increased their body weight. Group 2, however, deteriorated and eventually died.

When Kurkela analysed the heated oil and other unsaturated oil, he found they were filled with numerous poisonous compounds. Some of the substances found were powerful oxidisers, known for causing damage by altering the structure of cell membranes, cell nuclei and amino acids. Some other substances were cancer inducing. One such substance he discovered was malonaldehyde. Eliminate cooked fat!

ALPHA LINOLENIC ACID (ALA)

ALA is an omega-3 fatty acid found in the oils of various plants that slows down the activity of delta 6 desaturase. Oils such as stone-pressed extra virgin olive oil is a good choice, high in monounsaturated fats with no ALA. Flaxseed oil is high in ALA, which is why I recommend using the use of ground flax meal instead of the pure oil as you are less likely to use too much. Remember the story of Udo Erasmus, author of 'Fats That Heal, Fat That Kill', who used too much flax oil and ended up dry scaly skin. That's an example of poor eicosanoid control. Many sufferers of arthritis consume flaxseed oil to help their condition, and may be a little confused at this point. The reason flaxseed works is because it inhibits all eicosanoid formation. It knocks out the bad ones which are causing the problem, but at the expense of preventing the formation of the good ones. This action is similar to that of aspirin.

STRESS

Stress is a word that means many things to many people. Regardless of what many authorities tend to believe, there are means and ways of accessing calm, relaxed, focused and alert states of minds without the presence of stress. Not only are there techniques that can be learned, but there are also machines that assist you in accessing peak performance brain states.

When you stop and think about it, why would you want to control stress? If you control it, the pre-supposition is that it still exists. You wouldn't want to control a dangerous old car with bad brakes and unreliable steering would you? Once you knew about its condition, you'd want a new one, or at least get it repaired. Learning to create peak performance states of mind at will, whether it be on your own, or using some of the latest brain enhancing/peak performance mind machines, is where you need to place your attention. When you use these devices or techniques, not only do you eliminate stress (a potential delta 6 desaturase inhibitor), but you also condition states of mind that can be used productively to increase the quality of your life. The hormonal benefits of relaxation training/mind machines will be covered later in chapters 11 and 12.

Back to the chase. Take a look at how stress can cause biochemical havoc in your body by overproducing the two menacing hormones...

CORTISOL AND ADRENALINE:
A PAIR OF MENACING DELTA 6 DESATURASE INHIBITORS

Stress elevates blood levels of the hormones adrenaline and cortisol.

◆ Adrenaline decreases the activity of delta 6 desaturase, and that in turn decreases the production of good eicosanoids.
◆ Cortisol increases insulin levels, leading to an over production of bad eicosanoids.

Are you beginning to see that you can be doing everything right nutritionally, but if you don't take time to relax and be quiet on the inside, you'll never master AGGRESSIVE HEALTH?

Research from Harvard Medical School with 1623 cardiac patients strongly suggests that angry outbursts more than double the risk of a heart attack in the following two hours. Eliminating negative stress is a major factor in the quest to mastering eicosanoid production.

In a study carried out at the Seattle Pacific Northwest Research Foundation, hundreds of rats were bred to be susceptible to breast cancer. They were then subjected to varying amounts of stress, whilst carefully monitored. The rate of cancer increased from between 7% and 92% depending on amount of stress the rats experienced.

In one interesting study, scientists took the saliva from a man who was experiencing rage. Upon analysis they were shocked to find that the composition of his saliva matched the composition of a rattle snake's venom. To test the potency, they injected some of the saliva into a group of small animals and each one died.

So once again, don't underestimate stress, especially with respect to eicosanoids. Some people eat poorly all their life, but manage to stay relaxed and calm, and in good spirits and live a long fun-filled life.

STRESS HORMONES AND
HORMONAL COMMUNICATION BREAKDOWN

Cortisol is the most abundant corticosteroid synthesised by your body. In excessive amounts it can accelerate ageing and cause widespread damage. The neurons in your brain are incredibly sensitive to cortisol and if exposed to increasing levels within the bloodstream, can die! If this happens continuously, the powerful feedback mechanism that controls the release of cortisol gradually breaks down and increasing amounts of cortisol are released from the adrenal glands exacerbating the problem. When someone continues to damage the cortisol-sensitive neurons in their brain, cortisol secretion gradually overwhelms the body. The result: Inhibited eicosanoid formation.

Ask anyone who has taken synthetic corticosteroids for more than 30 days. After this amount of time their body goes haywire and deteriorates rapidly because they prevent any formation of eicosanoids, good or bad! Synthetic corticosteroids may appear to be doing some good initially because they knock out the production of 'bad' eicosanoids (the cause of the problem), but eventually they cause death!

DISEASE

Disease is usually a sign that your body has been under-functioning for some time. Many of the principles of AGGRESSIVE HEALTH direct your attention to maintaining stable pH balance through powerful nutritional principles and deep cleansing. If you haven't been taking good care of yourself, you may have created an internal environment that has fostered the over growth of unwanted organism in the form of yeast, fungus and mold. If you've created an environment of weakness, a viral infection may have run you down. Viruses inhibit the action of the delta-6-desaturase enzyme. The eicosanoid PGE1, is an incredibly powerful protector against viral infections, highlighting why prevention is better than cure. Viruses cause a roadblock in the eicosanoid pipeline inhibiting the activity of the delta 6-desaturase enzyme, and ultimately the production of PGE1 and other 'good' eicosanoids. For an immediate victory against viruses in your body, turn to the systemic enzyme formulation Vitälzym™ . It has been shown to reduce viral load in the body dramatically by eating away at the exterior coating rendering viruses inert. Ultimately, you are less likely to suffer a viral infection if you engage in habits that optimise the balance of favourable eicosanoids to unfavourable eicosanoids.

EMBRACE THE BUILDING BLOCKS OF IMMUNITY

If you want to resist and recover fast from infection you need to supply the raw materials necessary for your body to produce antibodies. The materials in question are globulin proteins. Go straight to the source – hemp seeds. Another excellent food to focus on is…

THE MIRACLE OF COCONUT OIL

Take a look at some of the powerful effect coconut oil can have on your body:

♦ Kills viruses that cause mononucleosis, influenza, hepatitis C, measles, herpes, AIDS and other illnesses
♦ Kills bacteria that cause pneumonia, earache, throat infections, dental cavities, food poisoning, urinary tract infections, meningitis, gonorrhea, and dozens of other diseases.
♦ Kills fungi and yeast that cause candida, jock itch, ringworm, athletes foot, thrush, diaper rash and other infections
♦ Expels or kills tape worms, lice, giardia, and other parasite
♦ Helps to protect the body from harmful free radicals that promote premature aging and degenerative disease
♦ Does not deplete the body's antioxidant reserves like other oils do

---

AGEING

As people age, the activity of delta 6 desaturase begins to slow down, especially after 30, leaving it up to you to take responsibility to keep it active.

Age doesn't just relate to the number of years that you've been alive, it also relates to a number of other factors. There are in fact three distinct and separate ways to measure your age:

1. Chronological age – How old you are by the calendar.
2. Biological age – How old your body is in terms of critical life signs and cellular processes.
3. Psychological age – How old you feel.

Imagine being in a group of people all of similar chronological age. What would you see? Would they all look similar? Would they all act the same and have the same outlook on life? Of course not, It doesn't take a genius to realise that some people are ageing faster than normal.

HOW DO YOU SLOW DOWN THE AGEING PROCESS?

It is safe to say that you can't change your chronological age, but you can change your biological age. All you need to do is take a look at the list of biological parameters that determine how fast various systems of your body are ageing, and then reverse these parameters. Through the process of ageing the following biological markers alter to some degree. Take a look for yourself:

◆   Insulin resistance increases.
◆   Systolic blood pressure increases.
◆   Body fat percentage and lipid ratios increase.
◆   Glucose tolerance decreases.
◆   Aerobic capacity decreases.
◆   Muscle mass and strength decreases.
◆   Temperature regulation decreases in efficiency.
◆   Immune function diminishes.

It's worth pointing out that this fairly broad list of physiological changes can all be related to one single factor – excess insulin production. Need I say more! By combining the very best nutritional principles present within these pages, backed up with aerobic exercise, anaerobic exercise and the use of the latest developments in mind technology, you'll live a long youthful life, maintaining an optimal eicosanoid balance.

Psychological age is also a very powerful factor, which is influenced by many interweaving personal and social factors. Here is a list of questions you may like to ask yourself. Regardless of your answers, it would be worth asking yourself how you could improve each one and therefore increase the level of your psychological health.

How happy are you in your marriage or existing relationship?
How happy are you within your present job?
How happy are you within yourself?
How satisfying is your sex life?
How good is your ability to make and keep close friends?
How regular is your daily routine?
How regular is your work routine?
Do you take at least one week's vacation per year?
How much control do you feel you have over your personal life?
How much do you enjoy leisure time and your hobbies?
How easy do you find it to express your feelings?
How optimistic are you about the future?
How financially secure are you?
How much do you enjoy living within your means?

When you read chapter 17 – The Parameters of Success, you'll read an amazing story of how a group of people reversed every biological marker of ageing simply by changing their environment and their perception of reality! But for now let's get back to the eicosanoid production pipeline.

ZINC DEFICIENCY

Zinc deficiency, which is widespread, slows down the delta 6-desaturase enzyme. Every vital nutrient must be included in your diet to prevent viral infections, weak tissues and a weak immune system. The importance of having a base-line standard where you consume nutrient rich raw foods, minimising cellular stress and maximising waste elimination, can never be under-estimated. If you have white spots on your nails it's likely you have zinc deficiency. The best way to increase your zinc uptake is to include E3Live in your diet. Dr Gillian McKeith, in her book 'Miracle Superfood: Wild Blue-Green Algae' tells the remarkable story of how zinc capsules, tablets, lozenges or zinc liquid did nothing to improve her condition of zinc deficiency. The only food that eliminated the white spots and restored her zinc levels to normal was AFA blue-green algae. I suggest you buy the book and begin to use E3Live daily.

LET THE STRUGGLE COME TO A GRINDING HALT

You've covered just about everything that inhibits Delta 6 desaturase. You should now have a fair idea why many people struggle with their health. They live in stress, eat a high carbohydrate diet, use margarine and other foods with high levels of trans-fatty acids and cook oil causing it to become carcinogenic.

By applying the principle of AGGRESSIVE HEALTH, you'll eat a variety of sprouted foods, green leafy vegetables, raw plant fats, fibrous fruits and vegetables along with other superfoods. It's hard to feel stress when your body is operating so perfectly!

Take a look at the table again and get a sense of what you've just discovered. It's easy to see why many people engage in habits that result in the inactivity of the enzyme delta 6 desaturase.

VARIABLES THAT GOVERN THE ACTIVITY OF DELTA 6 DESATURASE

SPEEDS UP DELTA 6 DESATURASE	*SLOWS DOWN* DELTA 6 DESATURASE
1.Dietary Protein	1.High carbohydrate diet/sugar
	2.Trans fatty acids
	3.Alpha linoleic acid
	4.Stress
	5.Disease
	6.Ageing
	7.Zinc deficiency

At this point I suggest you take a break. You've learned a great deal already and it's worth re-reading the first part of this chapter or at least skimming over it to refresh your memory. Essentially, linoleic acid is supplied via raw plant fats and transported via LDL cholesterol into the eicosanoid production pathway. Linoleic acid needs to be converted into gamma linoleic acid (GLA) and the activity of the enzyme delta-6 desaturase determines how fast this conversion takes place. The activity is controlled by the factors in the previous table. The next stages of eicosanoid production are critical, so when you come back from your well-earned break, prepare for...

THE VITAL CONVERSION:
LINOLEIC ACID – TO – GAMMA LINOLEIC ACID (GLA)

So far we've done everything to maximise the activity of delta 6 desaturase. We've taken the abundant amounts of Linoleic acid and followed some simple guidelines to keep the gatekeeper 'delta 6 desaturase' active. Linoleic acid has now burst into the eicosanoid production pathway and is ready for action!

At this point delta 6 desaturase converts the linoleic acid into a more metabolically activated fatty acid known as gamma linoleic acid (GLA). What is so special about GLA? GLA is the result of the body's first biochemical step, transforming the essential fatty acids into eicosanoids. GLA is an activated essential fatty acid, and tiny amounts enter the metabolic pipelines allowing the body to make other activated essential fatty acids. Your body's metabolic pipeline must be filled with enough GLA to allow eicosanoid production to be efficient.

HEMP SEED, AFA ALGAE AND THE GLA CONNECTION

If delta 6 desaturase is inhibited, you can supply GLA directly to your cells by including hemp seed and its oil in your diet along with E3Live. This is a key factor why these two foods keep cropping up, over and over again in AGGRESSIVE HEALTH. Usually when eicosanoid production is compromised, illness and disease are given the chance to run rampant, but with the inclusion of GLA, the eicosanoid production pathway can continue to some degree.

SUCKLING ON THE BOSOM OF HEALTH:
THE MOTHER'S MILK CONNECTION

Since delta 6 desaturase doesn't reach full activity until six months after birth, how does a baby ensure their eicosanoid production runs smoothly? Answer: By drinking mother's milk! In fact figures published by the World Health Organisation show that mother's milk contains about 4.4% fat, of which an average of 8% is LA. It has little GLA but does contain the fatty acid that GLA converts to next – DGLA. Rather than get confused simply remember that whether you've just given birth or are planning a pregnancy, the quality of the milk you supply your offspring makes a tremendous difference to the quality of their health. Hempseed is a galactagogue (milk stimulator) and will nourish yourself and your baby via your milk. Remember a healthy baby is a happy baby! Note: If you are pregnant, wait until your baby is born before you begin the use of E3Live. If you don't take this advice, ensure you only use ¼ teaspoon daily.

So where are you now in your level of understanding?

♦ LDL cholesterol transports linoleic acid into cells.
♦ The gatekeeper enzyme, delta 6 desaturase allows linoleic acid to be converted to gamma linolenic acid (GLA) and AFA algae contains GLA helping the equation.
♦ The next stage in the pipeline is for GLA to be converted to another fatty acid dihomo gamma linolenic acid (DGLA). This is a rapid process if you have enough GLA in your system to begin with, so we'll move swiftly on!

Now you are at a critical cross-roads. Your decision about what to eat will determine whether you make 'good' eicosanoids or 'bad' eicosanoids.

STANDING AT THE CROSSROADS
WITH DELTA 5 DESATURASE

Having followed the process meticulously up until now, there are two potential routes that DGLA can take. One path will lead to the production of 'good' eicosanoids and the other path will lead to the production of 'bad' eicosanoids. The key factor that determines which metabolic pathway will be chosen is controlled by another enzyme. The enzyme is called delta 5 desaturase.

♦ If delta 5 desaturase is activated, DGLA will be converted into another activated essential fatty acid: arachidonic acid (AA), and then towards 'bad' eicosanoid formation.
♦ If delta 5 desaturase is inhibited, your body will produce more DGLA and form 'good' eicosanoids.

In the early stages you wanted to increase the activity of delta 6 desaturase. Now you want to minimise the activity of delta 5 desaturase. Confused? You ought to be!

Now, if you can inhibit delta 5 desaturase and promote the production of 'good' eicosanoids you can…

PREPARE FOR THE UNLIMITED
HEALTH BENEFITS OF PGE1

The series 1 prostaglandins made from DGLA are the most famous eicosanoids. Although they've all been studied in depth, the most famous one is prostaglandin E1, or PGE1. PGE1 has a myriad of important functions in your body. To begin with, it keeps blood platelets from sticking together, helping to prevent heart attacks and strokes caused by blood clots in the arteries. It assists the kidneys by helping to remove fluid from the body, acting as a diuretic. It opens up blood vessels, improves circulation and helps to relieve angina. It slows down cholesterol production. It prevents inflammation and controls arthritis. It makes insulin work more effectively, helping diabetics. It improves nerve function and will give you a consistent emotional high. It regulates calcium metabolism. It is involved in the functioning of the T-cells of the immune system, which destroy foreign cell invasions. It may also help to prevent cancer cell growth by regulating the rate of cell division.

THE CRITICAL INSULIN AND GLUCAGON LINK: INHIBITING DELTA 5 DESATURASE

If you want to ensure you get all the benefits from PGE1 and the other favourable eicosanoids, your goal: Inhibit delta 5 desaturase. How? Disengage any habits that allow the over production of insulin.

SAVE MONEY ON OVER-HYPED FISH OILS BY MASTERING THE SECRETS TO ENHANCE EPA PRODUCTION

You may or may not be aware that EPA and DHA are the two famous fatty acids that are found in the oil of certain fish. Some authorities claim that unless you take regular fish oil supplements you'll never get enough EPA or DHA. The debate will never end!

When you include the right raw materials from regular use of hemp seed and its oil, your body creates EPA. Hemp seed contains Stearidonic acid (an omega 3 fatty acid derivative) needed for stage one of EPA production. Production does rely to a large degree on the inclusion of certain co-factors such as vitamins B3, B6, C and minerals magnesium and zinc. Bee Pollen as you know is an exceptional food source of the B vitamins and vitamin C. Magnesium and zinc will be easy to come by with a high raw diet rich in wheatgrass, E3Live, Hemp seeds, sprouted foods and everything else discussed so far.

According to Udo Erasmus, author of 'Fats That Heal, Fats That Kill' with the regular inclusion of flax meal and hemp seeds/oil, your body can make the equivalent EPA and DHA found in two large fish oil capsules. My suggestion is to master the basics of AGGRESSIVE HEALTH and if you're still not satisfied begin your investigations into the use of EPA/DHA rich fish oil.

EPA directly inhibits the activity of delta 5 desaturase. Let's re-cap:

- ◆ Insulin activates delta 5 desaturase. It's up to you to control its production!
- ◆ Glucagon inhibits delta 5 desaturase. Ensure you eat quality protein sources to stimulate glucagon!
- ◆ The omega-3 essential fatty acid EPA also inhibits delta 5 desaturase. It can be found in E3Live.

Need I say more! The positive balance of DGLA to AA sets up whether or not 'good' or 'bad' eicosanoids predominate. By following the principles of AGGRESSIVE HEALTH you'll be maximising the dynamic balance of eicosanoids and ensuring a vital life.

WHERE THE FORK IN THE CROSS-ROADS TAKES YOU
AND WHY ARACHIDONIC ACID IS YOUR BIOLOGICAL NIGHTMARE

You were at the crossroads. One path took you towards more DGLA and good eicosanoids, such as PGE1. The other path took you towards arachidonic acid and bad eicosanoids. Let's discover more about the effects of arachidonic acid (AA). Just as AA is essential to life, it is also destructive in excessive amounts. It is so dangerous that when injected into laboratory animals, they die within minutes. Other fatty acids can be injected into the same laboratory animals with no ill effects. AA is the precursor of bad eicosanoids.

WHERE CAN YOU FIND ARACHIDONIC ACID?

AA is found in all meats, especially red meats and organ meats and in egg yolks. These foods get a hard time for their saturated fat and cholesterol content. But most of the problems actually stem from the AA content – especially to those individuals who are sensitive to it.

Too much AA (or a distinct sensitivity to it) can cause a variety of symptoms such as chronic fatigue, poor sleep, grogginess upon awakening, brittle hair and nails, constipation, minor rashes and dry, flaking skin. For athletes however, AA could prove to be a powerful anabolic factor necessary for gains in muscular size and strength and is one of the reasons that meat and eggs are considered the most anabolic foods. Some people who need purine-rich protein will eat AA rich foods and be fine. At this point, you have to make the decision. There will never be one perfect diet, but through knowledge and curiosity, you will discover how to dance between principles to create balance and harmony. Much of your success will come in figuring out your ideal fuel mix. Once you have, and you build it on a foundation of raw living foods, you'll success will be obvious. If you are on the road to recovery from disease or illness, you may need to focus more on omega-3 fatty acids – many of the testimonials for those who use flax, hemp and fish oil are from the sick, dis-eased or those suffering insulin resistance.

If you wish to maximise growth and engage in a lot of strength training or athletics, you may want to experiment with a higher omega-6 to omega-3 fatty acid ration as high as 5:1. Many athletes feel eggs and meat help produce the best gains in size and strength. If you are a vegan and you're looking for a role model for strength take a look at Mike Mahler www.mikemahler.com. He proves that a vegan diet can still be an excellent foundation for gains in size, if your body type is demands it. Mike Mahler takes protein very seriously – many vegans don't.

FINDING YOUR OWN MASTER FORMULA FOR AGGRESSIVE HEALTH

If you want to learn more about the importance of eicosanoid control, read 'The Zone' books by Dr Barry Sears. These are some of the finest nutritional books on the market, and will reinforce the principles of nutrition for hormonal control.

Barry Sears recommends a 40:30:30 ratio for carbohydrate, fat and protein respectively, I don't believe one size fits all. Many people instinctively know that their diet should be balanced, but it's finding the correct fuel mix that really makes the difference. Even for those who thrive on a higher carbohydrate diet, protein intake should never really drop below 25%. For those who thrive on a higher protein diet, protein content should really never exceed 40 – 50%. Then there comes protein selection. Which foods work best for you? Purine-rich proteins such as organ meats, anchovies, sardines, herring and caviar, or lighter protein sources such as chicken, eggs and cottage cheese? A raw foundation is critical and protein rich hemp seeds, flax seeds and sprouted foods are all a must. How you build on top of that will be down to you. Remember, most dieting 'success stories' are from those who've unknowingly found their correct fuel mix. But where there are success stories, there are millions of people who feel like they've failed because 'the new diet approach' didn't work for them. For more information on finding out which foods may work best for you, contact www.aggressivehealth.co.uk.

ARE YOU READY FOR THE CHALLENGE?

I want you to have a reason – why you eat – what you eat – when you eat it. With this knowledge you'll be able to anticipate and design the result you want, leading to mastery. Some people say it's too technical, but so is driving a car until you master it. People never question learning to drive because their life depends on it. I think your life depends more on your diet and health than your ability to move a metal box around a strip of tarmac. Some people say it takes the spontaneity out of eating, yet 90% of their meals are probably the same week in and week out, they just don't notice it because they don't pay attention to it.

I appreciate this was not the easiest of chapters to read and will take you time to master, so here is a re-cap.

♦ Eicosanoids control all of your body functions including your cardiovascular system, immune system, and how much fat you store!

♦ Most prescription drugs have a direct effect on eicosanoid production. The reason aspirin is so powerful and effective is because of its eicosanoid modulating capabilities.

♦ Heart attack victims are making more 'bad' eicosanoids (that promote platelet aggregation and vasoconstriction) and not enough 'good' ones (that prevent platelet aggregation and promote vasodilation).

♦ High blood pressure victims are making more 'bad' eicosanoids (vasoconstrictors) and not enough 'good' ones (vasodilators).

♦ Arthritis sufferers are making more bad eicosanoids (pro-inflammatory) and fewer 'good' ones (anti-inflammatory).

♦ Cancer victims are making more 'bad' eicosanoids (immune depressing) and too few 'good' ones (immune stimulating).

♦ Sufferers of Type II diabetes, are making more 'bad' eicosanoids (that stimulate insulin secretion) and fewer 'good' ones (that inhibit insulin secretion).

♦ Essential fatty acids are the basic raw materials needed to produce eicosanoids. Essential fatty acids can't be manufactured in the body, so therefore have to be present in the food that you eat.

♦ Linoleic acid is your starting point. It's an omega 6 essential fatty acid and found in virtually every food. With enough in your diet the part of cholesterol known as low-density lipoproteins (LDLs) will transport it to the eicosanoid production pipeline. An enzyme known as delta 6 desaturase determines whether or not linoleic acid enters the eicosanoid production pathway, acting like a gatekeeper. Speed up its activity and you are on your way to unassailable health. Slow it down and the problems begin. Protein is critical – the secret is in selection.

♦ Delta 6 desaturase also converts the linoleic acid into a more metabolically activated fatty acid known as gamma linolenic acid (GLA). To obtain this directly from food there are only a few sources - hemp and E3Live are both a good choice. Babies don't produce GLA until they are six months old.

♦ GLA then gets converted into another fatty acid known as Dihomo Gamma Linolenic acid (DGLA – a substance found in mothers' milk). This is a rapid process if you have enough GLA in your system.

♦ You are now at the crossroads: If delta 5 desaturase is activated, DGLA will be converted into another activated essential fatty acid: arachidonic acid (AA), and then towards bad eicosanoid formation.

♦ If delta 5 desaturase is inhibited, your body will produce more DGLA and form 'good' eicosanoids. Your goal: Inhibit this enzyme by controlling insulin and glucagon.

♦ The Omega-3 essential fatty acid EPA also inhibits delta 5 desaturase. So with enough raw materials from hemp seed and it's oil along with flax meal, you can expect your body to make enough EPA to do the job.

♦ The whole process can be enhanced with the inclusion of foods rich in vitamins B3, B6 and C and the minerals magnesium and zinc. Bee pollen is an exceptional superfood to add to your arsenal to keep the production pathway flowing.

♦ If you want to ensure your mineral intake is optimal remember this. The hemp plant reaches 10 feet below the earths surface drawing out vital minerals that can powerfully impact your health. Whether you need is for more phosphorus, potassium, sodium, magnesium, sulfur, calcium, iron, or zinc, the hemp seed delivers.

So there you have it. The distinctions in this chapter can catapult you to unprecedented success. YOUR health is in YOUR hands. Make your choices wisely and a life of freedom awaits you.

THE AGGRESSIVE HEALTH EVALUATION:
Are you eating a healthy supply of raw plant fats?
Are you doing all you can to keep delta 6 desaturase active?
Are you doing all you can to keep delta 5 desaturase inactive?

CHAPTER 9

TWO KILLER SUBSTANCES CAN WRECK YOUR HEALTH FOREVER CREATING ABNORMAL BLOOD PRESSURE, OBESITY, HIGH CHOLESTEROL, DIABETES, AND OUTRAGIOUS WEIGHT GAIN

Imagine a society free from obesity. Imagine if diabetes and blood sugar abnormalities no longer plagued millions of people. Imagine no-one suffering from elevated cholesterol levels. Imagine if high blood pressure was a problem of the past and the number 1 killer, heart disease, was eradicated for good! Do you think this is a crazy dream? It isn't when you realise that they are all symptoms of one problem: insulin excess. Each of these so-called health disorders are nothing but messages from your body telling you to STOP ENGAGING IN HABITS THAT OVER-STIMULATE INSULIN – STOP EATING REFINED SUGAR AND COOKED FAT. Each and every day, advertisers are attempting to influence you to eat more sugar rich foods, drink more alcohol and eat convenience foods loaded with cooked fat and transfatty acids! Moderation is one thing, addiction is another! If you don't use what you've learnt in this book to expand and extend the range of your own healthy habits, recreational foods will become the mainstay of your diet and insulin will rob you of your health. Be warned!

Due to the complexity of this chapter, I suggest you come back to it later to further your knowledge of how devastating insulin can be when over stimulated. If you're suffering from obesity, diabetes, high blood pressure, heart disease, high cholesterol or need ANOTHER reminder of how deadly refined sugar and cooked fat can be – read on. Otherwise move onto the next section. I believe section 3 is the most important part of AGGRESSIVE HEALTH and will open your mind to what is possible now that your brain and body are beginning to work at their very best. ENJOY.

THE DEADLY JOURNEY FROM INSULIN RESISTANCE TO TYPE II DIABETES

If you continue to eat a high sugar, high cooked fat diet and over-stimulate insulin you put yourself at risk of developing Type II diabetes. It's not something you develop overnight, it's more insidious than that. Rather than call it a disease, or even a symptom of hyperinsulinemia, think of it as a last ditch effort from your body to communicate to you that your current habits are destroying your health! It's up to you to...

HEAR THE MESSAGE AND RESPOND

A genetically susceptible person may spend their childhood consuming all kinds of insulin-inducing junk, (sweets, crisps, chocolate, fizzy drinks) and look fine on the outside! But as time goes by, the onslaught of sugar, saturated fat and toxicity is doing nothing but laying the foundation for a future of disastrous health! A child or teenager may appear to be riding 'high' on a diet of recreational foods, but with insulin occupying their bloodstream morning, noon and night, the foundation is set for future problems. As the insulin sensors in their tissues become overwhelmed by the constant influx of insulin, gradually they develop a mild form of insulin-resistance. Their sensitivity to insulin begins to weaken and their pancreas has to produce more and more to keep blood sugar levels under control.

Remember when your blood sugar level is normal, it falls into a range of between 60mg/dl to 120mg/dl (mg/dl = milligrams of glucose in 100 millilitres of blood). The higher your blood sugar level the more it can damage your brain. If it was to rise as high as 800mg/dl, you could end up in a coma and die. Need I say more? Insulin prevents blood sugar levels from rising too high, making it an important part of your hormonal balancing act, but as you know, this is only half the story.

OVER-TIRED AND STRESSED? ARE YOU FIGHTING THE BATTLE OF BLOOD-SUGAR ABNORMALITIES?

Have you ever wondered why overweight people are tired so much of the time? As more and more insulin is secreted in response to a high sugar diet, the insulin receptors on the surfaces of the cells become blocked from transferring glucose to the cells for energy use.

If this story sounds 'a little too close to home', pay attention. There is another factor to consider...

MEDICAL STUDENTS HIGHLIGHT THE DANGERS OF COOKED FAT

Back in the 1920s, Dr S. Sweeney conducted a 48hour study. He took his class of medical students (none of which showed any signs of diabetes) and fed them a diet very high in cooked vegetable oil. ONLY 48hours later and they all had signs of the disease. The reason…

COOKED FAT DAMAGES THE INSULIN RECEPTOR

Think of insulin as the key that fits the lock (receptor) on your cells that opens the door to allow glucose to enter. If you damage the lock, insulin has trouble opening the door. The result: glucose and other nutrients have difficulty entering cells. As the medical students found out, a diet excessive in cooked fat can damage the lock. Let's summarise:

As the lock becomes degraded – the key no longer works as well – the door remains shut – glucose is left occupying the bloodstream – your cells stop getting their required fuel – you begin to feel more tired – the extra sugar left in your bloodstream converts to triglycerides – and if not used for energy ends up being stored as fat.

The problem continues as tiredness creeps in. People find themselves reaching for that chocolate bar or fizzy drink for a much needed 'lift/beta-endorphin high', but end up stimulating even more insulin production. If you are highly sensitive to sugar your body will a massive quantity of insulin driving blood sugar levels through the floor. It's these consistent 'lows' that create the foundation for hazy thinking, poor memory, confusion, perpetual tiredness, restlessness and emotional turmoil.

Not only are obese people tired because their cells are not effectively taking in energy, but throughout the day, they are the victims of hypoglycaemia, the ironic consequence of consuming *too* much sugar! Ask yourself the question: What would my blood sugar level look like if I plotted it on a graph throughout the day? Would it be constant or would it fluctuate? Your energy and mood are good indicators. Remember, the first step to mastery is paying attention.

If you know of anyone with diabetes, turn them onto coconut oil. You don't need an excessive amount, but it does help regulate blood sugar, lessening the effects of the disease. The Nauru people consumed large amounts of coconut oil for generations without any signs of diabetes. But guess what? As soon as they adopted the addictive Western diet their good health disappeared almost overnight. According to Mary Enig, Ph.D., when monkeys were fed transfatty acids from margarine, the ability of their red blood cells to bind insulin began to malfunction. Coconut butter is different. It lessens the stress on the pancreas, doesn't require excessive output of enzymes or insulin for absorption and has been shown to improve insulin secretion and utilisation of blood glucose. Flax meal lowers the amount of insulin required by diabetics. This should come as no surprise since it has a rich fatty acid content along with fibre, vital nutrients and protein. Marvellous.

WARNING: INSULIN EXCESS CAN EXCITE
THE DEADLY STRESS HORMONE

Excess insulin also inhibits the release of glucagon. Glucagon's job is to restore blood sugar levels for optimal brain function. If glucagon secretion is inhibited, your body has to release cortisol from the adrenal glands in an effort to restore blood glucose levels. If this cycle continues the adrenal glands can burn out, your ability to deal with stress weakens and your ability to raise blood sugar levels declines, resulting in hypoglycaemia again! The picture isn't pretty is it!? Eliminate refined sugars!

AN UGLY SITUATION: REACHING BURNOUT

When severe insulin resistance takes hold of its victim, the pancreas is forced to release copious amounts of insulin in an effort to regulate blood sugar levels. If the situation worsens and the insulin sensors continue to malfunction, there comes a point when their pancreas is working at maximum capacity. This is the critical point. If nothing is done to improve the situation the insulin sensors continue to lose sensitivity and eventually the pancreas can't produce enough insulin to control blood sugar levels. Gradually the patient's blood sugar status reaches diabetic levels. At this point Type II diabetes is just around the corner. We'll get back to that shortly. For now...

A BRIEF INSIGHT INTO TYPE I DIABETES

Just to sidetrack for a moment. In type I diabetes, a virus or other toxic substance destroys the insulin-producing cells in the pancreas, and the victim requires treatment with insulin injections. It usually develops in childhood or adolescence. You can imagine what happens can't you? With no insulin being produced, glucagon causes fat to pour rapidly out of the fat cells and into the blood, putting a heavy burden on the liver. In contrast to other cells, liver mitochondria process fatty acids differently. They don't burn the fatty acids for energy, but instead partially break them down into molecules called ketone bodies, and release them into circulation. Ketone bodies are a good source of fuel for the brain and can also be burned for energy by muscle and other tissues, or eliminated via bladder, bowels or breath. Ketone bodies, however, are acids and if too many accumulate in the blood, the blood becomes more and more acidic, throwing the acid/alkaline balance into turmoil. If this continues untreated, the victim experiences the metabolic nightmare known as diabetic ketoacidosis, often leading to coma and death. With this kind of metabolic disaster it's easy to see why an undiagnosed victim can lose 30 or 40 pounds in a month or two, regardless of their increased food intake. They will often experience uncontrollable hunger.

The similarities that exist between Type I and Type II diabetes, include:

◆ Sugar spillage into the urine.
◆ Frequent urination.
◆ A great thirst.
◆ Increased blood glucose, which causes degenerative complications of the eyes, nerves, kidneys, and blood vessels.

THE LINK BETWEEN TYPE I AND TYPE II DIABETES

Back to Type II diabetes. When someone has spent a lifetime eating an abundance of insulin inducing foods (refined carbohydrates and convenience 'junk' food) their chronic blood-insulin levels eventually dampen the sensitivity of the insulin sensors. This continual cycle pushes the pancreas to its limit. It can no longer produce enough insulin to restore optimal blood glucose levels. Glucose at high blood concentrations is toxic to the brain and many other tissues, including the pancreatic beta cells that produce the insulin. After many years, if excessive glucose has over-stimulated the insulin producing beta cells, they can eventually burn out and ultimately stop producing insulin altogether.

THIS IS WHERE BIOCHEMICAL TURMOIL REALLY SETS IN

As long as the beta cells can produce insulin, the deadly ketoacidosis of Type I diabetes is avoided. But if enough beta cells fatigue and insulin production falls sufficiently, glucagon takes the reins and the balance shifts in the opposite direction causing the problems of Type I diabetes to prevail. In normal circumstances the beta cells continue to produce just enough insulin to keep ketoacidosis at bay.

Under the supervision of a physician, even those with Type I diabetes can significantly lower their insulin doses and attain much better control over their blood sugar levels by concentrating on raw, enzyme rich foods. They must also eliminate the 'nutritionally suicidal foods' that caused the blood sugar highs and lows in the first place. Many people have completely regenerated their pancreas with the use of raw food and over time eliminated the need for insulin!

AGGRESSIVE HEALTH HEALS
THE PERILS OF A COOKED DIET

Raw chlorophyll has been used to treat diabetes. It acts as a catalyst allowing for greater absorption of nutrients essential for metabolising sugar. Acidic blood can be a serious problem for sufferers of diabetes and is usually the result of a diet excessive in recreational foods. Chlorophyll has a strong alkalising effect, helping to combat this condition. With a weakened pancreas, if chlorophyll is derived from E3Live or wheatgrass juice, it will also contain blood sugar balancing nutrients like chromium, magnesium and zinc. Both E3Live and wheatgrass juice encourage cell renewal for the restoration of the weakened pancreas. The three nutrients chromium, magnesium and zinc also help to restore the sensitivity of insulin receptor sites that need to remain highly sensitive in order to assist in the regulation of insulin.

ENZYME RICH RAW FOODS CONTROL INSULIN
RESTORING OPTIMAL HEALTH

The great Albert Schweitzer was a severe diabetic and when he decided to get help from the raw food pioneer Max Gerson, he was incredibly ill and injecting mega doses of insulin. The first change Gerson made to Schwietzer's diet was to eliminate cooked protein. Excessive protein relies on enzymes produced by the pancreas for its breakdown. The pancreas also secretes insulin and glucagon. In this case it needed to be rested and given the chance to regenerate, so its functions could be restored. A poorly functioning pancreas plays a significant role in diabetes. To restore flagging enzyme levels and put even less strain on the pancreas Gerson put Schweitzer on a regime of fresh raw vegetables and lots of vegetable juices. Only ten days after this intervention, Gerson judged it safe to reduce his patient's insulin intake by half and only one month later Schwietzer needed no insulin at all. His diabetes never returned and he remained healthy and very active until his death in 1965 at the age of 92. Raw foods help clear the body of waste allowing hormonal communication to tighten and become efficient. They also help maintain stable blood sugar levels, minimising insulin excess.

USING JUICING TO YOUR ADVANTAGE

Juicing is a very powerful tool in your raw food arsenal. There are many juicers on the market. When buying one, choose one that is easy it is to clean! Complicated juicers may extract more nutrients, but if you can't be bothered to use it, it'll be a waste of space.

If you haven't heard of Jay Kordich, you need to buy his book immediately, entitled 'The Juiceman'. In the late 1940s, he conducted an experiment on 65 prisoners suffering from stomach ulcers. The majority of his treatment involved feeding them cabbage juice, which is saturated with the amino acid glutamine. Within only three weeks, 63 of his subjects were completely cured and the other two only had minimal symptoms. Cabbage has sometimes been called the king of the cruciferous family. It is alkalinising, cleansing, rejuvenating, contains substantial amounts of sulphur, iodine, iron, vitamins C and E. It also happens to be one of the cheapest vegetables. Always over-estimate the power of juicing! Back to the chase...

WHERE ELSE CAN HYPERINSULINEMIA CHIP AWAY AT HEALTH?
INSULIN INCREASES THE PRESSURE

Hypertension is the term used for high blood pressure, and once again, excess insulin is the cause. If you've ever suffered with high blood pressure, treat it as a message that your health is in need of repair. There are three ways that hyperinsulinemia causes hypertension.

1. Hyperinsulinemia causes fluid retention

Imagine the bloodstream as a superhighway that runs throughout the body delivering nutrients to cells, whilst simultaneously assisting in the elimination of waste. What most people fail to realise is that the blood also bathes cells with electrolytes allowing the critical functions of the cell to operate as effortlessly as possible. Sodium, potassium, chloride, bicarbonate, and other substances must be maintained within a strict zone to maintain optimal cellular function. But how is this done? In step the kidneys. They act like filters and ensure that waste products are removed and the concentration of electrolytes remains balanced.

THE INCREDIBLE BALANCING ACT

If too much sodium is present at any one time in the blood, the kidneys filter it out. It gets sent to the bladder to be removed via your urine. If there isn't enough sodium, your kidneys hold onto as much of it as they can, whilst removing enough fluid to encourage optimal blood sodium concentration.

The role of diuretics is to force the kidneys to eliminate more sodium than usual, which then causes excess fluid to be eliminated allowing blood concentrations of sodium to remain in a tight zone.

Insulin, however, forces the kidneys to retain sodium no matter what the circumstances, and since the sodium concentration must be kept in a tight zone, the kidneys retain excess fluid in order to dilute the excess sodium. The equation is simple: More insulin = more sodium retention = more fluid retention. With body fluids rising and blood volume increasing, it's easy to see how blood pressure increases, reaching dangerous levels. Diuretics are often used in these circumstances, causing the release of sodium and fluid as blood pressure is returned to normal levels. But this treatment just scratches the surface of an insulin disorder that runs very deep. The irony is that even though excess insulin causes fluid retention, diuretics actually stimulate insulin! Crazy isn't it? Save yourself from death by shooting yourself in the head!

2. Hyperinsulinemia alters the mechanics of the blood vessels

In excess, insulin has the power to make arteries less elastic. It also acts as a growth hormone on smooth muscle cells in the walls of the arteries, causing them to increase in thickness, become stiffer and less supple, while at the same time decreasing the volume within the arteries. Is it any wonder blood pressure rises as the heart begins to struggle, forcing blood through these narrow, more rigid arteries?

3. Hyperinsulinemia increases nervous stimulation of the arterial system

The third way insulin causes elevated blood pressure is by raising blood levels of the neurotransmitter norepinephrine. You'll learn a lot about this adrenaline-like substance in a later chapter. It is critical for the formation of memories and heightened states of awareness, yet too much can prevent the laying down of new memories, and can interfere with rational thought and decision making. Just as stress, excitement or intense fear can radically alter your physiological response, it's the adrenaline that causes your heart to beat faster and give you that shaky, uncomfortable feeling. By engaging in habits that over-stimulate insulin, norepinephrine is released into the blood, helping to keep blood pressure high and heart rate above normal. All these factors put unnecessary stress on the heart.

A COMMON TALE OF INSULIN EXCESS

A patient may gain weight and in the process develop high blood pressure. Their doctor may prescribe a mild diuretic and low salt to lower their blood pressure. A few weeks later the patient returns. Their blood pressure has improved but their cholesterol level is elevated (another by-product of insulin excess, as you'll learn shortly). The doctor decides to put the patient on a low fat-high carbohydrate diet, expecting a drop in weight and lowered cholesterol levels, but insulin levels remain high. One month later the patient returns, they're still overweight (due to excess insulin production) with similar cholesterol problems, but this time their triglycerides or blood sugar levels have increased. If the doctor had looked beyond the symptoms they'd have discovered insulin excess was the root of all the problems.

The actual medications used to regulate blood pressure (Beta-blockers) also stimulate insulin. Can you believe doctors prescribe such drugs to lower blood pressure that actually fuel the original cause? There isn't a medication on the market that lowers insulin, although many stimulate it. Your only chance is to take control of your diet. Let raw foods heal the misery caused by cooked foods and medications.

So there you have it. Insulin excess stimulates high blood pressure in three unique, yet complementary ways. It stimulates the kidneys, causing water retention. This increase in pressure exerts its force on the artery walls, which have been thickened and stripped of their elasticity – again due to insulin. And to top it all off, unbalanced levels of norepinephrine constricts the flow of blood and the pressure heightens. It isn't exactly the ideal way to run your biochemistry is it? With the right use of food, the problem of water retention and high blood pressure can be corrected within a few short weeks. Make sure you use them otherwise...

EXCESS INSULIN CAN PAVE THE WAY
FOR HEART DISEASE

Your heart is immortal if it is supplied with oxygen rich blood via the coronary arteries. If something occludes a coronary artery, compromising blood flow to the heart, such as the formation of plaque, blood can be reduced or cut off completely. The main culprits are cholesterol filled fibrous growths, which may develop on the inner linings of coronary arteries, over a long period of time.

THE DEADLY REALITY OF INSULIN EXCESS

In the early 1960s, Dr Anatolio Cruz and his research team demonstrated the danger of chronically elevated insulin levels. Each day for eight months, they injected insulin into one leg of a large group of dogs. As a control, they injected another leg with a sterile saline solution. The result: No change in the arteries injected with the saline solution, but in the arteries that had been exposed to excess insulin three main developments occurred:

1. The accumulation of cholesterol.
2. The accumulation of fatty acids.
3. Arterial thickening.

Each of these factors compromised blood flow, demonstrating the dangers of engaging in habits that continuously stimulate insulin. The amount of insulin administered to the dogs was relatively small! Can you imagine what happens to individuals who eat and drink in such a way that their bloodstream is never free from insulin? This experiment didn't even last for a year and most people are stimulating excessive amounts of insulin for a lifetime. Take a look at the history books if you haven't yet made the link between recreational food eating (high sugar consumption) and heart disease.

THE INCREASE OF SUGAR CONSUMPTION LEADS DIRECTLY TO HEART DISEASE

In 1865, human beings consumed about 40 pounds of refined sugar per year and death from cardiovascular disease was extremely rare. By 1900 sugar consumption had risen to 85 pounds per person per year and today it stands at over 120 pounds per person per year. The first heart attack case was not described until 1912. In 1930, heart attacks caused no more that three thousand deaths in the United States. Cardiovascular disease used to kill 1 in 7 people back in the early 1900s but now kills 1 in 2. Are you getting the point?

The occurrence of diabetes has risen at a similar rate, and today accounts for 1 death in 20. Obesity affects about 30% of adults in Western society today, and is highly correlated with cardiovascular disease, diabetes, allergies, cancer, and a host of other ailments. Excessive sugar consumption causes hyperinsulinemia and hyperinsulinemia kills.

HOMOCYSTEINE: VITAMIN DEFICIENCY AND HEART DISEASE

Homocysteine is produced in the body when the amino acid methionine is metabolised. Usually it is cleared rapidly from your blood before it can damage your arteries. Many heart disease studies point the finger at high levels of homocysteine for the cause of 10% of coronary deaths and a somewhat greater proportion of stroke deaths. This accounts for more than one hundred thousand deaths in the United States every year.

Elevated homocysteine is the result of vitamin deficiency, in particular sub-optimal blood levels of the B complex vitamins, especially folic acid, B6 and/or B12. You need these vitamins to make the enzymes that remove homocysteine efficiently from your body. You discovered in chapter 4 that a high fat diet eats away vitamin B6 levels and that bee pollen is a great source of this vital vitamin. Bee pollen and AFA algae found in E3Live are excellent sources of all the B vitamins, but remember if you don't eliminate refined sugar, you'll never eliminate the true cause of the problem. Sugar eats away at B vitamins. Eliminate it!

THE HORRIBLE TRUTH ABOUT INSULIN AND CHOLESTEROL

Imagine knowing more useful facts about cholesterol than the majority of the medical profession. Imagine never having to pop any pills or take any special formulas in order to stabilise your cholesterol within a perfect zone. If you are interested, you need to...

LEARN HOW TO OPERATE YOUR
CHOLESTEROL MANUFACTURING MACHINERY

If you are one of the unfortunate few who have been attempting to lower your cholesterol levels by restricting cholesterol in your diet, you're fighting a losing battle.

Think of how many products you've seen with the infamous words 'cholesterol free' or 'contains no cholesterol'. People don't even know what it is. If you think cholesterol is a fat then you are wrong! It's a pearly white waxy alcohol with a soapy feel. Maybe you've been lead to believe that cholesterol is a deadly killer and leads to heart disease and death. Again, you've been misinformed. As long as you control your cholesterol regulation system, it won't matter if you increase the amount of cholesterol in your diet or decrease it. Your body will adjust accordingly! Concentrating on cholesterol consumption alone could be your biggest downfall, since the cholesterol you eat only accounts for as little as 20% of the total cholesterol in your bloodstream. The other 80% is produced primarily in your liver. It is also produced in your intestines and skin. Each and every cell in your body can make cholesterol, so if you eliminate it from your diet, your liver will produce whatever else is needed to keep your system running smoothly. If you consume large quantities of cholesterol your cell production making machinery will ease up on production.

MANY DOCTORS ARE THROWING
A SPANNER IN THE WORKS!

Many doctors still prescribe a low fat, high carbohydrate diet for lowering dangerously high cholesterol levels, but all this does is stimulate more of the hormone insulin, causing the cells of your body to manufacture more cholesterol. That's the equation: More insulin – More cholesterol synthesis. You'll find out why shortly.

Cholesterol is critical to life, which is why you must learn what it is, where it comes from, how to reduce it (if it is dangerously high) and finally how to control it. You won't have to take any drugs and you certainly won't have to eat a low fat diet. Rather than concentrating on your intake, you'll learn how to control the complex cholesterol regulation system and keep it running smoothly. For now, take a look at the importance of cholesterol. You'll soon discover the endless advantages of keeping blood cholesterol levels optimal.

♦ Each and every cell in your body requires cholesterol to maintain the structural integrity of its cell membrane. This controls the flow of water and nutrients into the cell and regulates the disposal of waste.
♦ Your brain and central nervous system need cholesterol for normal growth and development and optimal electrical signal transmission. Cholesterol coats the nerves and makes the transmission of nerve impulses possible.
♦ Cholesterol is the building block for many important hormones. For example, the adrenal hormone aldosterone helps to regulate blood pressure, whilst hydrocortisone has a natural steroid type effect. Both are built from cholesterol. The sex hormones (oestrogen and testosterone) are also made from cholesterol.
♦ Your digestion relies heavily on bile acids, especially for the digestion of fats. Cholesterol is the main component of these acids and without it you wouldn't be able to absorb the critical fat-soluble vitamins A, D, E and K.
♦ Cholesterol gives skin its ability to shed water and is a precursor of vitamin D in the skin, essential for protection in the sun.
♦ Triglycerides allow fat to circulate through the blood and cholesterol plays a major role in this transportation process.

THE SECRET OF CHOLESTEROL CONTROL:
KEEPING CHOLESTEROL LEVELS IN A STRICT ZONE

Blood cholesterol levels may vary from one person to the next, but inside each and every one of your cells, cholesterol levels are always kept in a strict zone. The level of cholesterol within each cell is so important to your health that each one has its own feedback mechanism that informs the cell of the current cholesterol levels. Your bloodstream doesn't possess such a mechanism which explains why the majority of cholesterol problems are due to a build up of plaque within artery walls, rather than a lack of cholesterol at a cellular level.

RESTRICTIVE DIETS, CHOLESTEROL AND CANCER

Very restrictive diets may limit cholesterol intake but more importantly limit the essential nutrients needed for the production of cholesterol. If cells can't take cholesterol from the bloodstream, and the liver is unable to manufacture enough cholesterol, low cell-cholesterol levels cause cells to lose their strength and stability, putting them at risk of infection and malignancy. Rock bottom cholesterol levels can lead to the development of cancer or crippling arthritis.

If you get it right, you can indirectly control cholesterol within the blood and prevent the unnecessary build up of plaque within artery walls, as long as you supply all the necessary nutrients to allow cholesterol formation to continue effortlessly. Let's look in more detail at how you can do this…

REGULATING CHOLESTEROL LEVELS
AND MAINTAINING THE BALANCE

Each and every cell in your body requires a steady supply of cholesterol to sustain health. In order to meet the demands of your cells, cholesterol is supplied in two ways.

1. It's either extracted from the bloodstream, or
2. The cells make their own (or both).

The sensors on the inside of the cells detect the cholesterol level within the cell. If levels fall within the cell, the sensors fire off a series of chemical reactions that cause the cholesterol production line to crank out more cholesterol, or journey to the bloodstream to extract it from the blood. The aim: To restore balance within the cell. This explains why increased levels of cholesterol in the blood can clog the walls of the arteries that supply the heart, body and brain, whilst individual cells are unaffected. As far as individual cells are concerned, the bloodstream is there to supply cholesterol! The cells aren't directly concerned whether levels are too high within the blood. It's up to you to take responsibility for your diet if you want to keep blood cholesterol levels within a healthy zone. That's where we're headed!

CONTROL THE LOW-DENSITY LIPOPROTEINS (LDLs)

Even though cholesterol occupies your bloodstream, it isn't soluble in your blood. Question: How does it get transported around? Answer: By the lipoproteins. Lipoproteins act like envelopes, encasing cholesterol and triglycerides allowing them to be transported to the target cells.

There are many varieties of lipoproteins, but for the purpose of this section, concern yourself with only low-density lipoproteins (LDLs). They have been given a bad name since they are known to be the no. 1 villain responsible for developing coronary artery disease. If you can prevent the excessive build up of LDLs in the bloodstream you've got the secret to cholesterol control! Remember, some LDLs are needed to transport linoleic acid into your cells for eicosanoid production.

THE SECRET OF THE LDL RECEPTORS

If a cell is in need of cholesterol, it sends LDL receptors to the surface of the cell, where they lie in wait for cholesterol-filled LDL particles in the blood. When a cholesterol-filled LDL particle passes an LDL receptor, the receptor grabs it and pulls it into the cell. At this point cholesterol has been taken from the blood and transported into the cell where it is needed. Once the LDL receptor has released the LDL particle it heads back to the surface of the cell if more is needed. Blood cholesterol levels are lowered and forces within the cell extract the cholesterol from the LDL particle and utilise the cholesterol for various cellular functions.

If you've had problems with high LDL-blood levels in the past, an increase in these tiny scavengers (LDL receptors) will prevent the excessive build up of LDL cholesterol in your bloodstream, instantly bringing cholesterol into a safe and healthy zone.

THE POWER OF THE LDL RECEPTORS

Researchers discovered that people who develop heart disease in their teens or early twenties have a genetic disorder preventing their cells from making adequate LDL receptors. Thus LDL removal from the blood is incredibly limited causing levels to remain elevated. If LDL levels remain too high for too long, the chances of plaque formation and blockages in coronary arteries increase tremendously. The message: do whatever you can to ensure that your cells are teeming with the hardworking LDL receptors and you'll keep blood LDLs within the normal range reducing the risk of heart disease.

In fact even if your diet was high in saturated fat and cholesterol, as long as you crank out as many LDL receptors as possible, you could keep your blood cholesterol levels optimal.

MIRACLE MICE CRANK OUT FIVE TIMES MORE LDL RECEPTORS PREVENTING THE PERILS OF HEART DISEASE

Through careful research and experimentation, a group of scientists were able to breed a selection of mice that cranked out five times more LDL receptors in their livers than a control group of mice. The result: The super-mice were able to maintain blood cholesterol levels 50% lower than the mice in the control group.

Even if the researchers fed the mice diets high in saturated fat and cholesterol, the LDL values in the control group went through the roof, whilst the super-mice maintained normal LDL levels similar to the previous diet.

THE SECRET: INCREASE THE PRODUCTION OF THE LDL RECEPTORS AND WAVE GOOD-BYE TO CHOLESTEROL PROBLEMS ONCE AND FOR ALL!

The trick to increasing LDL receptor production is to limit cholesterol production inside the cells. That way it is inevitable that the cell would have no other option than to increase the number of LDL receptors and send them to the cell surface to scavenge cholesterol from the blood. It may come as no surprise that a drug exists to do just that. Its name is lovastatin (Mevacor) and it is an incredibly potent cholesterol-lowering drug. The reason it is so successful is because it slows down the activity of an enzyme known as 3-hydroxy-3-methylglutaryl-coenzyme A reductase (HMG-CoA reductase). Now there's a mouthful!

LIMIT HMG-CoA REDUCTASE AND YOU HAVE THE ANSWER TO YOUR CHOLESTEROL LOWERING PRAYERS

If you limit the production of this enzyme, you reduce cholesterol synthesis inside of each cell. Less cholesterol synthesis forces the cell to manufacture more LDL receptors, which scavenge LDLs from the blood and thus deliver cholesterol to the cells. As with many powerful drugs you can expect side effects! The term 'side-effect' is a term used by the medical profession to hide the truth. What they really mean is 'toxic-effects'. 'Side-effects' presuppose the primary effects are beneficial. All drugs, medicines, pills and potions are poisons. Rashes, muscular disorders, liver problems, gallbladder disorders and psychiatric disturbances are hardly just 'side effects'. They are poisonous toxic effects of a substance your body tries desperately to eliminate. So how do you limit the production of HMG-CoA reductase without drugs?

THE MASTER HORMONES OF ENERGY METABOLISM ARE BACK!

Two hormones determine the activity of the enzyme HMG-CoA reductase – insulin and glucagon. Insulin stimulates HMG-CoA reductase. Glucagon inhibits it. Insulin is the key to increased cellular cholesterol, basically killing any chances of maintaining healthy blood cholesterol levels.

Glucagon inhibits the activity of HMG-CoA and as a result is just as powerful as lovastatin. Increase glucagon and you decrease the cholesterol producing machinery inside the cells, forcing LDL receptors to rush to the cell surface in an effort to pull cholesterol from the blood, restoring the appropriate balance.

REDUCE INSULIN AND SILENCE CHOLESTEROL PRODUCTION

Insulin speeds up the workers within the cholesterol manufacturing pipeline, leading to a build up and surplus within each cell. At this point there is no need for the cell to retrieve any from the bloodstream and hey presto, as if like magic, cholesterol begins to build up in the blood. If you want potentially life threatening levels of cholesterol in your blood, increase your insulin levels.

Reduce insulin and immediately the signal that causes an increase in cholesterol synthesis is silenced and the cells begin to harvest the necessary cholesterol directly from the blood, causing blood levels to drop. Even if your diet was rich in red meats, egg yolk, cheese, butter and cream, as long as you keep insulin and glucagon balanced, you'll maintain healthy cholesterol levels, somewhere between 180 to 200mg/dl. Your LDL/HDL ratio will be under 3 and any extra fat will simply raise levels of HDLs (high-density lipoproteins). LDLs have a reputation for causing ill health because they are the main culprits in the development of coronary artery disease. HDLs have a reputation for being 'good' because they scavenge cholesterol from the tissues, including the lining of the coronary arteries, and transport it back to the cells of the liver where it is disposed of.

PARAMETERS OF CHOLESTEROL SUCCESS

Your risk of heart disease increases if LDL levels are above normal. But the real key to optimal cholesterol levels is keeping an eye on these parameters.

1. Total cholesterol divided by HDL should be below 4.
2. LDL divided by HDL should be below 3.
3. Total cholesterol should be kept between 180-200mg/dl range.

As blood cholesterol levels rise, so do your chances for heart disease. As blood cholesterol levels fall, cell cholesterol levels can drop to dangerous levels, increasing your chances of cerebral haemorrhage, gallbladder disease and cancer. Nutrient deficiencies can lead to sub-optimal manufacture of cholesterol, so eat a wide variety of life-enhancing raw plant foods and take control of the insulin/glucagon balancing act. Your health is at risk if you don't.

THE DEADLY POTENTIAL OF REFINED SUGAR

Sugar is the enemy! It over-stimulates insulin causing biochemical destruction whilst stripping your body of vital nutrients and destroying any chance of perfect health. Memorise the following 21 reasons why you should avoid it like the plague:

1. Refined sugar inhibits the release of linoleic acid from fat storage, causing essential fatty acid deficiency.
2. Refined sugar interferes with the function of essential fatty acids.
3. Refined sugar promotes bacterial invasion, as in rheumatism, inflammation of the heart and the more publicised tooth decay.
4. Refined sugar feeds bacteria, yeast, fungus, and cancer cells, causing fermentation in the alimentary canal.
5. Refined sugar prevents the body from absorbing calcium. It also pulls calcium, chromium and other minerals from the body.
6. Refined sugar interferes with vitamin C transport and therefore with immune function (The colds we get right after Christmas? They're from eating chocolate, sweets, and cake and from drinking too much alcohol, all of which are full of sugar!)
7. If refined sugar is consumed just before bedtime, it destroys the body's immune system's ability to build antibodies, which normally occurs an hour and a half into sleep.
8. Refined sugar may, during the filtering process, have carcinogenic impurities introduced into it.

9. Refined sugar plays havoc with blood sugar levels by raising them temporarily and then lowering them to dangerous levels if they cannot be stored.
10. Refined sugar prevents B complex vitamins and other nutrients from being absorbed.
11. Refined sugar causes red blood cells to lose their flexibility and become more rigid.
12. Refined sugar produces an acid that etches the protective tooth enamel and fosters gum disease.
13. Refined sugar interferes with insulin function causing the pancreas to produce excess amounts of insulin.
14. Refined sugar can increase adrenaline production by up to four times, making it a very powerful internal stressor. This stress reaction increases the production of both cholesterol and cortisone. Cortisone inhibits immune function.
15. Refined sugar is physically habit forming. It causes a shift in brain functioning by 'priming' beta-endorphin receptors in the brain. The short-lived beta-endorphin high leads to perpetual craving cycles. It has been theorised that the addiction to refined sugar, which begins in youth, is the basis of all addictive behaviour lasting throughout a lifetime.
16. Refined sugar cross-links proteins and speeds up ageing.
17. As little as six teaspoons of sugar a day can suppress the immune system by up to 25%, with the suppressing effect beginning almost immediately and lasting for up to five hours. How easy is it to eat six teaspoons? Very easy! One chocolate bar would be enough. A 12oz can of cola contains nine teaspoons. Eliminate sugar!
18. Refined sugar inhibits the production of the enzymes needed for detoxification weakening liver function. Strengthen these enzymes with the juice from cruciferous vegetables, such as kale. Kale is rich in sulforaphane that helps your liver convert toxins into non-toxic wastes that can easily be removed.
19. Rats live twice as long when sugar is cut from their diet. With the addition of chromium their lifespan increases by as much as 33%.

FREE YOURSELF FROM HYPERINSULINEMIA
FREE YOURSELF FROM AN EARLY GRAVE

Education gives you the knowledge to make decisions with confidence. Take what you've learned and do what most doctors fail to do – take control of the underlying problem of hyperinsulinemia and listen to the silence as the messages of detrimental health (obesity, diabetes, hypertension, problematical cholesterol and heart disease) begin to fade away.

THE AGGRESSIVE HEALTH EVALUATION:
Do you realise how detrimental excess insulin production can be to your health?
Have you consciously eliminated refined sugar and cooked fat?
Are you doing everything in your power to control insulin production with the foods you eat?

In order to stand out from the crowd and become a shining example of PHYSICAL MASTERY you need more than a gym membership! If you want to unleash a cascade of youth enhancing hormones on your body, whilst developing REAL WORLD functional strength, it's time you discovered the exercises that separate the elite from the average.

CHAPTER 10

SCULPT YOUR BODY WITH OLD SCHOOL – CUTTING EDGE SOLUTIONS AND UNLEASH POWERFUL YOUTH ENHANCING HORMONES

Just stop for a moment and look at the front cover. What you'll see is the 21st Century Vitruvian Man in all his glory. One hand clasps a Clubbell®. Another crush-grips a kettlebell, whist two others squeeze the life out of a set of gymnastics rings

A STRANGE COMBINATION OF CONDITIONING TOOLS?

Certainly not. And as this chapter unfolds, you'll discover that you've arrived at a crossroads. You can either continue to walk the path you've been walking, maybe pushing a few weights, throwing a few dumbbells around or remain hypnotised to brain numbing T.V. whilst your body downgrades into an old, frail, weak, flabby version of a former you. Or... you can take a new direction – a direction that invites rapid whole body evolution, a direction that will maintain joint integrity as well as strength, a direction that will lead you to a place where your great grandchildren will look at you with awe and respect.

Many people arrive at the gym and push themselves to the limit with the 'NO PAIN – NO GAIN' mentality engraved into their consciousness. They spend 60 – 90 minutes grunting, sweating and moaning in an effort to reach a personal best. The reality – many are taking one step closer to 'burn-out'.

A few pages from now, this 'die-hard' mentality will be a small, distant memory as you embrace a colourful, bright, inspiring future that teeters on the precipice of peak performance. Let me hack away the garbage that most fitness instructors teach, and target your attention on the key principles that'll catapult your results into the stratosphere. Let's get to it.

REASONS COME FIRST, ROUTINES COME SECOND

Before I introduce you to the 'tools of the AGGRESSIVE HEALTH trade' let's discover why they are going to be your allies in the quest to master your body and master your health.

FOUNTAIN OF YOUTH BREAKTHROUGH

In a moment you are going to read about an amazing anti-aging substance that could help you turn back the hands of time and regain your youth. I'll call it substance X for now, but will shortly reveal its true identity.

In 1990, The New England Journal of Medicine produced a very interesting report. Daniel Rudman, M. D., and his research group at the Medical College of Wisconsin produced some amazing results when they injected substance X in a group of elderly males between the ages of 61 and 81. Dr. Rudman's group showed that tiny amounts of substance X injected just beneath the skin produced almost unbelievable results in less than six months. They reported that:

√   Lean body mass increased by 8.8%.
√   Body fat decreased by 14.4%.
√   Bone density increased in the lumbar spinal bones.
√   Skin thickness increased by 7.1% (thin, brittle skin is one of the consequences of ageing).

Every result was directly influenced by the injections of substance X alone – no dietary or exercise regimes were suggested. In Dr Rudmens words, "The changes were equivalent in magnitude to the changes incurred during 10 to 20 years of reverse ageing."

The impact caused a wave of clinics to start showing up in Mexico and other less medically regulated countries to administer substance X.

HAVE I GOT YOUR ATTENTION?

Do you want to know what substance X is? Of course you do! But first, let me give you another example of how powerful it really is. Then I'll share with you the secret to jacking up production in your body naturally.

A study performed at the University of New Mexico, demonstrated that in a six week period, weight lifters injected with substance X lost four times more body fat, and gained four times more lean body mass, compared to those who received only a placebo.

WARNING: Injections of substance X are a difficult and dangerous way to trim fat and build muscle, and are only used to treat unusually small children under medical supervision. Any other use is illegal; the side effects can be very destructive. People who do inject substance X increase their body's chances of shutting down its own natural release, increasing the chances of diabetes!

So there you have it. One side of the equation is appealing, the other side – life threatening.

YOU'VE WAITED LONG ENOUGH - LET'S RAISE THE CURTAIN AND REVEAL SUBSTANCE X'S TRUE IDENTITY

Substance X – the fountain of youth – is human growth hormone (HGH). It is a profound tissue building (anabolic) hormone produced in the pituitary gland (a small gland located at the base of the skull) and is secreted at intervals throughout the day. HGH stimulates tissue growth, increases muscle tone and lean mass, enhances flexibility, thickens muscles, stimulates the growth of bones and organs, mobilizes fat stores, shifts the metabolism to the preferential use of fat, and helps maintain healthy tissues. But the all important question remains…

HOW DO YOU STIMULATE IT NATURALLY?

Forget injections to increase HGH levels, there exists a much safer, natural way to regenerate your youth with HGH. Take a look at the body of a world class sprinter, a conditioned gymnast or a world class fighter. Their lean, toned bodies highlight the remarkable effect of HGH. They have embraced strength training as part of their routine to gain the edge in their chosen profession, and so can you. It won't be long before you are looking back on the 'old days' remembering what 'being flabby' used to be like. It won't be long before you see a toned, well sculpted body, knowing that on the inside, where it counts, you've unleashed a cascade of youth enhancing hormones. How do you begin? Patience my friend – we'll get to the drills shortly.

MAXIMISINGE THE RELEASE OF GROWTH HORMONE?

When you were a teenager, you released a lot of growth hormone naturally. You could even fill your face with 'junk food' without affecting growth hormone production. But life is a little different now. Blood samples show that the older you are the less growth hormone you produce. HGH is released into your blood stream at two specific times.

1. About 90 minutes after you go to sleep, and
2. Once before you wake up in the morning.

High levels of HGH naturally drop over time. By age sixty, about 30 % of men produce little or none of the substance. It is assumed that women continue to secrete growth hormone into their old age, and thus live longer.

LET THIS PATTERN COME TO A GRINDING HALT

The reason you may not produce as much as you used to, isn't because you can't, but because you are more sensitive to the factors that prevent its release. Everyone has the potential to release more HGH into the bloodstream, but is everyone creating this environment? Absolutely not. Guess what controls the release of human growth hormone from the pituitary gland? The super hormones you learned about in chapter 8 - good eicosanoids. Here's a comprehensive list of the factors that stimulate the release of growth hormone:

√ Decreased blood glucose levels - easy if you limit high carbohydrate 'junk' and focus on mineral rich vegetables and sprouts.

√ Foods rich in the amino acid arginine – easy if you increase your consumption of activated nuts and seeds which are all rich in arginine, along with other high protein foods.

√ Carbohydrate restricted diet - Easy when you understand the previous chapters of AGGRESSIVE HEALTH

√ Fasting – As insulin levels drop and glucagons levels rise, HGH begins to peak. People have successfully completed mini fasts themselves without any harm. Longer fasts should always be under the supervision of a healthcare professional.

√ Optimal pH – HGH is deactivated in an unbalanced acidic environment. If your body is under functioning, you may wish to book an appointment with me for a biological terrain analysis to ensure you bring the 'numbers of health' back into alignment. More about this later.

√ Increased protein diet - easy if you are taking protein seriously. Once you've figured out your ideal fuel mix you'll know what is best for you - hemp, flax, sprouted beans, eggs, fish, meat etc.

√ Free fatty acid decrease – easy if you select your fats wisely.

√ PGE1 (a good eicosanoid) – easy if you apply the hormonal distinctions in chapter 8.

√ Stage 4 sleep - Growth hormone is secreted in a pulsatile surge during stages 3 and 4 of sleep, just prior to REM (Rapid Eye Movement – the first hour or two after reaching deep sleep.) The better your quality of sleep, the more growth hormone you'll release.

√ Mind Technology – see chapter 12.

√ Anaerobic Exercise – Finally, the nuts and bolts of this chapter.

YOU ARE ALWAYS YOUNG ENOUGH
TO START LIFTING WEIGHTS

When it comes to anaerobic exercise, there are no excuses. Laboratory tests in Miami, Florida have produced exciting results. People in their sixties who've spent at least ten to fifteen years with minimal muscle tone are learning to lift weights and create muscle mass equivalent to that of twenty-one-year-olds, with energy levels to match. Yes! You can be as strong in your seventies and eighties as you were in your twenties and thirties! Strength training also stimulates the release of the hormone testosterone – growth hormone's comrade in arms. It is a vital hormone for muscular development, health and sexual potency. It is an aphrodisiac, increasing libido in both males and females. Don't leave home without it!

STRESS INTERFERES WITH TESTOSTERONE PRODUCTION:
THE PERILS OF OVER TRAINING

Most of the negative effects of over-training can be attributed to excess cortisol production, increased Interleukin-6 production and a decrease in DHEA. Professor Patrick Bouic, co-author of 'The Immune System Cure' and other researchers have discovered that the function of the T-cells (the generals of our immune army) and natural killer cells (our cancer fighting cells) is suppressed by over-training. In addition, testosterone levels begin to drop as more precursors (building blocks) of testosterone are diverted to facilitate increased cortisol production in response to exercise-related stress. Testosterone is anabolic, building strength and health. Cortisol is catabolic and breaks down tissue, running you down. The more you reduce excess cortisol, the greater your chance of unleashing the anabolic benefits of testosterone.

MIND TECHNOLOGY IS YOUR WEAPON
AGAINST THE RAVAGES OF STRESS

Relaxation and rest are both critical in triggering large quantities of both HGH and testosterone. Professional body builders such as Frank Zane use mind machines immediately after a workout to promote the release of these powerful youth enhancing hormones. See chapter 12 – The Electrifying Power Of Mind Technology to learn more about these amazing peak performance/relaxation tools.

Together, HGH and testosterone join forces and create a powerful fat-burning environment in your body. Fat burning and energy production takes place in the mitochondria of muscle cells. As you sculpt your body with strength training, you increase the number of these little energy factories and simultaneously increase your fat-burning potential. Awesome.

GRAB HOLD OF SOME IRON
AND BOOST MITOCHONDRIAL DENSITY

With all the talk of 'diet' to boost energy levels, how many health care professionals are motivating you to pick up some iron and boost your mitochondrial density? Dr William Wong, who specializes in helping people with fibromyalgia and Chronic Fatigue talks about how his patients can often find themselves in a downward spiral. As fibrosis increases and a lack of activity through tiredness causes muscular wastage, mitochondrial density decreases. As mitochondrial density decreases so does the potential to generate energy. In this situation motivation to exercise diminishes and the person feels trapped.

PLAN YOUR ESCAPE NOW!

Through systemic enzyme therapy and the use of ribose – which naturally boosts ATP (assisting the natural role of the mitochondria), a person can escape this trap and begin to strength train. In the process of strength training, their mitochondrial density increases as does the production of youth enhancing hormones. Escaping the trap sounds simple – but takes time and patience. Remember, if your muscles are wasting and your mitochondrial density is in decline, you may get worse as life passes you by. The key is in breaking the cycle. Start with systemic enzymes such as Vitälzym along with ribose and if you eat well from the principles of AGGRESSIVE HEALTH you may find yourself strong enough to begin strength training. Good luck.

A long-term study of 17300 Harvard alumni, published in the New England Journal of Medicine, concluded that intense exercise could add years to your life and life to your years. It showed that people who participated in intense exercise lived the longest.

PULL OUT THE TOOLS OF YOUR 'AGGRESSIVE HEALTH' TRADE AND LET THE GAMES BEGIN

OK. Enough theory – Let's get down to business. When it comes to developing strength there are three areas you need to be concerned with, and one very important pre-requisite - Joint Mobility. You can get all excited about HGH, testosterone and the cascade of youth enhancing hormones that your body releases in response to effective strength training. But unless you recover the mobility of your joints, you may suffer at the mercy of the weight you are wielding. If you want to be the best, you need to consult with the best. Get hold of Warrior Wellness™ today from www.aggressivehealth.co.uk and begin your quest to a better life. Coach Scott Sonnon, via his joint mobility program Warrior Wellness™ will show you how to recover, co-ordinate and refine movement through 6 degrees of freedom. Simply put, you'll develop the most powerful platform possible before loading your joints with clubbells®, kettlebells and other bodyweight conditioning exercises. Enough. When it comes to strength we're going to concern ourselves with three key areas.

1. **Circular Strength Training™ with Clubbells®.** CST™ as it is referred to will develop strength through 360°. You can't build 360° strength any other way. Thanks to Scott Sonnon, US National Coach, Master of Sports and creator of the Clubbell®, you can take your physical evolution to a level that most people dream about. More about this shortly. Initially, many people think CST™ is just about swinging clubbells®. That's like saying a car is just about the wheels! CST™ is a doorway to a complete physical culture that has to be experienced to be believed. Grasp the handle, turn it, and open the door if you think you're ready to enter the world of advanced mental and physical conditioning. For more information go to www.clubbellwarrior.com.

2. **Linear/Ballistic Strength Training with kettlebells.** Kettlebells are superior to free weights. Their offset centre of gravity will force your body to work harder than ever before maximizing shoulder strength and stability through a healthy range of motion. Popularized in the UK by award winning coach Lee Hadden, and Pavel Tsatsouline, ballistic kettlebell exercises and other more familiar presses and pulls will be an essential ingredient in your 'AGGRESSIVE HEALTH' strength training cocktail. For more information goto www.worldclasskettlebells.com

3. **Bodyweight conditioning.** Being able to use your own strength and structure to move more fluidly through the world is a unique benefit most people never acquire. Ring Training will bring this back creating the unrivalled upper body strength of a champion gymnast. Lower body drills such 1 legged squates (pistols) for strength will give you superior development and more functional strength than you may ever need. Beyond strength and joint mobility is the ability to move through the world gracefully, with zero stress and maximum flow. Body-Flow™, an all important dimension of CST™ addresses this facet of body evolution and will be discussed in chapter 13.

These three key areas all involve old fashioned, compound joint, strength work. We're not interested in isolating the triceps, or targeting just the deltoids. We want complete, usable strength we can transfer to the real world of activity and sport.

Most people lose 10% of muscle mass EVERY year between the ages of 50 and 60. In the process, everything in life becomes a struggle – getting up from the toilet, lifting a heavy pan or suitcase. Life should get easier as you age. Strength training is the answer.

It's impossible to cover all the training secrets of CST™, Kettlebells and bodyweight/ring training in this book alone. For now let me give you a taster of what you can accomplish as you embrace these powerful tools. This chapter is designed to open your mind to what is possible. For more information on how to train with these tools, contact www.aggressivehealth.co.uk

Circular Strength Training™ with Clubbells® - THE MILL

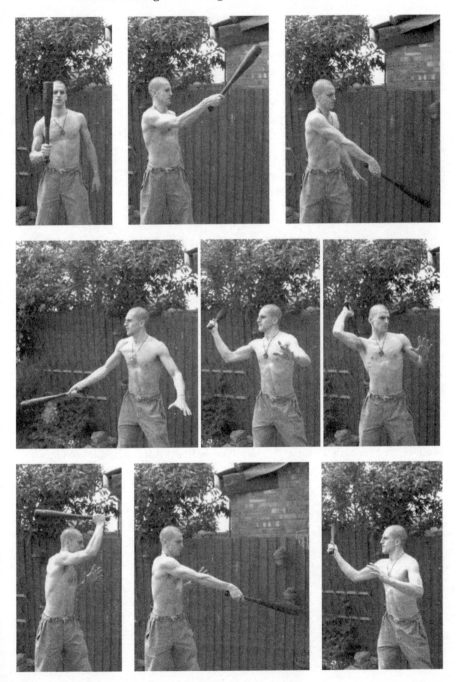

Circular Strength Training™ with Clubbells® - THE SWIPE

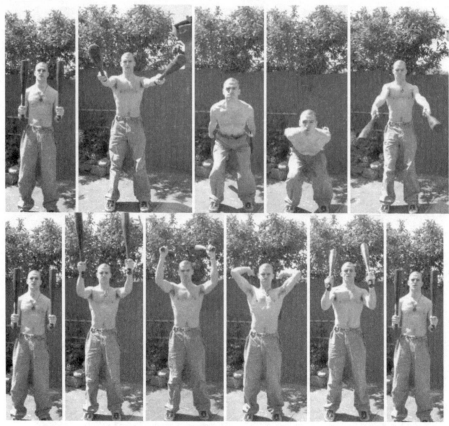

Circular Strength Training™ with Clubbells® - THE ARMSWING

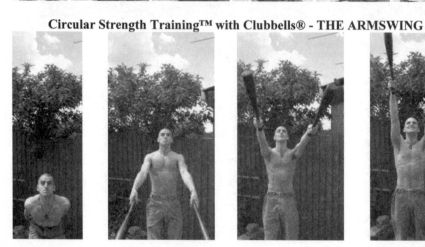

Kettlebell Training – THE TWO HANDED SWING

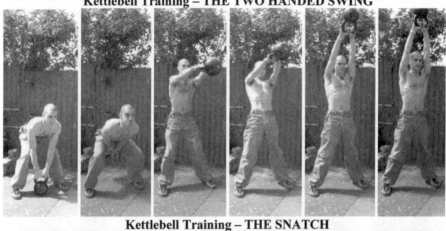

Kettlebell Training – THE SNATCH

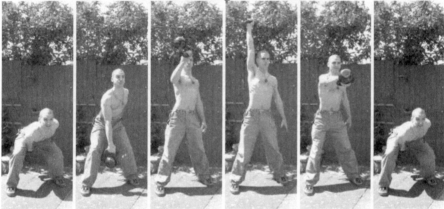

Kettlebell Training – THE WINDMILL

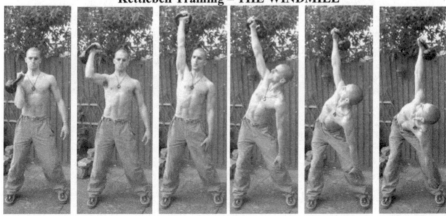

For comprehensive training instruction by the founder of the legendary clubbell® - Scott Sonnon, visit www.aggressivehealth.co.uk and seek out Clubbell® Training For Circular Strength (book and DVD). For the ultimate workout with kettlebells, order Kettlebell Training – Strength And Conditioning – Volume 1 by awarding winning coach Lee Hadden. Other resources are available at www.aggressivehealth.co.uk.

Ring Training – THE MUSCLE UP

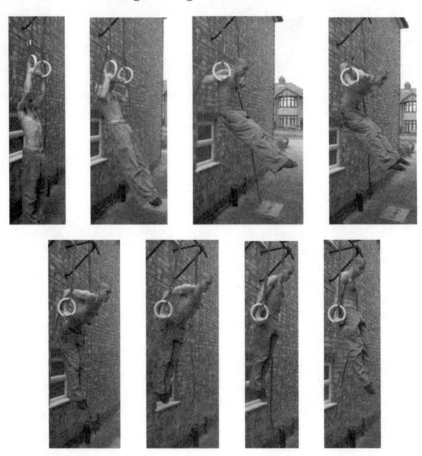

Begin with pull ups and dips before you attempt the muscle up. Both exercises are safer and more gruelling on the rings because of the lack of stability. Those who take up gymnastics will do more on the rings, such as swings, rolls, levers etc. Gymnastics rings and the Jayebe fitness bar (featured in the above picture) can both be purchased from www.aggressivehealth.co.uk. Note: The Jayebe fitness bar allows you to hang a punch bag from it.

Ring Training – THE HANDSTAND PUSH UP

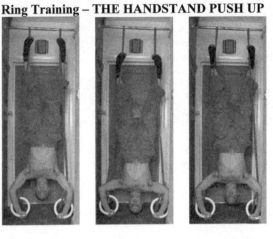

There a many more exercises to perform with clubbells®, kettlebells and on the rings. The DVD ring strength, featuring Jordan Jovtchev, 2003 gold medallist will take your ring training workouts to a different level.

The great thing about these rings is their portability. Simply find a beam, throw them up there and you're ready for one of the most gruelling strength workouts you'll ever have. And don't think that the legs get off lightly. 1 legged squats, talked about in length in Pavel Tsatsoulines 'The Naked Warrior', will take you leg conditioning to a whole new level.

Bodyweight Drills – The PISTOL (ONE LEGGED SQUAT)

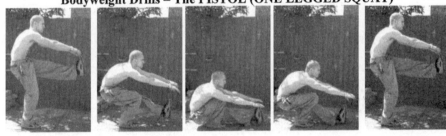

Just stop for a moment. Imagine being able to knock off 5 muscle ups in a row! Imagine being able to pick up 40kg of kettlebell iron and do 10 'rock-bottom' pistols. Imagine having the superior muscular and joint strength to be able to weild 25lb clubbells® around your head. Now picture yourself performing 24 snatches with 24kg of kettlebell iron – a necessary requirement for kettlebell certification. If you thought strength training was all about building those biceps with endless curls, now is the time to rethink your routine. All of these drills are to do with strength. What would you prefer to be able to do – crush grip a set of gymnastics rings and perform an inverted iron cross (an unbelievable demonstration of strength, power and skill) – or stand on stage, in a posers pouch with balls the size peanuts, dripping with oil as you flex your monster biceps? Select you role models wisely. This chapter is about functional strength, NOT bodybuilding. This chapter is about tapping into your central nervous system and muscle software, NOT getting bigger and heavier through bodybuilding and steroid abuse.

Note: If you love bodybuilding and it is your passion, do it! Your progress will accelerate once clubbells®, kettlebells and ring training weave their way into your routine.

Ok. You're ready to train for strength, but how do you begin? What approach do you take? Do you train to failure, and thus fail, or do you approach your training with a different goal?

ELECTRIFYING STRENGTH THROUGH CNS STIMULTION

As an avid golfer, I know that if a storm is brewing, it's time to get off the course. If I stayed out and risked being electrocuted by lightening, I would expect the surge of electricity to cause my tendons to rip off of their attachments, my bones to break, leaving me in a mangled heap on the fairway, tee or green. Why? When muscles are fully activated by electricity their contractile potential reaches levels you cannot imagine.

Although it's impossible to rev up your central nervous system to the point where you'd be able to pull your body to pieces, it is possible to consciously increase the electrical charge sent to your muscles and increase your strength immediately. Within a few short sessions, you can train your central nervous system to contract your muscles harder than ever before. The formula is simple. The more 'nerve force' you can send to a muscle, the harder it will contract. The harder it contracts, the more tension you generate. The more tension you can generate the stronger you become and the more you can lift.

THE BODYBUILDER – V – THE GYMNAST

Side by side, a professional bodybuilder would dwarf a professional gymnast. But looks can be deceiving. Larger biceps, huge flaring lats and a chest many women would be proud of, still doesn't compare to the jaw dropping strength that a gymnast demonstrates when tackling the rings, parallel bars or pommel horse. Even many power-lifters are able to maintain a low body weight and size, but demonstrate amazing feats of strength and power with jaw dropping poundage's.

GYMNASTS AND POWERLIFTER ARE MASTERS OF THEIR CENTRAL NERVOUS SYSTEM

Right now, with no training of your nervous system, you may only be able to contract 20-30% of any one muscle. An elite powerlifter or gymnast may develop the neurological efficiency to tap into as much as 50%. All you need to do is learn how to generate more tension.

THE TENSION/RELAXATION CONTINUUM

For the purposes of rest, recovery and total body relaxation – you need to learn how to release tension and let go. For the purposes of developing strength, you need to learn how to direct more 'nerve force' to muscles through high tension generation.

The secret is in understanding the law of irradiation, best summarized by Pavel Tsatsouline in his books, 'The Naked Warrior' and 'Power to the People' (both available at www.aggressivehealth.co.uk). The law states that as you increase the load on a muscle, it will recruit surrounding muscles to amplify total strength. Pavel uses the word 'cheering' to describe what happens as neighboring muscle groups begin to assist in the development of tension. With this knowledge, you can power out of the blocks before the sound of the gun. What do I mean by this? By stimulating neighbouring muscles to 'begin cheering' before you lift, you give yourself a head start. Arm wrestlers use this technique to maximum effect. They begin tensing their entire body before they even sit down and clasp hands! Before performing a muscle up, I'll crush grip the rings and allow this tension to spread down my forearms, shoulders, chest and back, torso, glutes, legs and toes before beginning the movement. Try it. The results will astound you.

RING TRAINING WILL TEACH YOU THIS
WITHOUT YOU EVEN KNOWING IT

It only takes a few weeks of training on the gymnastics rings to realize what happens if you don't stay tight and under high tension. The moment you slacken off, you fall to the ground in a heap. It doesn't matter how you learn the lesson, just make sure you learn it.

Let's recap. If you want to develop awesome strength, you must select exercises that impose high levels of tension on the muscles involved. If doing 1000s of press ups turns you on – fine. But strength comes from tension. Tension is stimulated with load. Heavy load can be defined as something you can only move a few times, no more than 5 or 6. For example, if you can nail 10 chin ups; you might want to hang a kettlebell around your waist. You'll do fewer reps, but your strength will increase dramatically. The increased load leads to increased tension (which you can control by activating neighboring muscle groups), which leads to increased strength. The options are endless.

OVERTRAINING – V – STAYING FRESH

Have you ever been told that in order to develop your body you have to push to failure in every set? Well, take a deep breath, pay attention and prepare for a revelation that could cause you to get results so fast, your peers may suspect you've been taking a wonder drug.

DO LESS – SO YOU CAN DO MORE

If you remember one idea from this chapter, remember this. Strength is a skill. It's your goal to master this skill and like any skill, the more you practice – the faster the results. "But how can you practice often, and not burn out?" I hear you cry. The answer is simple. By doing sub-maximal sets and training your central nervous system to generate more tension.

For example, if you can do a maximum of 10 chin-ups, try doing just 3-5reps every 1 or 2 hours during the course of a day. Do this for a few weeks, have a few days rest and then test for a personal best. The increased volume of work may seem like it's going to tire you, but by doing sub-maximal sets you embrace two very powerful principles of strength development

1. You stay fresh, because you never reach failure.
2. You train your nervous system to contract harder because of the frequency of your practice.

Have you ever noticed that a hod carrier or brick layer is strong and defined? They're not lifting to failure when they pick up heavy load, but during the day they are lifting – a few bricks here, a few bricks there. It all adds up. When you read 'The Naked Warrior' and 'Power To The People' by Pavel Tsatsouline, you'll read about the principle 'Greasing The Groove: How to get superstrong without a routine'. The essence of this methodology is to do as much work as possible whilst being as fresh as possible. Never train to failure unless you are chasing a personal best. Training is different to practice. When you practice you want to limit the number of exercises so you can stay focused.

STRENGTH PRACTICE CODE OF CONDUCT:

1. I only select one or two strength exercises to focus on.
2. I practice my strength exercises regularly to train my nervous system.
3. I never train to failure unless going for a personal best.
4. I pay attention to technique, smooth movement and high tension.
5. I have long rests between sets in order to stay fresh.
6. I know when I'm practicing correctly because I feel energized not drained.

ELIMINATE BOREDOM WITH
HIGH LOAD/LOW REP/LONG REST TRAINING

The formula is simple for high tension strength development. You design your sessions around exercises you can only perform between 1 and 5 times. You move slowly under high tension and you employ long rest periods between sets. If the rest period is between 3-5 minutes you'll get a lot of work done in a short period of time. If the rest period is 1-2 hours (yes I did say hours!) you'll get your practice done over the course of a day.

For example when I first started doing muscle ups it was tough. I could do pull ups and I could do dips, but combining the two was a challenge. Once I learned the skill I began employing the techniques of maximal tension and practicing 1 rep every hour or so throughout the day, it wasn't long before I sharpened my technique, creating awesome strength.

THE MAGIC OF 1 REP

Exercises like muscle-ups, pistols, 1 arm/1 legged push-ups are all body weight drills that demand maximum tension and focus. If you can't do them, focus on doing whatever it takes to master 1 rep.

For example, when I started doing handstand push-ups I couldn't even hold a handstand for longer than a few seconds. Through hourly practice, it only took a few days before I could hold a handstand for a couple of minutes. I then moved onto lowering my self just 1 inch, then 2 inches, then 3 until I could do 1 full handstand push-up. As time trickled by I kept practicing and making sure I didn't over do it.
After a few weeks I was in a hotel room in Chicago and it dawned on me that I had been neglecting my routine. Eager to know if I'd lost my touch, I got into position against the wall. To my surprise I nailed 12 'head to floor' handstand push ups with ease. The rest period that I hadn't scheduled gave me the preparation time to attempt a personal best. This example shows how I'd trained my nerves to become superconductors.

STRENGTH TRAINING IS FOR EVERYONE

Everett Smith, director of biogerontology laboratories at the University of Wisconsin, reported in 1993 that a group of middle-aged women, who did nothing more than hoist 5-pound weights, once a week for over four years, slowed the loss of bone mass in their arms by a staggering 50%. Can you imagine what the results would have been if they'd been trained in the art of handstand push ups?

A loss of bone mass is one of the leading causes of fractures in the elderly, particularly in women after the onset of the menopause. In worst cases, bones are so weak that the act of stepping off a high curb can lead to fracture. Every year, 1000s of elderly people die from the complications following hip fractures. 5lb weights may be a good start, but by embracing Circular Strength Training™, kettlebell swinging, and bodyweight conditioning, worries of osteoporosis will be banished forever.

EXPECT TO REACH PLATEAUS

Initially you'll be training to avoid osteoporosis and muscle wastage, but a few weeks into your routine and you'll have more inspiring objectives. Treat your strength training as an adventure. Where you have weaknesses you can now create strengths. Fall in love with the 'tools of the AGGRESSIVE HEALTH trade' and learn how to master your body. This is only a beginning. Remember, when it comes to strength training, unless you are targeting your practice for your chosen sport, treat it as play time. You will reach plateaus, but if you make the decision that you're in it for the long haul, not just for the overnight results you'll be sure to succeed. Embrace the 3 steps forward, two steps back approach. You don't have to be driving forward in 5th gear all the time, drop back down to 4th and 3rd. Enjoy rest and recovery – it is JUST as important as pushing the limits.

I took my son to an adventure playground recently and it dawned on me why all of this 'training/practice' was so worthwhile. I was the biggest kid there. I was swinging, jumping, and bounding around with more vigor and enthusiasm than ever before. It is my intention to be doing the same with my grandchildren and great grandchildren. Think about the future from time to time and ensure you have purpose in your daily practice.

LOCKING ONTO YOUR VISION AND FOLLOW THE PATH OF YOUR ROLE MODEL

When I saw gold medal winning gymnast Jordan Jovtchev demonstrate his power on the gymnastics rings I knew my training was about to change forever. His demonstration of ring training exercises (found on the DVD 'Ring Strength') highlighted the amazing strength and body awareness needed to master this amazing discipline. I knew I'd never step in his gold medal winning shoes, and neither did I want to, but that didn't stop me from wanting to train the same way he does.

Many a young gymnast has been poached by another sports coach because their conditioning is so advanced. I know 8 and 9 year olds that make me look like a bumbling idiot at the gymnastics centre, but what I want to do is shine the light of possibility down on those who think they're too old to succeed. I see all shapes and sizes of people at the gymnastics centre, so if it appeals to you, go for it.

WARNING: WEIGHT-BEARING EXERCISE INCREASES BONE DENSITY – BUT NOT WITHOUT A GOOD DIET

According to Dr Robert Schulze, a daily walk of 45 minutes can cause dramatic increases in bone density, but don't just stop there! Mineralization is laid into bones along axial lines of stress. What this means is that when you tug, yank, push and press on a bone you strengthen your bones and simultaneously strengthen your muscles.

Coconut oil, olive oil, flax oil, hemp oil, avocados etc all improve calcium and magnesium absorption and supports the development of strong bones and teeth. One of the reasons MCFAs (medium chain fatty acids found in coconut oil) are used in baby formula is that they help with the absorption of other nutrients. The absorption of calcium, magnesium and amino acids increases when coconut oil is included in their diet. MCFAs are also used to treat children suffering with rickets which involves a demineralisation and softening of the bones similar to osteoporosis in adults. Bone cells will not grow bone from processed junk food or soft drinks. These foods have been shown to degenerate and eliminate all the usable calcium from the body. Without quality nutrition, it doesn't matter how much exercise you do, you're just going to build brittle bone, or no bone at all

THE PERILS OF PASTEURISATION

Many people still think of pasteurization as one of the most important discoveries of the 20th Century, but a study in the British Medical Journal (Vol. 14, No. 10) written in 1960 clearly highlights the dangers of milk pasteurisation. Entitled...

'The Effect of Heat Treatment on the Nutritive Value of Milk for the Young Calf: The effect of Ultra-High Temperature Treatment and of Pasteurisation'

In this study, researchers fed a group of calves their mother's milk, after it had been cooked, and in nine out of ten cases the calf died before reaching maturity. Can you believe this? Can you believe advertisers spend millions in an effort to convince us it is a near perfect food! It can't even sustain life in the animal it was designed for, so how is it supposed to help you build health?! Conclusion: Cooked milk is a poison. Science has proved it. What does your common sense tell you? Think about it! The dairy council advises children to drink lots of milk to grow up big and strong. What they don't tell you is the enzyme necessary for the digestion of milk is lactase, and 20% of Caucasian children and 80% of black children have no lactase in their intestines.

INCREASE YOUR BONE DENSITY WITH SUPER-NUTRIENT NON-DAIRY FOODS ...AND LET THE X-RAYS PROVE IT!

Medical Herbalist Dr Richard Schulz, renowned for his success with so-called impossible patients, used carrot juice regularly with his patients to build strong bones, especially if they were calcium deficient. Take a look at these figures and you'll see why.

♦ An 8-oz. glass of fortified milk has about 250 mg of calcium – with a very low assimilation percentage.
♦ An 8-oz. glass of carrot juice has 100-400 mg of calcium (depending on the quality of the carrots), and you'll assimilate all the calcium!

Many of Dr Schulze's patients were able to dramatically increase their own bone density, from the simple inclusion of a few daily glasses of fresh carrot juice and other naturally high calcium foods, without calcium tablets.

One lady he treated sustained severe injuries after a nasty fall. She broke a wrist on one hand, her elbow on the other, and also fractured her hip! Doctors tested her bone density and were so concerned about the frailty of her bones, they wanted to put steel pins in her limbs in case of future accidents. The lady refused the operations and decided she wanted the bones to heal. She consulted Dr Schulze who put her on a program of increased exercise, and a diet of fresh juices high in calcium, whilst reducing protein.

If you mix green leafy vegetables such as parsley, kale and chard with a carrot juice base, your calcium intake will skyrocket. Add some nuts or an avocado, to slow the release of the sugar from the carrots into the bloodstream (carrots are hybrid foods) and you're on your way to AGGRESSIVE HEALTH! Sea vegetables such as seaweed and kelp are also an excellent source of calcium, as is AFA algae found in E3 Live. Sesame seeds are another food source often underestimated for their potent calcium content. Anyway...

WHAT HAPPENED TO THE LADY?

After following the program for two months, with no hormone replacement or calcium tablets, her bone density was checked again. The doctors' jaws dropped in amazement! The bone X-rays in front of them looked no different than those of a teenager!

MINERAL DEPLETION:
THE DANGERS OF PUSHING THE LIMITS

Have you ever heard of professional athletes dropping dead on the sports field? According to the Centre for Disease Control in Atlanta, 100,000 youngsters/sports professionals die each year from cardiovascular disorders. Almost half of this number played basketball. The intensity of basketball causes players to sweat profusely leading to electrolyte loss, which if not replaced, can eventually lead to chronic deficiency and maybe even death.

If you think a simple sports drink will replace nutrients lost during exertion, then think again! The majority of sports drinks are loaded with salt, potassium, food colouring and sugar, further depleting valuable minerals and upsetting the acid/alkaline balance.

Healthy blood falls into a very narrow range on the pH scale of between 7.3 and 7.45. This may not appear to be a big difference, but in terms of oxygen content, tenths and hundredths of a point make a huge difference. Blood with a pH of 7.45 contains 64.7% more oxygen than blood with a pH of 7.3. Values above or below this range have drastic, potentially fatal, consequences.

DESTROYERS OF HEALTH ARE EVERYWHERE

An example of how easy it is to upset your alkaline balance is illustrated here. By pouring a single 8-ounce glass of cola into 10 gallons of water slashes the water's pH from 7.4 to 4.6, a value that's considered very acidic. Can you believe that? Can you believe some people spend their lives drinking such waste?

Your body consists of about 10 gallons of water, which is supposed to be slightly alkaline. Although the body goes to every length to maintain a balance and keep its fluids at an acceptable pH, you can imagine the impossibility of the task if you drink cola. Here are the pH values for various drinks. Remember, numbers lower than 7.0 are acidic; higher numbers represent better alkalinity.

Cola	2.5
Diet soft drink	3.2
Beer	4.7
Reverse Osmosis filtered water	5.4
Distilled water	5.2
Bottled water	7.8
Ionised alkaline water	10.0

So what should you drink?

THE ULTIMATE RAW MINERAL RE-HYDRATION

A great formula for athletes after their workouts is the all-powerful green juice made from kale, celery, and cucumber. Kale provides the heavy 'muscle nourishing' minerals and has high alkaline properties that neutralise lactic acid build up. Cucumber provides excellent fluids and soluble fibre. Celery (the favourite of the gorilla) should be eaten and/or juiced often to provide the sodium necessary to balance out the high potassium content of fruit. It's also excellent for replacing fluid losses through excessive perspiration. Other sources of sodium are raw olives, kale, dandelion, spinach, and sea vegetables (laver and dulse). Sodium is a vital mineral that needs replacing if you exercise often as it can be lost heavily through sweat. My post recovery meals may include a vegetable juice which is celery, greens, cucumber based, followed by an either some hemp seeds, almonds, eggs on my 'non-raw days' or fish. Wheatgrass juice and AFA Algae are also excellent foods for athletes as they are rich in vital nutrients. Protein is also essential when you've finished working out, and small protein recovery meals will be easily digested in an efficient, clean system.

ENERGISE YOUR BLOOD AND BUILD A POWERFUL BODY

An excellent formula for energising the blood and building a powerful body involves the use of young coconut water and freshly made green juice. If you are a body builder or an athlete, this formula is a must! Young coconut water and green juice directly targets the blood. Here's why:

1. In the plant world young fresh coconut water is virtually identical in structure to human blood plasma, which makes up 55% of your blood. It is also the highest source of natural electrolytes (electrically conductive charged minerals in solution that directly nourish the tissues).

2. Chlorophyll found in green juice, is the closest substance to human haemoglobin in the plant world.

Put these two together and you have the ultimate blood building/revitalising formula. Remember the Golden Rule: When you rebuild your blood you rebuild your body.

These distinctions separate those who seem to make continual progress from those who never seem to get out of the blocks. Use them and you'll join the elite group of people who don't have to spend all day at the gym to produce incredible results. Good Luck!

ARE YOU READY FOR THE CHALLENGE?

It's up to you to use food to your advantage! High levels of insulin generated by too much carbohydrate will decrease the production of good eicosanoids and increase the production of bad ones. With the balance tipping from favourable eicosanoids to unfavourable, you won't as efficiently access body fat during exercise, and your oxygen transfer rate will be dramatically reduced. In this state exercise will feel like an up hill battle, rather than a paddle downstream! If you want results, control your insulin levels!

♦ High tension exercises increase your amino acid uptake. High volume training will pack on size. Low volume/high tension training will create amazing muscular tone, ideal for those wanting to keep bodyweight low but strength high.

♦ Boredom leads to laziness, laziness leads to inactivity, inactivity leads to bone and muscle wastage. Design your body by practicing high tension, high load, low rep exercises.

♦ Daily practice yields the best gains in strength. If you want to master a skill such as a pull up, muscle up, press up, 1 legged squat, 1 arm press up. Focus on it daily until you can do 1 rep.

♦ A German Study showed that practicing your chosen strength exercise every other day causes a 20% drop in your potential compared to daily practice. Elite Russian and Bulgarian weightlifters have up to twenty-eight sessions a week.

♦ Many young gymnasts are poached by other sports coaches because they have the best overall physical conditioning. Be prepared to be humbled when you arrive at your local gymnastics centre, but it may be the best decision you ever make.

♦ Electrolytes used up during stress and exercise. See stress chapter for when minerals drop due to stress. Ensure you link back to this chapter when talking exercise recovery and stress. People need to appreciate nutrient rich foods protein and carbs and fat are all key to help recover from exercise and stress as is deep relaxation through mind technology.

♦ Exercise on an empty stomach before you have eaten a meal is a most effective way to accelerate the activation of an anabolic state while forcing the body to burn fat and inhibit fat gain.Add to exercise bit - Liver detoxification is critical for the proper production of the steroid hormone and for the proper utilisation of food and energy and maximum growth Mention the important of a cleansed liver, go back to wheatgrass, AFA Algae and notice how chlorophyll has a powerful effect on the liver for steroid hormone formation.

♦ Exercise chapter - Most cancer drugs, if not all, act as growth inhibitors. In fact, all anti-inflammatory drugs, including nonsteroidal anti-inflammatory drugs (NSAIDS) such as aspirin or ibuprofen, and blood pressure drugs such as beta blockers are also inhibitors of hormones and enzymes that stimulate growth.

♦ Put in strength training section – Many body builders consider meat and eggs to be the most anabolic foods. Vegetarians should focus on beans and nuts to reclaim their virility and potency and assume anabolic potential. Nuts, especially almonds, have been considered an aphrodisiac food from the time of antiquity. With superior nutrition content, almonds should be considered one of the most important anabolic supporting foods.

♦ If you need to lose unwanted fat then strength training will help stoke the fire of your fat burning metabolism by increasing the density of your muscles.

♦ In an effort to burn as many calories as possible, many people workout too hard, yet the calorie content of their next meal usually replaces what they've just expended through exercise! It's not calories that are important but the hormonal cascade you set in motion before and after you exercise that determines the benefits you get from your workout.

♦ The most efficient source of energy is fat. It is more plentiful, and supplies more than twice the energy of carbohydrates. When exercising, carbohydrate or fats are needed to replenish the supplies of ATP essential for muscle contraction. No ATP – No muscle contraction! Fat is most efficient at replenishing ATP.

♦ rH2 is measurement I take when conducting bioterrain analysis. It is a combination of pH and ORP (oxidation/reduction potential) and can indicate cells ability to communicate effective on a biochemical level. If rH2 readings aren't balanced, there may be an early incapacity to produce ATP somewhere in the krebs cycle, which ultimately effects energy production. Live blood analysis may also show warped red blood cells when ATP is low. If you have severe problems with energy, even after much intervention, you may wish to book a bioterrain analysis session. Contact www.aggressivehealth.co.uk for more details.

♦ After you've exercised, eat a small protein rich recovery meal with mineral rich greens, raw plant fats and low stimulating carbohydrates. Glycogen levels will be replenished at a faster rate than if you were to eat carbohydrate alone!

♦ A great formula for athletes is the all-powerful green juice made from kale, celery, and cucumber. Another excellent juice to devour after a heavy workout is celery/apple juice as it has the perfect sodium-potassium ratio (1:5) which helps prevent and relieve muscle cramping and fatigue.

♦ Celery (the favourite of the gorilla) should be eaten and/or juiced often to provide the necessary sodium to balance out the high potassium content of fruit.

♦ Everett Smith, director of biogerontology laboratories at the University of Wisconsin, reported in 1993 that a group of middle-aged women, who did nothing more than hoist 5-pound weights, once a week, for over four years, slowed the loss of bone mass in their arms by a staggering 50%.

♦ According to Dr Robert Schulze, a daily walk of 45 mins can cause dramatic increases in bone density. But to build bone, your bone cells also need nutrition.

♦ An 8-oz. glass of carrot juice has 100-400mg of calcium and you'll assimilate all the calcium. Add some nuts or an avocado, to slow the release of the carrots sugars (since it is a hybrid food) and you're on your way to AGGRESSIVE HEALTH!

♦ Parasitic infections can cause emaciation and prevent the gaining of weight. The best way to prevent this is to have a series of colonics and include garlic, onions, hot peppers, ginger, and spicy wild greens (wild mustard is excellent) in your diet. These foods will burn out a parasitic infection.

♦ Nuts are acidic – EAT THEM IN VERY SMALL QUANTITIES. For every 10g of nuts, eat/blend/juice 100g of green leafy vegetables.

♦ Human growth hormone can be seen as 'the fountain of youth'. It is a profound tissue building (anabolic) hormone produced in the pituitary, a small gland located at the base of the skull, and secreted at intervals throughout the day. HGH stimulates tissue growth, increases muscle tone and lean mass, enhances flexibility, thickens muscles, stimulates the growth of bones and organs, mobilises fat stores, shifts the metabolism to the preferential use of fat, and helps maintain healthy tissues.

♦ If you have children you'll know how pleasurable it is to hug and caress them. When you do their levels of growth hormone increase and the protective coating of the motor nerves (myelin sheath) becomes thicker. Your loving urge to cuddle your offspring translates directly into life-sustaining biochemical reactions. Babies deprived of loving attention can become emotionally stunted or dysfunctional.

♦ HGH is released into your blood 90 minutes after you go to sleep and once before you wake up in the morning. To increase the release of human growth hormone from your pituitary gland, decrease your blood glucose levels, increase your blood protein levels, restrict carbohydrates in your diet, fast from time to time, eliminate cooked fats, engage in habits that increase PGE1 (a good eicosanoid), get a good night's sleep, rest often, and finally, exercise!

♦ People who eat sweet, starchy, or otherwise carbohydrate laden foods before they go to bed, inhibit the normal shot of growth hormone released an hour or so after falling asleep. The same goes for people who eat high carbohydrate foods before or immediately after a workout. The pulse of growth hormone released by exercise generally hits the circulation towards the end of the workout and immediately after. To inhibit this growth hormone surge, people only have to eat a power bar, chocolate bar or drink a fizzy soft drink.

♦ By strengthening and developing your muscles, you immediately build a bigger dumping ground for blood sugar, causing your body to store less fat. Think about muscle as an enormous protective barrier against rising blood sugar levels. Intense exercise can add years to your life and life to your years.

- People in their sixties are learning to lift weights and create the muscle mass and energy levels equivalent to that of twenty-one-year-olds.
- For comprehensive information on strength training routines, either sign up for my 4 day boot camp or purchase one of the many books found at www.aggressivehealth.co.uk. Coach Sonnons Clubbell Training For Circular Strength, Pavels 'Power To The People' and 'Naked Warrior' are excellent additions to your peak performance library.
- Any horse vet will tell you, if you want to kill a horse, keep it locked up in a stable! Most vets know that if you let it get out and run around, it will probably get better. The fastest way to kill a senior citizen is to do the same – trap them in room or a home where movement is limited.

It doesn't matter what your background is, whether you're looking to lose a few pounds or win a title fight, whether you are a professional golfer or a seasoned powerlifter you'll find incredible benefit in beginning to train with heavy loads. Now you now have a clear and concise battle plan of how to fit the principles of strength practice into your daily routine, the results are there for the taking. The tools to carve out a body that is hormonally balanced, superstrong and fully charged are all waiting for you. Go for it.

THE AGGRESSIVE HEALTH EVALUTATION
Do you use clubbells®, kettlebells and bodyweight/ring training to develop the body of your dreams?
Do you maximise your chances of releasing HGH?
Have you employed the strength training principles of the super strong to maximise your strength gains?

PART THREE

ELIMINATE UNWANTED STRESS *FOREVER*, USE MIND TECHNOLOGY TO SUPERCHARGE YOUR BRAIN AND CHARGE TOWARDS AN AWESOME EXISTENCE

Every cell in your body is crackling with energy. You feel you can conquer the world, and in an effort to do so, your life has become incredibly busy. BUT BEWARE! Constantly pushing yourself to the limits without taking adequate rest may expose you to a never-ending cycle of stress. Although stress can be useful at times, too much can cause biochemical destruction.

CHAPTER 11

DISCOVER THE SECRETS OF REMAINING CALM AND ALERT IN A WORLD OF CHAOS: ELIMINATE STRESS

Congratulations! If you've read every chapter so far, you'll have discovered what it takes to create incredible energy levels and maintain tight control over the subtle hormonal balancing act that governs your health and vitality. But beware! Many people find that with their newfound energy and desire to achieve their dreams, comes increased stress as they burn the midnight oil and push themselves to the limit. The purpose of this chapter is show you what happens when stress hormone imbalances take hold of your body, and then guide you towards the ultimate solution. Cycles of activity and stress are necessary for the achievement of your deepest desires, but if not backed up with cycles of deep, profound relaxation, chronic imbalances can develop.Like the smoker who dies of lung cancer after 40 years of continual smoking, stress hormone imbalances can gradually strangle your health in much the same way. Fortunately, research has been carried out in the area of neuroscience, highlighting how easy it is to restore balance to a flagging system. That's where we're headed, so strap in and prepare for the most powerful distinctions AGGRESSIVE HEALTH can offer.

THE ULTIMATE POWER OF CORTISOL

In the animal kingdom, no journey is more dramatic than that of Pacific salmon as they overcome powerful currents, leap past dams, battle against waterfalls, and fight their way upstream to return to their birth site to spawn. But do salmon thrive after such an adventure? Certainly not. After spawning, they begin to age at an accelerated rate and usually end up dying within days. What causes this accelerated ageing? Cortisol. That's right, the hormone that allowed them to reach their birth site against all odds is now the cause of their death. Put simply, the mechanism that usually monitors cortisol production becomes exhausted, leading to a massive outpouring of the hormone. When the adrenal glands are exhausted from the overproduction, the salmon's finely tuned hormonal communication system completely breaks down.

At this point the immune system is virtually destroyed leading to incredible weakness and vulnerability to disease, whilst parasites and infections begin to invade the salmon with tremendous ferocity.

HOW MANY SALMON DO YOU KNOW?

Can you think of anyone who seems to work excessively, is always stressed and never seems to relax? You don't have to be a genius to see that they are putting tremendous strain on their brain, body and nervous system. I suggest you take a look at your own life and ask yourself whether or not you think you experience too much stress. I hope you don't, but if you do, I'm glad I brought it to your attention. In the right amounts, cortisol helps to increase your capacity to withstand stress. It assists in the metabolism of fat, protein and carbohydrate and thus energy production. It also helps thyroid activity, muscle and joint function, the rate of bone turnover, immunity to infection, quality of sleep, and the health of your skin. If over-stimulated, cortisol can destroy you both mentally and physically. That is the secret – To understand that everything in your body has power and purpose, but if one hormone is chronically inhibited or activated, imbalances can often lead to metabolic catastrophe.

STRESS: THE TICKING TIME BOMB

Three stages make up 'the general adaptation syndrome', a term used by Hans Selye, author of 'The Stress of Life' and leading expert in the area of stress and health. Take a look for yourself and you'll see how over-exposure to stress can eventually kill!

STAGE 1 – THE ALARM REACTION
In the first stage you secrete adrenaline, cortisol and DHEA, as your whole physiology reacts and prepare for the threat of pain, whether, physical, verbal or even mental. Your body responds by increasing heart rate, breathing rate and muscle tension. Stress is perceived differently by different people, highlighting the fact that it is only the perception of threat that causes stress rather than the threat itself. Manipulating your perception and conditioning your nervous system to remain calm and alert is one of the most powerful and rewarding skills you can learn. Contact www.aggressivehealth.co.uk for details of upcoming seminars.

STAGE 2 – THE RESISTANCE STAGE
Prolonged stress promotes the increased release of cortisol, which in turn causes an immune factor, Interleukin-6 (IL-6) to be secreted.

Abnormal levels of IL-6 are associated with autoimmune conditions, inflammatory diseases and allergies. IL-6 also causes calcium to be pulled from the bones, increasing the chances of osteoporosis.

DHEA is a precursor of the stress hormones adrenaline and cortisol. Every time the body makes these hormones, DHEA levels are depleted. When cortisol and IL-6 levels rise, DHEA production dwindles. The real problem begins when the natural cortisol shut off mechanism becomes disrupted, damaging a part of the brain called the hippocampus.

Let me explain. Usually when the threat/stressor has vanished, the hippocampus tells the system to stop producing cortisol, but in cases of extreme stress, excess cortisol damages the hippocampus and it fails to register the elevated levels. The damage turns what is supposed to be a feedback mechanism into a feedforward mechanism. Rather than shutting down cortisol production the brain allows it to continue, even in the absence of any threat. As your body adapts to the stress your brain structure begins to alter until finally, hormonal imbalances become the norm.

Overexposure to stress also inhibits the delta 6 desaturase enzyme and knocks out the production of good eicosanoids, predisposing its victim to many illnesses including depression, ulcers, premature ageing, cancer, heart disease, skin diseases, Alzheimer's disease, hypertension, diabetes, multiple sclerosis and Parkinson's disease.

You'd think by removing the stimulus, stress hormones would decline and return to normal, but at the end of this second stage the threat could have vanished and a person can still have high levels of the stress hormones in their bloodstream. Have you ever seen anyone go on holiday and find it hard to relax because they are so used to being busy? Stress hormones make you pursue activities rather than rest.

STAGE 3 –THE PHASE OF EXHAUSTION
This is the most evil stage of all. The chosen organs that continue to fight the battle against the stressor gradually weaken. As they wear out, the body turns to other organs. This drafting in of other organs causes another surge of adrenaline and cortisol secretion.

Eventually not enough stress hormones are produced and low levels are detected in the blood. The adrenal glands enlarge, the thymus, spleen, and lymph nodes shrink, and the number of white blood cells diminish in number resulting in chronic fatigue and susceptibility to infections, as the immune system is weakened. Even excess stomach acid is secreted as blood pressure rises and sex hormones decline. Hardly an advert for AGGRESSIVE HEALTH is it? I hope what you're reading is motivating you to take control. The place to begin is by increasing the production of...

THE ANTI-AGEING HORMONE: DHEA

In the late 1980s Arthur Schwartz, a biochemist at Temple University, administered DHEA to mice. He observed a remarkable reversal of ageing: Old mice regained their sleek, glossy coats and youthful vigour, cancers disappeared (whether naturally occurring or induced by artificial means), obese mice returned to normal weight, diabetes improved, and immunity to disease increased.

Under normal circumstances, between 10 and 20mg of cortisol is produced by the body on a daily basis. DHEA production ranges from between 25 to 30mg, making it the most abundant steroid in your body. Both are produced at different levels during the day and it's the rhythm between the two that is critical. Cortisol is usually higher in the morning and lower at night. If any one factor disturbs this synchronicity, health can be compromised. Too much stress and not enough relaxation/recuperation eventually upsets the fine hormonal balancing act, causing an increase in cortisol output. Think of excess cortisol production as the first step to dropping your 'immunity' guard, inviting the one-two punch of infection and disease.

DHEA is critical! It prevents cortisol from causing widespread damage by binding to its receptor sites, ultimately protecting part of the eicosanoid production pathway by preventing cortisol from inhibiting delta 6 desaturase. As you'll remember, delta 6 desaturase is the enzyme that allows linoleic acid to flow freely into the eicosanoid production pipeline. DHEA indirectly keeps delta 6 desaturase active. Without it you'd have no mechanism to prevent the devastating effect of excess cortisol on eicosanoid production.

ARE YOU BEGINNING TO SEE
HOW ALL THIS FITS TOGETHER?

1.   Excess Insulin production = increase in cortisol output
2.   Excess stress = increase in cortisol production

When cortisol levels increase, DHEA binds to cortisol receptor sites protecting part of the eicosanoid production pathway. But if cortisol continues to increase, the ratio of cortisol to DHEA increases – eicosanoid balance suffers – insulin rises even more – and health gradually spirals downwards. At this point the hormonal philharmonic isn't sounding too terribly good and accelerated ageing is too often the result!

A decrease in DHEA, with a corresponding increase in cortisol can cause biochemical destruction. Let this destruction happen to someone else, not you! It's your responsibility to maintain optimal DHEA levels by:

1.   Preventing the secretion of excess insulin by eliminating refined sugar and cooked fat! Excess insulin interferes with an enzyme that helps produce DHEA. Experiments with rhesus monkeys that were put on calorie-restricted diets caused DHEA levels to rise, whilst simultaneously lowering insulin levels. (See Chapter 15 – Maximise Your Lifespan)

2. Take 200mcg of chromium daily! Studies have shown that patients' levels of DHEA drop by an average of 10% after they discontinue to take the supplement. Eat foods such as pulses, nuts, seeds and asparagus to keep your chromium levels topped up.

STIMULATE DHEA AND BOOST YOUR IMMUNE SYSTEM

DHEA controls age-related disorders, helps repair and maintain tissues, reduces arteriosclerosis, increases insulin sensitivity, controls allergic reaction, and most importantly, balances the immune system. Low levels of DHEA cause sexual dysfunction, muscle shrinkage, memory loss, degenerative diseases and poor immune function. Research has found DHEA to help reduce obesity, ageing, and cancer (particularly breast cancer).

TRACKING THE DECLINE OF DHEA

DHEA production is naturally high (regardless of diet) until about age 30, highlighting why young people are less prone to disease. At age 30 in many people (not all) there is a decline in production. In fact, no other age-related hormone declines as fast as DHEA, with the average drop being from about 30mg per day at age 20 to less than 6mg per day at age 80. It isn't unusual for sufferers of cancer, heart disease, atherosclerosis and Alzheimers to all have low levels of DHEA in their blood. Stimulate DHEA and you also trigger the release of human growth hormone (HGH), the true elixir of youth!

A twelve-year study looking at hundreds of ageing humans highlights the importance of maintaining adequate blood DHEA levels. When DHEA levels dropped, mortality increased. According to Dr. William Regelson of the Medical Collage of Virginia, DHEA is "one of the best biochemical biomarkers for chronological age."

MAXIMISE DHEA AND BOOST YOUR BRAIN POWER TODAY

In an experiment with brain cell tissue cultures, anti-ageing researcher Dr. Eugene Roberts discovered that even very low concentrations of DHEA will "increase the number of neurons in the brain, improve their ability to establish connections and their differentiation." He concludes that DHEA plays "a significant role in normal function of neuronal cells". By actively keeping your DHEA levels adequate/high, evidence suggests that your ability to learn and remember will increase and you'll enhance every aspect of your mental performance.

ENHANCE YOUR BRAIN POWER FURTHER
AND CEMENT YOUR MEMORIES

Chronic stress also depletes the stimulating neurotransmitter norepinephrine (see chapter 14 – Food For Thought). Take a look at how a simple neurotransmitter imbalance can sabotage your mental health:

♦ As norepinephrine is depleted, a deficit is created in the frontal lobe of the neocortex, where much abstract thinking takes place.
♦ Norepinephrine is used to cement memories, without it your ability to remember declines. Students with chronic stress scored 13% lower on IQ tests than students with low stress in one revealing study. Excess cortisol causes learning ability and concentration to hit rock bottom!
♦ Norepinephrine plays a critical role in keeping you happy and in good spirits. Chronic stress causes norepinephrine to be shunted away from your limbic system (part of your brain that controls your emotions). With a lack of norepinephrine in the emotional centre of your brain, people often experience a biological depression leading to feelings of anxiety and malaise.

DO YOU WANT TO MAXIMISE YOUR PLEASURE PATHWAYS OR
DISRUPT THEM?

If brain chemistry is disrupted for too long a period, the disruption can lead to a condition known as anhedonia, the inability to feel pleasure. Anhedonia leaves its victim biochemically incapable of being excited, joyous or happy and is very common among chronic abusers of stimulating drugs such as cocaine.

Have you noticed how those who abuse drugs, alcohol and sugar foods, eventually need more of the stimulant to feel satisfied? One of the reasons is because their brain down regulates. Down regulation is a process in which the number of neuroreceptors for a certain brain chemical decreases to compensate for an increases in the number of neurotransmitters carrying that chemical.

Simply imagine that the drug abuser has supplied so much artificial stimulation to their brain via the drug, that in order to maintain balance their brain has responded by decreasing the number of neuroreceptors. Imagine your house as a brain cell and all of your friends and familys houses as brain cells. Now imagine you send a welcomed invite to a party. The postman (neurotransmitter) posts the invite (information) to each of the houses through the letter box (the neuroreceptor). Now imagine you start sending out 1000s of junk mails to your friends, so much so that some of them start to seal up their letter box. That's what happens when you start introducing too much 'stimulating junk' to your diet. The problem is that when you stop supplying the stimulant and your body starts to produce its own pleasure chemicals such as norepinephrine (a critical ingredient in the pursuit of unlimited happiness) and other stimulating catecholamine neurotransmitters, the brain has downregluated (the letter boxes are sealed temporarily) and the addict experiences the low associated with withdrawal.

HAVE YOU EVER FELT NUMB AFTER COMPLETING A LONG STRETCH OF WORK?

Many people experience a mild form of anhedonia after completing a long, stressful piece of work. When they finally finish, they know they should feel ecstatic, but end up feeling numb. Their brain's happiness chemicals were burned up by excessive stress.

The great advantage of training in N.L.P. or hypnosis is that you can begin to train yourself to experience more pleasure and joy on a day to day basis for absolutely no reason. People think this is crazy, but it's not as crazy as getting stressed for no reason – and there are millions of people doing that every minute of every day. The more pleasure you experience on a day to day basis, the less you will physically react to stress. The less you react to stress, the less you will damage your brain with cortisol! Simple.

IF YOUR BRAIN ISN'T HAPPY, YOU WON'T BE HAPPY!
THREE POINTS WHERE STRESS CAN DESTROY YOUR BRAIN

There are essentially three ways that stress can destroy optimal function of the brain.

♦ Stress disrupts the supply of the brain's only source of fuel, glucose
Firstly, your ability to adapt and deal with the unpredictable nature of life will determine whether you perceive situations as stressful or not. If you find yourself relaxed and in total control, then congratulations. But if you've been stressed at times when a more relaxed state of mind was appropriate, you are risking the integrity of your brainpower!

Stress causes cortisol and adrenaline to be released from the adrenals, inhibiting the uptake of blood sugar from part of your brain called the hippocampus. The hippocampus happens to be the brain's primary memory centre and without enough blood sugar it suffers an energy shortage. This energy shortage means the brain has no way to chemically lay down a memory, leading directly to short and long term memory problems.

The importance of conditioning relaxed states of mind cannot be overemphasised, especially if you want to learn something like a new language or a new skill. Another unwanted mental effect of chronic stress is its influence on brain waves. A person experiencing stress has a predominance of "uptight" beta brain waves, rather than 'calm' alpha and theta waves. More about this in chapter 12.

♦   Stress interferes with the function of neurotransmitters
Imagine what happens in a freak snowstorm when all the power cables are down. The telephone, television or computer won't work and the weather is too bad to travel. What do you have? Complete communication breakdown. This is the kind of effect stress and cortisol has on the mind. It prevents neurotransmitters from sending information between various areas of the brain, causing problems with concentration

and focus. Can you see why people are often so muddled and confused in stressful situations?

Have you ever wondered why hypnosis is used for memory retrieval? Quite simply, a skilled hypnotist can access a relaxed/lucid state of consciousness, increasing the chances of memory retrieval.

One of the reasons we need sleep is to rebalance brain chemistry and re-establish neurotransmitter equilibrium. If you can actively learn to maintain optimal neurotransmitter equilibrium you'll maintain a magical mind and powerful brain for the rest of your life. You'll learn more about neurotransmitter equilibrium in chapters 12 and 14.

◆ **Stress causes the eventual death of neurons, by creating free-radical molecules**

Cortisol allows excessive amounts of calcium to enter the brain cells, increasing free radical formation. Excess free radical formation can lead to brain cell death. Antioxidants protect you from aggressive free-radical attack, highlighting the importance of a diet based around raw, living foods and nutrient dense superfoods.

Half the dry weight of your brain is fat and a third of that is made from polyunsaturated essential fatty acids making it incredibly vulnerable to free radical attack. Eicosanoids are made from polyunsaturated fatty acids and since they're easy targets for free radicals, it's up to you to protect them with antioxidants.

I FOUND MY FREEDOM ON BLUEBERRY HILL

Scientists have found that the antioxidants within blueberries can actually reverse the effects of the passing years and help retain optimal health. For example, rodents begin to lose their balance and co-ordination at 12 months and according to researchers, by 19 months (human equivalent – 65 to 75 years old) the time they can balance on a narrow rod falls from 13 seconds to 5 seconds. However, when the researchers gave the rodents daily doses of blueberry extract for eight weeks (equivalent to half a cup of berries for humans) their times dramatically improved, returning to an average of 11 seconds. Their ability to find their way around a maze, a test of short-term memory, also improved.

Imagine that! By including a daily cup full of the berries into your diet you could benefit from improved balance, improved co-ordination and a more powerful short-term memory! With their low sugar load and high antioxidant potential, berries are the fruits of choice for students of AGGRESSIVE HEALTH. For other antioxidant rich superfoods, see Appendix 1.

ELIMINATING QUICK FIX
REFINED 'EMPTY CALORIE' FOODS

Is it a habit of yours to reach for a chocolate bar or cup of coffee in order to raise your energy level and mood? Stop! This habit could be killing you! If it's coffee you choose, the reason it wakes you up is because the caffeine latches onto the adenosine receptor site in your body and brain. Adenosine is a neurochemical responsible for quietening the mind, but if it's 'calming message' cannot get through because it is blocked by caffeine you're likely to feel sharp and alert. You may think there's no harm in this, but caffeine also stimulates the same reward centres of the brain as amphetamines and cocaine. Now you can see why so many people are addicted to caffeine!

The high sugar content of stimulating foods is perceived by your body as a threat and it mobilises unnaturally high levels of insulin along with the stress hormone cortisol and adrenaline to restore blood sugar levels. If you hammer your body morning, noon and night with these kind of stimulants, you can expect adrenal fatigue. The best analogy for this situation can be found in the ground breaking book 'Potatoes Not Prozac' by Kathleen DesMaisons PhD.

> "Think of the adrenals as a volunteer firefighter who has been working overtime for three months. He is totally exhausted. The alarm bell rings at three in the morning. Instead of leaping out of bed, he vaguely hears the alarm, struggles to focus, finally recognises that it is the bell ring rather than his dream, stumbles out of bed, gropes for his boots, walks to his truck, slumps at the wheel, then finally gets mobilised to turn the motor and get to the fire. He used to leap from his bed, drop his feet into his boots in an instant and be out the door before the bell had finished ringing. But his fatigue is clobbering his response time."

If that doesn't wake you up to the dangers of adrenal fatigue, go and buy the book Potatoes Not Prozac today. Adrenaline exerts such a powerful force on the body in response to sugar, blood sugar levels take a steep nose dive, forcing you to reach for the next stimulant. If wild blood sugar levels and crazy mood swings are what you want, along with adrenal fatigue and hormonal disturbances throughout your body – sugar and stress is the answer!

STRESS EATS AWAY AT STORED VITAL NUTRIENTS

Stress places the same demands on your body as exercise. It magnifies your nutritional needs and burns up extra nutrients very rapidly. Whether you think you suffer from stress or not, you need to benefit from both cycles of activity and cycles of profound relaxation.

A fascinating study by the U.S. Department of Agriculture shed more light on this phenomenon. Researchers created a scenario where subjects were given more work than usual, with very strict deadlines. When they completed the work, blood samples showed a 33% drop in mineral content.

When cortisol is released in response to stress, it causes the mineral magnesium to be excreted in excessive amounts. The irony is that magnesium happens to be a calming mineral and low levels increase your vulnerability to stress. This is how the downward spiral continues, stress causes magnesium loss –

magnesium loss increases your chances of perceiving situations as more stressful – cortisol is released and magnesium is excreted – stress increases etc. etc.

THE POWER OF TRANSCENDENTAL MEDITATION

Before I whisk you away on a wonderful journey into the world of neuroscience and brain technology, I want you to take a look at the power of meditation – specifically Transcendental Meditation (TM). More than 500 studies and research projects have highlighted the incredible power of this discipline. Here are just a few:

♦ TM consistently produces a significant lowering of blood pressure – typically around 10mm Hg for systolic blood. This could have a major significance for the health of the world, as hypertension is the main risk factor for stroke and a major factor in coronary heart disease.

♦ TM has been shown to produce positive health, including increased creativity and intelligence, more satisfaction from relationships, a feeling of mental and physical rejuvenation and a dramatically increased ability to manage depression, insomnia, migraines and irritable bowel.

♦ The act of meditating allows you to slow your metabolism down to the point where you reach a hypometabolic state. The only other time this state is reached is during sleep or hibernation. When you enter the hypometabolic state your consumption of oxygen decreases rapidly. To be more precise, sleep causes an 8% drop in oxygen consumption, but meditation can cause a decrease of between 10% and 20%, highlighting the deeply relaxed state that it creates. In this state your entire physical system is rejuvenated.

♦ Meditation influences your body on many different levels. To begin with it causes a decrease in blood lactate. Lactate is secreted by muscles and can cause mild anxiety. Researchers demonstrated the power of lactate in an interesting study with a group of patients, all suffering anxiety disorders. The group was split in two. One half received a placebo injection, the other group received an injection with lactate. As you can imagine, the first group had no response, but the second group quickly experienced an anxiety attack. As you meditate, you can expect blood lactate levels to drop significantly within as little as ten minutes.

♦ One of the main benefits of meditation is that it causes a decline in cortisol production, which will stay with you long after your meditation session ends. If you meditate on a regular basis you can expect cortisol levels to remain low, day after day, week after week. This is another reason why meditation significantly slows the ageing process, increasing lifespan and health span.

♦ Meditation is known to decrease ageing. You only have to look at the DHEA levels of meditators compared to those of non-meditators. When you're 20 years old, your DHEA level is about 800. When you're 40, it's about 300. And when you're 70, it's about 2. People who practice TM regularly have been shown to have much higher levels of DHEA than average people of the same age. Levels of DHEA normally decrease with age and high levels are directly linked to a low risk of heart disease, cardiovascular disease, osteoporosis, and breast cancer.

♦ The sleep hormone melatonin is increased by meditation. Studies at the University of Massachusetts Medical Centre have shown that meditators produce significantly more melatonin than non-meditators on a regular basis, offering people exceptional relief from insomnia.

♦ A study of 2000 people practising Transcendental Meditation showed that they had fewer than half the number of doctor visits and days in hospital than a control group. They needed less medical and surgical treatment in all 17-disease categories, including 87% fewer hospitalisations for cardio-vascular disease, 55% fewer for tumours, 73% fewer nose, throat and lung problems and fewer disorders of the nervous system.

♦ Because DHEA is an adrenal steroidal hormone, it is part of the body's response mechanism to stress. Generally, stress (excess cortisol production) depletes DHEA. In fact, many clinicians monitor DHEA levels as a measure of long term stress. If DHEA levels are low, it can indicate that the patient suffered long-term, chronic stress. If you can keep cortisol secretion to a minimum, using meditation and other techniques that induce the 'relaxation response' you automatically protect DHEA. Another study of meditators showed that men over the age of 45 had on average 23% more DHEA than non-meditators, whilst women had a staggering 47% more!

♦ In one study, 242 men aged 50 to 79 were monitored for their DHEA Levels. Afterward their health was tracked for twelve years. Those with the highest levels of DHEA had the best long-term health, even if they smoked and had high cholesterol. For every 20% increase in DHEA levels in these men, there was a 48% decrease in heart disease, and a 36% decrease in death from any cause.

♦ Alzheimer's patients, however, invariably have much lower levels of DHEA than do non-Alzheimer's patients of the same age. One study indicated that Alzheimer's patients had 48% less DHEA than a matched control group.

♦ People who meditate and increase DHEA levels report renewed energy and sex drive, an increased sense of well-being, an elevated mood, and a greater ability to cope with stress. More importantly, DHEA has been shown to have immune-boosting properties. Research had shown, for example, that DHEA restores the cancer-fighting T cells and enhances the activity of the natural killer cells (NK cells).

♦ DHEA can reverse osteoporosis by increasing the activity of bone-building cells (osteoblasts), whilst inhibiting the activity of bone-destroying cells (osteoclasts). Although cortisol is only one of the many hormones secreted by the adrenal glands, it's secreted in response to stress. Like all hormones, moderate amounts prove to be anything but harmful, but when produced in excess, many problems can occur.

Amazing isn't it? But what's more amazing is that the marvellous effects of brain technology such as light/sound stimulation devices, the Alpha Stim and The Holosync

Solution® can produce good, if not better results than transcendental meditation (TM) and in less time! It's worth knowing how powerful meditation is before you learn about the power of mind machines. The point is simple: whether you choose to buy a mind machine or meditate, ensure you take time out every day to quiet the mind and go inside, allowing your whole body to relax and rejuvenate.

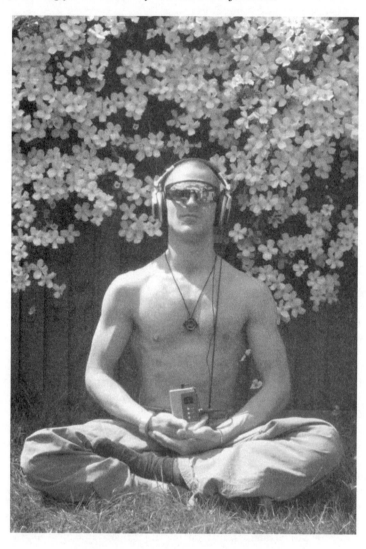

SOMETHING ELSE TO CONSIDER:
THE STRESS OF LONELINESS

Did you know that if an older person loses their spouse, they are ten times more likely to die within a year than if their spouse were to remain alive? Did you also know that when a person gets divorced, their chance of becoming ill over the course of the next year rises dramatically by 1200%? Those who are chronically stressed have higher chances of mortality and illness. This information may not inspire some people, but at least it highlights the importance of taking responsibility and doing everything in your power to maintain health and wellness. In this case start appreciating your partner and/or circle of friends/pets, they are as important to your health as your next meal!

If emotional pain from loss of a loved one or the break up of a relationship makes you turn to chocolate, ice-cream and other sugary foods for comfort, take note. Dr Elliot Blass has shown in experiments with 10-day-old albino rats that when taken away from their mothers they begin to cry over 300 times in a 6 minute period. But guess what? When sugar water was given to them, the rate of crying dropped to 75 times over the same time period. Sugar actually helps numb the pain by stimulating the beta-endorphin system, but at the expensive of causing hormonal chaos and leaching vital nutrients from your body needed to deal with the stressful event. You'll learn more about this phenomenon in chapter 14. Steer clear of sugar!

ARE YOU READY FOR THE CHALLENGE?

Although cortisol is only one of the many hormones secreted by the adrenal glands, it's secreted in response to stress. Like all hormones, moderate amounts prove to be anything but harmful, but when produced in excess, many problems can occur. Cortisol does have a positive role in your body, but like insulin, too much can lead you down a road you'd rather not travel. The importance of doing all you can to prevent stress from compromising your immune system is obvious when you're aware of the insulin-cortisol-IL-6-DHEA connection. It's up to you to safeguard yourself against stress by ensuring your body is abundant in all the vital nutrients that build and support life. Use the principles in these pages, enhance your own production of DHEA, and eliminate any habits that cause its production to dwindle. Set aside time in the day to relax, allowing your brain to recuperate. Continue to take responsibility. You've built a powerful foundation. Now is the time to excel yourself. Here's a re-cap:

♦ Cortisol can be incredibly toxic. If your brain is exposed to excessive levels of it, brain degeneration is usually the result. In fact, overexposure to cortisol is possibly the number one cause of brain degeneration.

♦ When cortisol is released in response to stress, it causes magnesium to be excreted in excessive amounts. Magnesium is a calming mineral and low levels increase your vulnerability to stress.

♦ In the wild, animals manufacture vitamin C out of glucose, and under times of stress they produce a phenomenal amount. If you are under stress, select foods and superfoods high in vitamin C. Vitamin C is crucial for reversing adrenal fatigue. Goto www.aggressivehealth.co.uk for more details.

♦ A fascinating study by the U.S. Department of Agriculture showed that when subjects were given more work than usual, with very strict deadlines, blood samples showed a 33% drop in mineral content.

♦ Cortisol is responsible for triggering the release of the brain chemical neuropeptide Y, which leads to carbohydrate cravings.

♦ High carbohydrate diets that stimulate too much insulin cause a rapid drop in blood-sugar levels resulting in poor brain function and cause the secretion of cortisol to increase blood sugar levels. Excess insulin also interferes with the enzyme that helps produce DHEA.

♦ DHEA prevents cortisol from causing widespread damage by binding to its receptor sites. It helps protect part of the eicosanoid production pathway by indirectly keeping delta 6 desaturase active. Without DHEA you'd have no mechanism to prevent the devastating effect of excess cortisol on eicosanoid production. The less stress you experience the more harmonious your eicosanoid status.

♦ DHEA acts as a buffer against stress related hormones (such as cortisol). If you don't actively do as much as you can to increase/maintain optimal levels of DHEA, as you age you'll make less, making you more susceptible to stress and disease.

♦ Recent research has found that eating some protein with carbohydrate provides additional adrenal support by reducing the stimulation of cortisol. Calorie restricted diets also cause DHEA to rise (as long as the diet isn't nutrient deficient). Sprouted beans supply an excellent source of both protein and carbohydrate and pre-digested making them easy for your body to break down.

♦ Dr. Eugene Roberts discovered that by actively keeping your DHEA levels high, evidence suggests you'll boost your ability to learn and remember, whilst enhancing mental performance.

♦ It isn't unusual for sufferers of cancer, heart disease, atherosclerosis and Alzheimers to have low levels of DHEA in their blood.

♦ Stimulate DHEA and you also trigger the release of growth hormone, the true elixir of youth!

♦ Dr. William Regelson of the Medical Collage of Virginia, states that DHEA is "one of the best bio-chemical biomarkers for chronological age." When DHEA levels drop, mortality increases!

♦ DHEA helps control stress, maintain optimal mineral balance, control the production of sex hormones, build lean body mass and burn fat by enhancing energy metabolism. You'll burn calories more easily as your energy levels rise.

♦ A trained body can cope with stress better than a sedentary one can. As you strengthen your body, cortisol waves will shorten in times of stress and you'll avoid high cortisol fluctuations associated with high stress.

♦ When you decrease cortisol production, testosterone levels increase. Testosterone is responsible for many health advantages including sex drive. High insulin levels retard testosterone production, because one of the steroid precursors (pregnenolone) required for testosterone production is diverted toward increased cortisol production.

♦ Laughter is such an effective form of stress diffusing exercise that it has been called inner jogging. Research has shown that people who laugh easily respond better to treatment for disease. Laughter prompts positive physiological changes that benefit the immune system.

♦ One last point. When you purposefully follow your passion and every day is a labour of love, you stand a greater chance of limiting stress in your life. Passion and purpose are fundamentals for a life of joy. If you can honestly say that you love what you do, love where you spend your time, love the people you surround yourself with, you're a greater success than you can imagine. When I talk of 'love', I'm not talking about sitting in a big circle holding hands and chanting, "We love herbal tea", I'm talking about grabbing life by the balls and loving every minute of it..

Master this chapter and soon you'll be looking in the mirror at someone who is not only slim, with clear beautiful skin and toned muscles, but who has an incredibly calm and powerful mind. The choice is yours, a lack of control and a stressful life, or total control and complete abundance.

THE AGGRESSIVE HEALTH EVALUATION:
Is your diet full of stress relieving/brain enhancing raw foods?
Do you control insulin and glucagon, optimising blood sugar levels and minimising cortisol output?
Do you take time to meditate or relax during the day?

Whether you choose meditation, hypnosis, biofeedback or any other proven system to alter your state of consciousness, make sure you use it and use it often. Each discipline allows you to experience profound relaxation and access incredibly resourceful states of mind. However, you can go one step further. Recent advances in neuroscience have opened the gateway to a range of machines that enhance peak performance brain states.

CHAPTER 12

OPEN THE GATEWAY TO EXPLOSIVE MIND POWER WITH THE MAGIC OF MIND TECHNOLOGY

As the young author sits busily writing his first best seller, his computer workstation is surrounded by many books. The subjects vary from hypnosis, nutrition and mind enhancing technologies to meditation and the mind/body connection. He's been working constantly for 40 minutes and feels he'd be more productive if he took a short break. He lies on his bed, grabs his Alpha Stim device, wets the electrodes, and attaches them to his ear lobes. Next he grabs his Mindlab and puts on the headphones and liteframe goggles (heavy-duty sunglasses with built in LEDs that flash at various frequencies, entraining brain wave frequency).

PREPARE FOR THE JOURNEY OF A LIFETIME – DAILY!

By pressing the 'on' button, the Alpha Stim starts to induce a kind of tingling in his ears, whilst stimulating his brain with electrical impulses. He then presses a button on the console of the Mindlab to engage a program of light and sound pulses.

For the next 20 minutes the hypnotic, pulsating tones capture his attention, whilst the rich variety of colours from the flashing lights of the goggles, move and swirl in front of his eyes. As he becomes totally engaged in the delights of the audio-visual experience provided by the Mindlab, the Alpha Stim sends micro-electrical current between his two ear lobes, stimulating various areas of his brain. He is spellbound and absorbed by the experience.

This may sound like something out of a science fiction movie, but elite athletes, sports professionals and business executives are using mind machines more and more frequently to combat stress and enhance peak performance – with exciting results – AND SO SHOULD YOU!

MIND TECHNOLOGY HAS THE POWER TO REVOLUTIONISE YOUR MENTAL HEALTH

When the 20 minutes are over, the Alpha Stim stops, the lights of the Mindlab fade, and the sound pulses gradually diminish to nothing. Silence. He can't believe that a mere 20 minutes ago he was feeling tired and overloaded by the task at hand. He now feels relaxed and alert, energised but calm. His brain is functioning far more effectively than it was before. The kinds of changes that have taken place at a neurological level are remarkable. Take a look for yourself and imagine reaping these benefits for yourself.

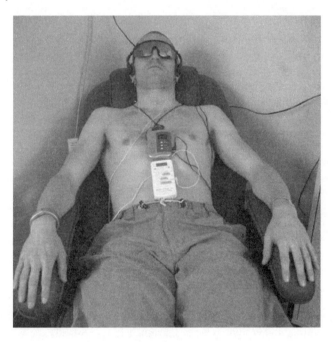

♦   **In the 20 minutes that passed, he exercised his brain making it healthier and more powerful.**
A wealth of brain research is proving that your brain, like your body, requires stimulation and challenge to function optimally. Just as your muscles grow stronger from physical exercise, by exposing your brain to stimulation that manipulates your brain waves, you exercise your brain and strengthen it.

Dr Marian Diamond, neuroanatomist and leader in the research of the physical effects of thinking on the brain, has proved that the more you think and challenge your intellect the bigger your brain becomes, and the better it functions.

Evidence suggests that mind machines can provide the kind of stimulation, challenge, and novelty that can strengthen your brain, increase the size and health of its neurons, produce peak performance states of mind, increase intelligence, and enhance well-being, regardless of your age.

Under the right conditions neurons can regenerate, suggesting that given the right type of stimulation your brain will continuously heal itself and replace lost cells, in much the same way as your skin can heal itself after it is cut.

One neuroscientist at the University of California at Los Angeles took specimens from over twenty human brains and analysed them under a microscope. He found a clear and definite relationship between the number of years of education and dendritic length. The more people had learned, the greater their dendritic length. Intellectual challenge has a direct physical effect on dendritic systems. With proper nutrition, your brain can create new dendrites, and forge new synaptic connections – indefinitely.

It doesn't matter whether you are young or old, your brain has the capacity to grow, and you have the capacity to become more intelligent. The more you learn, the greater your capacity for further learning. The more you put into your brain, the more open it becomes. But without sufficient stimulation, whatever your age, this capacity for growth will be limited.

The simple challenge presented by computer video games has proved to be enough to significantly improve the mental ability of the elderly. Mind machines can stimulate changes in brain wave frequency and access states of mind that are synonymous with accelerated learning.

♦ **In the 20 minutes that passed his memory has increased.**
Mind machines have been proven to improve both long-term and short-term memory. The Alpha Stim works by stimulating protein synthesis. For memories to become permanent in your brain, there has to be a process of nerve cell growth (protein synthesis) involving RNA (Ribonucleic acid). There is a greater concentration of RNA in your brain than anywhere else in your body. RNA synthesis is absolutely essential for the creation of memory and may even be a memory storage molecule itself. It declines naturally with age or illness suggesting why the elderly are known for their forgetfulness. RNA is such a powerful antioxidant and key to longevity that experiments with rats have shown it can increase life span by 20%.

AFA algae (E3Live) contains 4% RNA/DNA (nucleic acids). These are needed by the body to make new cells, repair damaged cells and for growth of body tissue. Without enough RNA/DNA, you may suffer the consequences of a weak immune system and ultimately age prematurely. Poor nutrition, pollution and stress can deplete your RNA/DNA. Ensure you use E3Live daily.

♦ **After the 20 minutes of stimulation he has a higher IQ.**
In several studies, subjects with learning disabilities have increased their IQ between 20 and 30 points with the use of mind machines. Other research suggests that mind machines can also dramatically boost the IQ of normal, healthy users.

♦ **His intelligence, creativity and problem solving ability has expanded after 20 minutes.**
Scores on several psychological tests measuring creativity show significant boosts when subjects used mind technology before the tests. If you stimulate different brainwave states with external stimulation, you may facilitate your ability to allow more variations in brain functioning by breaking up patterns of information flow at the neurological level. This can help you develop the ability to move rapidly from one state of mind to the other through increased neural flexibility. In fact, one of the useful by products of learning N.L.P. and hypnosis is developing the ability to create and alter your state of consciousness rapidly, allowing you to adapt more easily in any situation.

DISCOVERING THE MYRIAD OF MENTAL STATES
WITH MIND MACHINES

Every imaginable mental state you experience is the result of a specific pattern of electrical and chemical activity in your brain. Brain activity can be altered and shaped by external stimuli, including sounds, lights, electromagnetic fields, and physical movements. Mind machines can direct these stimuli to appropriate areas in your brain and reliably trigger specific brain states. When you use these technologies it's possible to guide yourself into such brain states as euphoria, reverie, recall of long-past experiences, stimulation of memories, sexual excitement, deep concentration, and heightened creativity – the list is endless. Studies by neurologists have now proved that in certain extraordinary mental states, such as deep meditation or intense creativity, both hemispheres begin to produce strong brain waves in a single, coherent rhythm, operating in unison. Scientists call this state of whole brain thinking synchrony, and it has recently become clear that certain brain stimulation devices can rapidly boost your brain into this beneficial state.

♦ **His brain's processing speed has increased after 20 minutes.**
In a variety of settings, subjects using mind technology have learned more, learned faster, and proven more adept at learning difficult and complex material than ordinary subjects. Accelerated learning is encouraged since brain cells can forge new, richer interconnections. Under the proper conditions, you can absorb, store, process, and recall vast amounts of information, given the right stimulation.

♦ **His body is now profoundly relaxed and the levels of adrenaline and other stress related substances in his body have decreased after 20 minutes.**
Evidence shows that various mind machines can dramatically reduce levels of stress-related neurochemicals, reduce muscle tension, lower high blood pressure, slow heart

rate, soothe jangled nerves, and quickly produce whole body levels of relaxation whilst increasing resistance to stress. This helps with the production of good eicosanoids. Remember, the delta 6-desaturase enzyme isn't inhibited along the eicosanoid production pathway when stress chemicals are minimised in the body.

♦ **His immune system is functioning more effectively after a mere 20 minutes.** Researchers are exploring the effects of mind machines on individual components of the immune system with healthy and sick subjects (including those with AIDS, chronic fatigue immune dysfunction syndrome, and cancer). They have found clear evidence that these devices can increase the power of the immune system to overcome existing diseases and boost its resistance to infection.

By reducing cortisol, your ability to produce favourable eicosanoids remains efficient, leading to a powerful immune system response!

CAN YOU BELIEVE THAT A MERE 20 MINUTES CAN MAKE SOMEONE INSTANTLY SMARTER AND HEALTHIER?

The story of this 20 minute break is the story of what it took for me to write this book. I frequently took these power breaks to boost my brain capacity, enter peak performance states of mind and condition relaxed, focused states of awareness. You may develop amazing energy levels by following the principles of AGGRESSIVE HEALTH, but make sure you set aside time to relax and recuperate. Cycles of activity and stimulation coupled with rest and relaxation will lead the healthiest most rewarding life.

BEGINNING TO SURF THE BRAIN WAVES

Beta Waves – In the waking state your brain is alert and busy. Beta waves are the most dominant and range from about 14 cycles per second (14Hz) to more than 100 Hz. Beta waves are associated with alertness, arousal, concentration, cognition, and in excess – anxiety.

Alpha Waves – As you relax, brain-wave activity slows down and you produce bursts of alpha waves. Alpha waves range in frequency from approximately 8 – 13 Hz. When your mind is unfocused and you're day dreaming or taking a break, alpha waves become dominant throughout your brain, producing a calm and pleasant sensation. Alpha activity can usually be found in those who are healthy and not under a great deal of stress. The lack of significant alpha activity can be a sign of anxiety, stress, brain damage or illness.

Theta Waves – The more relaxed you become, the deeper your state of drowsiness and the quicker your brain shifts to slower, more powerfully rhythmic theta waves. These waves range in frequency from about 4 – 8 Hz. They reflect the meditative state, which lies between wakefulness and sleep. Often, when people experience theta waves, they can access information otherwise out of their consciousness (unconscious retrieval). Hypnosis is very powerful and excellent for training its subjects to access theta brain activity. As you train your brain to access a theta state, you'll begin to experience deep personal insights, increased creativity and increased creative problem solving. Theta brain waves combine a pleasant, relaxed feeling with extreme alertness.

ZEN MONKS SPEND 20 YEARS IN ORDER TO MASTER THETA CONTROL – YOU CAN DO IT IN TEN MINUTES!

A series of EEG studies by Japanese scientists showed that the most skilled Zen monks sank right through alpha and began producing the slower theta waves when they went into deep meditative states. Even in the depths of theta where most people simply relax further and fall asleep, monks however, are extremely alert.

The more meditative experience monks had, the more theta they generated. If they had accumulated 20 years of meditative experience, they were able to access deep theta quickly. 20 years is a lot of training, but fortunately, through scientific breakthroughs in the field of neuroscience, scientists discovered it did not require years of training or any special meditative powers to produce such unique patterns of brain activity. They found that by using light stimulation in the way of flickering strobe lights combined with pulsating sound waves or even rhythmic physical movement, they could actually produce the same 'peak performance brain states' in ordinary people with no meditative experience at all. Over the last few years scientists and electronic engineers have used advanced technology to design a variety of mind machines that allow you to trigger these desired peak performance brain patterns at will!

Delta Waves – When you fall asleep delta waves become the dominant brain waves, ranging in frequency upto 4Hz.

With the possibilities of very advanced brain states and coherence, there exists evidence that individuals may be able to maintain consciousness while in a dominant delta state. This seems to be associated with certain deep trance-like states.

Within the delta state, your brain is triggered to release large quantities of human growth hormone (HGH). Professional body builders such as Frank Zane use mind machines immediately after a workout to promote the release of this powerful youth enhancing hormone. If you don't sleep much at night and retire late and wake up early, you may need regular siestas in the afternoon to stimulate HGH. By taking responsibility and cycling between states of aggressive activity and blissful relaxation you strengthen your ability to reach an anabolic state necessary for muscular development. Never underestimate rest! It is as important as any workout session. If exercise is the first step to the anabolic cycle, optimal nutrition and relaxation closes the loop facilitating growth and development. Take responsibility and the rewards will be there for the taking.

UNLEASHING THE MAGIC OF THE ALPHA-STIM

Electrical stimulation of your brain at the proper frequency, waveform and current can quickly and sharply increase the levels of many neurotransmitters in your brain, whilst smoothing over brain wave activity harmonising brain function.

77 SCIENTIFIC STUDIES OF CES: 90% POSITIVE

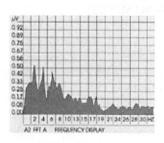 EEG [brainwave chart] before and after using the Alpha Stim for only 10 minutes. Notice how spiky they are in the first chart and how smooth they are in the second.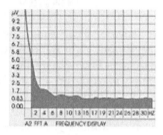

In total, there have been 77 scientific studies and 27 non-scientific studies on CES. 90% of the scientific studies seem to imply positive results — and 80% for the non-scientific studies. These studies have looked at CES's effects on anxiety, depression and insomnia.

NATURAL STIMULATION FOR AN ENDORPHIN HIGH

The Alpha Stim is most widely used for pain relief. If you were to experience pain in your neck for example, when the area of the pain is electrically stimulated at appropriate frequencies and amplitudes, your body responds with a flood of endorphins, alleviating the pain and in some cases leading to complete recovery.

There is evidence that this kind of direct stimulation to the neurons of your brain (by the use of electrodes that clip to the ears) has a profound optimising and normalising effect on brain functioning. The use of the Alpha Stim and other forms of Cranial Electro-Stimulation (CES) facilitate a re-balancing of brain chemistry. CES seems to act directly on the neurons to stimulate the release of neuropeptides, such as the endorphins, and other neurotransmitters, such as norepinephrine and dopamine (associated with memory and learning), as well as serotonin, adrenocorticotropic (ACTH) and cholinesterase. Researchers have found CES effective in the treatment of depression, chronic pain, migraine headaches, treatment of learning disabilities and the treatment of children with cerebral palsy. It's now easy to…

BOOST BRAIN JUICES FOR LEARNING AND ECSTASY

When you stimulate the reward centres in your brain, you immediately experience more pleasure due to the increased flow of catecholamines (including norepinephrine and dopamine). These neurotransmitters have a very similar effect on your brain to cocaine. Norepinephrine is so pleasurable that if a drug could be created to stimulate it on its own, without dopamine, it would produce undiluted ecstasy. Now there's a thought!

Low frequency currents induced by external electrodes from machines such as the Alpha Stim can dramatically speed up the production of various neurotransmitters in your brain, with different brain juices being triggered by different frequencies and waveforms. For example, a 10-Hz signal boosts the production and turnover rate of serotonin, as you'll see in chapter 14; this could be very significant for those suffering at the mercy of unbalanced brain biochemistry.

Each brain centre generates impulses at a specific frequency based on the predominant neurotransmitters it secretes. In other words, your brain's internal communication system is based on frequency. When you send in waves of electrical energy at 10Hz for example, certain cells in the lower brain stem respond because they normally fire within that frequency range. As a result, particular mood-altering chemicals associated with that region will be released.

MEMORY'S MATE – GLUTAMATE

Glutamate isn't as well understood as most of the other neurotransmitters, but is definitely essential to the formation of memories and the retrieval of old ones.

When experiments were conducted on rabbits and rats, researchers discovered that the formation of memories was directly related to the number of glutamate receptors in the brain. By using electrical stimulation at specific rhythms and amplitudes, the levels of glutamate can be dramatically altered, playing an important role in the formation of memories. Low levels of glutamate in your brain generally indicate decreased cognitive function. Furthermore, glutamate can be especially helpful in brain longevity programs because it inhibits the chronic stress response and, consequently, the over production of cortisol.

BALANCING BRAIN BOOSTING JUICES
FOR PEAK PERFORMANCE

The very slow 0.5Hz waves of the Alpha Stim, can act as a toner resonating and stimulating every one of your brain cells, restoring harmony and balance. This is critical for the following reasons:

♦ Too much norepinephrine can lead to anxiety, tension, and hyperactivity. Too little can impair memory and cause depression.

♦ Too much acetylcholine leads to lethargy. Too little leads to weakness and hallucination.

♦ Too much serotonin causes hallucinations and sleep. Too little brings depression, aggression, and insomnia.

Your brain functions at its best when the various neurotransmitters are within their optimal range. You wouldn't want a stereo that blasts out bass without any other frequency. You'd want balance. The same is true of your brain and your life.

By hooking yourself up to an Alpha Stim, you can activate your brain's learning pathways and enhance your ability to think, absorb new information, combine ideas in new and innovative ways, consolidate facts into memory, and recall information already stored in your brain. If you want to increase your ability to learn, think, create, imagine and explore, the only question is: how much and in what ways? Now, as you get excited at the infinite possibilities and potential, let me take you on another journey...

SENSORY PLEASURE WITH LIGHT-SOUND DEVICES

Modern scientific research into the effects of rhythmic light and sound began in the mid-1930s when scientists discovered that the electrical rhythms of the brain tended to assume the rhythm of a flashing light stimulus, a process called entrainment. For example, when they flashed a strobe light at a frequency of 10Hz into the eyes of a subject monitored by an electroencephalogram (EEG), the subject's brain waves tended to adopt a 10Hz frequency.

A flood of subsequent scientific research in the 1960s and 1970s revealed that such flicker effects at certain frequencies seemed to have amazing powers. Various scientists began discovering that photic-stimulation has a variety of beneficial effects, such as increasing IQ scores, enhancing intellectual functioning, and producing greater synchronisation between the two hemispheres of the brain. Other researchers found that the addition of rhythmic auditory signals dramatically increased the mind-enhancing effects. There is certainly more to light-sound machines than meets the eye.

THE HEALING POWER OF
'FORGOTTEN BRAIN NUTRIENTS'

Light and sound are brain nutrients that stimulate the electrical energy in your brain. They energise and heal. Light, falling on the photoreceptors of your eye, is translated into electrical impulses, which then, via the visual cortex and the hypothalamus, stimulates the entire brain. In addition, by stimulating the nerve endings in your ear (using pulses of sound), each pulse is translated into electrical impulses, which then stimulate the brain via the vestibular system, cerebellum, limbic system, and cortex. The most impressive way to send electrical impulses into your brain is by using the same rhythmic pulsation of electricity that naturally powers the brain cells. If light and sound are nutrients that enrich the brain with their electrical impulses, then the electrical impulses, if delivered in the correct form and at the correct intensity, are the purest nutrient. The Alpha Stim represents the best tool on the market to achieve this purity.

THE SOUND OF THE BINAURAL BEATS
HAS THE POWER TO ENTRAIN YOUR BRAIN

Robert Monroe, author of 'Journeys out of the Body', was the first person to really discover the power of stereo sound (played through stereo headphones) on the brain. For example, if you were to hear a signal of 200 cycles per second in your right ear, and a signal of 204 cycles per second in your left, the two hemispheres of your brain begin to function together and hear a phantom third signal. This signal, a binaural beat, is the difference in frequency between the two sound frequencies, in this case 4 cycles per second (4Hz). It isn't actually a beat, but an electrical signal created by both hemispheres of the brain when functioning harmoniously.

Monroe soon discovered that when precisely controlled tones are combined in the brain, the olivary nucleus begins to resonate sympathetically to this electrical signal/binaural beat. As this resonating/entrainment process begins to take place, signals are gradually sent into the cerebral cortex, mixing existing patterns of brain activity and causing profound state changes. By using certain frequencies, Monroe realised he could produce a unique and coherent brain state, known as hemispheric synchronisation.

ENDORPHINS, BINAURAL BEAT PATTERNS
AND BRAIN ENHANCEMENT

Scientists have also found that when the brain is exposed to alpha and theta binaural beat patterns, endorphins are released. Endorphins have a powerful strengthening effect on learning and memory, enhancing many mental functions, and have been known to reverse amnesia. Researcher David de Weid found that when rats were injected with endorphins their memory recall increased dramatically. 1977 Nobel Prize winner Andrew Schally found that when rats received injections of endorphins, their maze-running abilities immediately improved.

THE HOLOSYNC SOLUTION – THE MOST REVOLUTIONARY
BINAURAL BEAT MIND/BODY DEVELOPMENT PROGRAM EVER!

Embedded on cassette/CD beneath soothing music and environmental sounds, the Holosync sound technology will lead you into the deeper alpha, theta and delta brain wave patterns. By providing more input to the brain than it can handle, the Holosync sound technology causes the brain to respond by reorganising itself at higher levels of function. By doing this the brain begins to handle the additional input, creating new neural pathways and establishing communication between parts of the brain that were not previously communicating. If you don't get your hands on The Holosync Solution, developed by Bill Harris, you'll be missing out on one of the most powerful personal development tools in existence. To make it work, all you have to do is close your eyes and listen. It is an on-going personal development program utilising the Holosync® sound technology.

A recent study performed by Dr. Vincent Giampapa, M.D., of The Longevity Institute International and Vice President of The American Society of Anti-Ageing

Medicine, revealed that the Holosync audio technology had dramatic effects on the production of cortisol, DHEA, and melatonin.

Although you know a lot about cortisol and DHEA, melatonin is an equally important hormone. It helps create a blissful night's sleep, and as you age, unless you take effective action, your body may make less of it. Sleep is critical because many important rejuvenating substances are created in the brain. Optimal sleep leads to a rich and fulfilling life. Poor sleeping habits can accelerate the ageing process.

In a before and after study of 19 people using Holosync audio technology, the following changes were noted in levels of melatonin, DHEA and cortisol:

♦ In just three days over 68% of the group had increases in DHEA levels, with an average increase of 43%! Several people had increases of 50%, 60%, and even 90%! A study published in the New England Journal of Medicine (12/11/86) found that a 100 microgram per decilitre increase in DHEA blood levels corresponded with a 48% drop in death from cardiovascular disease – and an overall 36 % reduction in death from all causes.

♦ Cortisol levels were down an average of 46.5%, with several people experiencing decreases of 70 or 80%!

♦ Melatonin levels increased by an average of 97.8%, with positive changes happening in over 73% of the people! Many had improvements of 100%, 200%, and even 300%!

♦ Contact www.aggressivehealth.co.uk for all your peak performance mind machines, including The Holosync Solution.

ARE YOU READY FOR THE CHALLENGE?

The potential of the body and mind is limitless. Whether you find a brain gym in your local area or have to travel to find one, start investigating/investing in the following: PhotoReading by Paul Scheele, Light/Sound Machines, Cranial Electro-Stimulation (CES), EEG machines for biofeedback, binaural beat generators/CDs, motion machines, acoustic field generators, floatation tanks etc. I use an Alpha-Stim 100, a Mindlab Proteus and The Holosync Solution. I get fantastic results in mood enhancement, whilst conditioning peak performance brain states. I use this opportunity to utilise my training in N.L.P. and hypnosis to condition my brain and nervous system to experience more of what I want in life. In these states suggestibility heightens. Let's recap on some important points:

♦ Studies have shown that with proper stimulation your brain can continue to grow, increasing your intelligence, even after 70, 80 or 90 years. Under the right conditions neurons can regenerate, suggesting that given the right type of stimulation your brain will continuously heal itself and replace lost cells, in much the same way as your skin can heal itself after it has been cut.

♦ Mind machines have been proven to improve both long-term and short-term memory. The Alpha Stim works by stimulating protein synthesis.

♦ One neuroscientist at the University of California at Los Angeles took specimens from over twenty human brains and analysed them under his microscope. He found a clear and definite relationship between the number of years of education and the length of the dendrites in the subjects brain. The more people had learned, the greater their dendritic length.

♦ For memories to become permanent in the brain, there has to be a process of nerve cell growth (protein synthesis) involving RNA (Ribonucleic acid), of which there is a greater concentration in your brain than anywhere else in your body. E3Live is an excellent source of RNA/DNA (nucleic acids).

♦ In several studies, subjects with learning disabilities have shown average increases in IQ over 20 or 30 points. Other research suggests that mind machines can dramatically boost the IQ of normal, healthy users.

♦ In a variety of settings, subjects using mind technology have learned more, learned faster, and proven more adept at learning difficult and complex material than ordinary subjects. Accelerated learning is encouraged since brain cells can forge new, richer interconnections.

♦ By actively reducing cortisol production with the use of mind machines you may be doing all that is necessary to enhance your immune system. This is because cortisol/stress inhibits delta 6 desaturase and eicosanoid production.

♦ Evidence shows that various mind machines can reduce levels of stress-related neuro-chemicals, dramatically reduce muscle tension, lower high blood pressure, slow heart rate, soothe jangled nerves, and quickly produce whole body levels of relaxation. All these benefits increase resistance to stress.

♦ The use of the Alpha Stim (Cranial Electro-Stimulation (CES)) restores homeostasis in the brain. CES seems to act directly on the neurons to stimulate the release of neuropeptides, including endorphins, norepinephrine, dopamine, serotonin, adrenocorticotropic (ACTH) and cholinesterase.

♦ A 10Hz signal boosts the production and turnover rate of serotonin. Each brain centre generates impulses at a specific frequency based on the predominant neurotransmitters it secretes. In other words, the brain's internal communication system is based on frequency.

♦ By using electrical stimulation at specific rhythms and amplitudes to stimulate the brain, levels of glutamate can be dramatically altered, playing an important role in the formation of memory. A low level of glutamate in your brain indicates a decrease in cognitive function.

♦ By hooking yourself up to an Alpha Stim, you can activate your brain's learning pathways and enhance your ability to think, absorb new information, combine ideas in new innovative ways, consolidate facts into memory, and recall information in your brain.

♦ A flood of scientific research in the 1960s and 1970s revealed that flicker effects at certain frequencies seemed to have amazing powers on the brain. Subjects experienced increased IQ scores, enhanced intellectual functioning, and greater synchronisation between the two hemispheres of the brain. Other researchers found that the addition of rhythmic auditory signals dramatically increased the

mind-enhancing effects. There is more to light/sound machines than meets the eye.
♦ Cycles of activity and stimulation coupled with rest and relaxation will lead to the healthiest most rewarding life.

It's up to you to take this technology as far as you can. Combine it with a nutritional plan that kicks arse and regular exercise that allows you to evolve at an accelerated rate and you'll have an awesome future in front of you. Whether you're in sports, business or simply want to learn something new – Mind machines must play a part in your daily routine!

THE AGGRESSIVE HEALTH EVALUATION
Have you experimented with mind machines yet?
Have you purchased a mind machine yet?
Do you use your mind machine daily for peak performance/relaxation?

You know that over-exposure to stress can cause biochemical turmoil in your body. You know that Transcendental Meditation (TM) has the potential to restore harmony to your body. You know that mind machines, if used regularly can evolve your brain, allowing it to handle a greater degree of input. But where do you go from here...

CHAPTER 13

DISCOVER HOW EASY IT IS TO DEVELOP A BRAIN LIKE EINSTEIN WITH THE POWER OF ENRICHMENT

Although I'm sure you are excited about getting your hands on a mind machine, let me take you back in time – back in time when neuroscience was in its infancy. Back in time when brain science involved a laboratory and a group of rats! I'm not a great advocate of animal experimentation, but the results from these studies will certainly open your mind and expand your awareness to the unlimited power that resides within all of us.

A BRIEF HISTORY OF FINDINGS:
THE SECRETS EINSTEIN LEFT BEHIND

In the 1980s, Dr Marion Diamond, Neuroanatomist and leading expert in the area of brain research, was given the honour of dissecting and studying the brain of Albert Einstein. At the time, many of the members of the neurological sciences were eager to find out if the brains of geniuses had any distinguishing characteristics that separated them from so-called 'average' people.

When Einstein was alive, he used to explain that when he was in deep thought or day dreaming, his thoughts were simply a combination of 'certain signs and more or less clear images.' He used to think visually primarily, and said that words played no part in the process. Using this to her advantage, Dr Diamond chose to carefully examine the sections of Einstein's brain that were responsible for vivid imagery and abstract reasoning. These areas are known as the superior prefrontal and inferior parietal lobes.

To ensure her findings were as credible as possible, Diamond compared the results against a control group of brains, all of which were taken from intellectually average men, who had also died at age 76 in the same way Einstein did. What Dr Diamond discovered was that each of the brains, including Einstein's was almost physically identical, except for one distinguishing feature – The appearance of Area 39.

EXERCISE LIKE EINSTEIN – STIMULATE GLIAL CELLS AND IMPROVE THE FUNCTION OF AREA 39

The one distinguishing feature that made Einstein's brain stand out from the rest was the abundance of a particular type of cell in an area of his brain known as Area 39. If a person has lesions in Area 39, they have great difficulties with abstract imagery, memory, attention, and self-awareness, whilst showing a difficulty in integrating visual, auditory and kinaesthetic input. With problems in Area 39, a person can lose most of their higher intellect and display an inability to read, recognise letters, spell or do calculations.

The name of the cell that was in great abundance in Area 39 was the glial cell. Many people thought that glial cells were thinking cells, but it was discovered that they are actually 'house keeping' cells. Due to the intensity of Einstein's thinking, Area 39 needed a great deal of metabolic support, resulting in the accumulation of these cells, enlarging Einstein's Area 39.

Many people used to think Einstein was a 'born genius', with an efficient brain, but research is now proving that anyone can enlarge areas of their brain if they are willing to mentally exercise it. Einstein created his own genius, and you can do the same! The research continued, leading to…

MORE FINDINGS, MORE POTENTIAL, MORE EXCITEMENT

Biological Psychologists Mark Rosenzweig and colleagues at the University of California performed various experiments on rats in order to explore brain function. They had already discovered that the reason rats conquer mazes at different speeds is due to their learning ability. This ability to learn is primarily affected by a brain enzyme known as acetylcholinesterase (AChE). After various maze tests they found that the higher the level of AChE in the brain, the faster the rat learned. What they didn't know was whether this enzyme could be manipulated through stimulation, or whether its production was simply down to genetics. They decided to conduct a series of experiments. They took a group of genetically equal rats and divided them into three groups.

1. Group one was put in a standard environment – a mesh cage.
2. Group two was put in isolation. Each rat was subjected to a cage with three opaque walls, dim lights, little noise, minimal stimulation, and no chance to interact with other rats. This was the impoverished environment.
3. Group three was raised in play groups of ten to twelve rats, in large, well-lit, multi-levelled cages filled with swings, slides, ladders, bridges, an assortment of

toys, frequently changing stimuli, and a variety of challengers. This was called the enriched environment, suggesting you can...

STIMULATE AChE BY ENRICHING YOUR LIFE

After certain periods of time ranging from days to a number of months, the brains of the rats were removed and analysed. To their astonishment, researchers discovered that the rats raised in the enriched environment showed higher levels of AChE activity in their brain cortex than the rats raised in the standard and impoverished environments. (The cerebral cortex is a layer of nerve cells, where much of the thinking and higher intellectual activity of the brain takes place.) They found that cortical AChE activity isn't a fixed individual characteristic, but could be altered by experience!

Since AChE activity was directly linked to their ability to learn and process information, the rats in the enriched environment had developed a greater ability to learn and had become smarter than the other rats. Experience had altered intelligence. Now is the time to...

STIMULATE YOUR SENSES
AND PUT WEIGHT ON WHERE IT COUNTS!

As you might imagine, the researchers were more than just a little startled. What they accidentally stumbled across next was more than just remarkable, it challenged everything they believed about the brain up until that point. The way they measured AChE was by 'enzymatic activity per unit of tissue weight'. To do this they weighed brain samples, so they could measure chemical activity per unit of tissue weight. After two years of doing this they noticed that the actual weight of the brain samples also changed, the cortex of the rats in the enriched-environment had actually become heavier than the cortex of the other rats! Stimulating experiences had caused the rats' brains to grow. This finding sparked off a frenzy of studies and research that resulted in some groundbreaking findings in the field of neuroscience. In all cases, the rats raised in the enriched environment showed:

♦ An increase in the thickness and size of individual neurons in the cortex.
♦ An increase in protein levels, in alignment with increases in cortical weight. This proved that it was tissue growth and not an increased fluid level that was causing the weight gain.
♦ An increase in the amount of dendritic branching. Imagine your hand is the cell body of the neuron and your fingers are the dendrites. When stimulated with enriched environments your brain develops more branching. The nerve cells are designed to receive stimulation, so an increase in dendritic branching means an increase in possible connections.
♦ An increased number of dendritic spines per unit length of dendrite. The spines are the thousands of small projections that cover the surface of dendrites, each one marking the site of a synapse, the point where another neuron makes a

junction with this neuron. With an increase in the number of spines there exists a greater potential for interconnection between neurons.

♦ Increases in the number of synapses and in the size of synaptic contact areas. Synapses are the spots where different neurons are connected and by means of which communication amongst neurons takes place. By increasing their number and size, you increase the richness of communication in the cortex.

♦ An increase in the ratio between the weight of the cortex and the weight of the rest of the brain. The enriched environment is beneficial to the area that primarily controls thinking, learning and memory.

♦ A 15% increase in the number of glial cells. Out of all the cells in the brain these are the most numerous. They act like glue and hold together, support and nourish the brain neurons. They also act as guides for neural growth, assist in learning and also have a communicating network of their own. The message is clear...

ENRICH YOUR LIFE WITH AN ENRICHED ENVIRONMENT

Brain experiments were becoming increasingly fascinating and the potential of the brain – limitless. Dr Diamond continued her studies of Area 39. She was curious to find out whether it was the simple act of thinking that caused the unusual growth and she designed an experiment to test her theory. To begin with she built two totally different environments. The first one was a small box with nothing in it. The second one was filled with a variety of toys and games. Into the bare box Dr Diamond placed one rat and her three offspring. Into the second box she placed three female rats, with three offspring each.

Dr Diamond wasn't surprised to find that when the rats died, those that had spent their lives in the enriched environment had a 16% larger Area 39 than in the other rats. What she didn't expect to find was that other areas of their brains had also increased in size, by about 10%. She went on to find that this worked just as successfully with elderly rats, proving it's never too late to challenge and stimulate yourself. Now is the time for the critical question:

ARE YOU LIVING IN AN IMPOVERISHED ENVIRONMENT?

If you are still not sold on the idea of mentally stimulating yourself, think about this: Dr Diamond discovered that without enough thought provoking toys and an environment to match, the brains of rats could actually shrink. Could this be the reason for age-associated memory decline and cognitive impairment? Having been raised in a mentally impoverished environment, the dorsal cortex of the rats' brain shrunk by 9% and the entohorinal cortex, which is associated to memory, shrunk by 25%. It's up to you to stimulate yourself and...

DEVELOP WISDOM BY CREATING MORE
SIX SIDED DENDRITES

To delve even deeper into the intricacies of neuron development, Dr Diamond found that highly developed neurons responded better to enriched environments than less developed ones. During the developmental process, neurons reach out to other neurons with branch-like dendrites. As new information is assimilated, dendrites keep sending out new branches, and those branches send out more branches again. Dr Diamond discovered that the first, second, third, fourth and fifth dendrite didn't grow any longer even though exposed to an enriched environment, but the sixth branch did.

She explains that, "Whether we are young or old, we can continue to learn. The brain can change at any age. We began with a nerve cell, which starts in the embryo as just a sort of sphere. It sends its first branch out just to overcome ignorance. As it reaches out, it is gathering knowledge and it is becoming creative. Then we become a little more idealistic, generous, and altruistic; but it is our six-sided dendrites which give us wisdom."

CREATE SUPER ENRICHMENT – TODAY!

To follow these amazing findings, Argentinean researchers created a super-enriched environment and to their surprise found that it caused as much brain growth in four days as took place in thirty days in the ordinary enriched environments.

A short while later they found that four daily one-hour periods of enriched exposure significantly increased cortical growth. Then they went on to find that four daily exposures to an enriched environment, of only ten minutes, brought about significant increases in cortical weight! Other investigators found that a single forty-five minute session (where rats had to learn to choose various lighted alleys to avoid a nasty shock) resulted in significant brain changes, such as increases in the number and shape of some synapses. It got to the point where even short exposures to an enriched environment produced significant and long lasting effects on the cortex, sometimes within seconds of sensory stimulation! That's right – seconds!

HELPING THE AGED THROUGH STIMULATION

How would you describe nursing homes, hospitals and retirement homes? Would you call them enriched environments or impoverished environments? Obviously they have their uses, and in some cases are certainly the best option. Is it also possible to see them as the equivalent to 'impoverished environments'? Would it be fair to compare the lives of the elderly in retirement homes to the lives of rats who were placed in an impoverished environment, alone, cut off from challenges, change, companionship, and other sensory/intellectual stimulation? The rats experienced stunted brain growth and accompanying mental dullness/retardation. Could this also be one of the main reasons why humans placed in similarly impoverished environments lose their ability to think?

STIMULATE THE AGED AND REVERSE THE EFFECTS OF IMPOVERISHED ENVIRONMENTS

What is promising is that if the rats were taken out of their impoverished environments and placed in an enriched environment, the conditions of mental deterioration reverse almost immediately. For example, in one study, rats were isolated for 535 days until they reached middle age. Then they were presented with an enriched environment and quickly responded with rapid brain growth. This demonstrates one thing: It is never too late to make changes, and allow sharp and rapid development to be your birthright, no matter how dull the stimulation has been in the past.

BEGIN TO VALUE THE UNKNOWN AND WRESTLE WITH ENRICHMENT

The point is simple. If you continue to assimilate new information, if you continue to tackle challenges, if you continue to welcome change and new unpredictable experiences, you are assuring mental enhancement and complete mental health. To provide yourself with an enriched environment, your brain will continue to weave an ever richer, subtler and a more complex tapestry of neural connections, leading to increasing numbers of possible brain states. It is easy to see why communities such as the Hunzas who not only eat very healthfully but also challenge themselves physically and mentally, live incredibly long lives compared to most people in Western civilisation. The evidence indicates that it is not age that brings wisdom, but enriched environments.

Like the rats placed in the super-enriched environment (that showed as much brain growth in four hours, as the rats in the 'enriched environment' showed in a month), there exists a human equivalent. Mind machines – They subject the brain to intense amounts of stimulation and thus force-feed enrichment to your neurons, alter brain-wave activity, and trigger rapid brain growth.

HIGH PERFORMANCE, OPTIMAL PERFORMANCE, EXTRA-ORDINARY PERFORMANCE

The implications of these recent discoveries are quite clear: the brain is much more powerful, capable, and complex than had previously been imagined. What you think of as 'normal intelligence' is probably just a pale shadow of the brain's actual powers and faculties. Brain function can be substantially improved, provided the brain receives the right type of stimulation. Many mind machines are designed for exactly that, to increase mental power and stimulate actual growth of the physical brain. You now stand at a crossroads where you can make one of the most important decisions of your life...

GAZE INTO THE FUTURE
AND DREAM OF THE INFINITE POSSIBILITIES

Energy and matter are constantly flowing into your brain in the form of light, sound, sensations, information, oxygen and nutrients from your bloodstream. Whilst your brain is only about 2% of total body weight, it uses more than 20% of all oxygen taken into your body, making it the most prodigious energy consumer.

AGGRESSIVE HEALTH begins with the premise that in order to achieve greater than normal potential, and develop higher than ordinary capabilities, you must have energy. By operating your physiology optimally you set the foundation for a life of pleasure and discovery. Even though the mind machines I talk about have been used to stimulate the brains of people with a variety of neurological problems, including Down's Syndrome, mental retardation, and learning disabilities, think of them as your key to the doorway of peak performance. Extraordinary performance awaits you, giving you the chance to evolve as much as you choose through learning, growth and enriched experience. Remember the ultimate creative capacity of the brain may be, for all practical purposes, infinite.

ARE YOU READY FOR THE CHALLENGE?

When you've built incredible health and energy levels, you'll instinctively want to develop every aspect of your mind, body and emotions. You'll begin to avoid countless hours of mind numbing television as you search for new and exciting ways to add richness to your life. Whatever you choose to stimulate your higher thought processes, expect the kind of mental development that will serve your mind and emotions for the rest of your life. Let's recap:

♦ Einstein had a far greater abundance of a particular type of cell in an area of his brain known as Area 39. People with lesions in Area 39 have great difficulties with abstract imagery, memory, attention, and self-awareness, whilst showing a difficulty in integrating visual, auditory and kinaesthetic input. It's a very highly evolved area of the brain.

♦ Einstein spent many hours in deep thought, which is why Area 39 needed a great deal of metabolic support. Glial cells (house keeping cells) were abundant in this area of his brain, which accounted for its above average size.

♦ Create your own enriched environment with challenges and puzzles that stimulate you to think. Set yourself goals. Physical, mental, emotional, and even spiritual. When rats are raised in large, well-lit, multileveled cages, filled with swings, slides, ladders, bridges and an assortment of toys, they benefit from enrichment. Their brains mirror this.

♦ The ability to learn is primarily affected by a brain enzyme known as acetylcholinesterase (AChE). After various maze tests researchers found that rats with higher levels of AChE learned better than those with low levels. Cortical AChE activity isn't a fixed individual characteristic. You can alter it by stimulation!

- Stimulate your senses and put weight on where it counts. You can increase the thickness and size of individual neurons in the cortex of your brain, increase the amount of dendritic branching, increase the number of dendritic spines per unit length of a dendrite, increase the number of synapses and the size of synaptic contact areas and increase the ratio between the weight of the cortex and the weight of the rest of the brain. An enriched environment is beneficial to the area that primarily controls thinking, learning and memory.
- Dr Diamond discovered that the first, second, third, fourth and fifth dendrites didn't grow any longer even though exposed to an enriched environment, but the sixth branch did.
- Stimulate the aged and reverse the effects of impoverished environments. Enriched environments have been used to reverse mental deterioration in elderly rats, whilst simultaneously causing brain growth. Everyone has the potential to make changes, no matter how dull the stimulation has been in the past.
- Mind machines subject the brain to intense amounts of stimulation and thus force-feed enrichment to your neurons and trigger rapid brain growth.
- One hour of reading in your chosen field each day will make you an authority in that field in 3 years, a national authority in that field in 5 years, and an international authority in that field in 7 years. Invest in Paul Scheele's PhotoReading Personal Learning Course and contact www.aggressivehealth.co.uk. When you read about it you'll know why!

Many people stop learning when they leave school. They develop a phobia of books and of the unfamiliar. Let this be someone else, not you! Embrace the unknown and expand your mind. What have you always wanted to learn or master? Maybe you've always wanted to learn to play a musical instrument? Maybe you've always wanted to learn how to play golf, tennis, squash or snooker? Maybe you've always wanted to increase your memory and IQ? Whatever ignites the flame of desire within you, begin today. Forget about results and enjoy getting lost within the activity. The joy and development comes in the doing, not the outcome! If you find yourself struggling, it's because your brain is figuring out a way for you to succeed. Be patient, persist, and you will.

      The choice is yours: A dull brain and a lifeless body, or a brain that is charged with electricity, searching for challenge, enrichment and novelty.

THE AGGRESSIVE HEALTH EVALUATION:
Do you challenge yourself and stimulate your brain frequently?
Do you have a ferocious desire to learn?

Every day, millions of people rely on chocolate, coffee, cakes and biscuits to increase the stimulation in their lives, compromising the performance of their brain and body. They wonder why they can't get motivated, become inspired or reach any level of creativity. Many people live lives of quiet desperation, whilst their mind and emotions remain out of control.

CHAPTER 14

FOOD FOR THOUGHT: HOW TO DEVELOP AN UNCONQUERABLE MIND AND BODY BY NOURISHING YOUR BRAIN AND NEUROTRANSMITTERS

Just stop for a moment and flick through this chapter. At first glance what you are about to discover may seem quite complex, but the distinctions that await you are critical in completing your understanding of AGGRESSIVE HEALTH.

THE IMPORTANCE OF THE MINDBODY CHEMICALS: NEUROTRANSMITTERS

Your brain is composed of billions of brain cells that are constantly talking to each other. Between each brain cell is a space, and it's between this space where all the communication takes place. In a nutshell, when one of your brain cells wants to communicate, it releases a chemical messenger into this space which is then picked up by another brain cell. The chemical messengers that deliver the messages are called neurotransmitters, and for each neurotransmitter there is neuroreceptor on the receiving cell ready to accept the message.

As you can easily see, neurotransmitters are communicators of information. Each and every one of them has a profound and important impact upon your life. Without them you'd lose the ability to think, experience emotions, process information, and basically stay alive. They are critical to memory, focus, learning, energy, happiness etc. and controlling them is ultimately down to what you eat and when. If imbalances occur you can experience all sorts of problems from anxiety and depression to sugar craving and low self esteem. It's up to you to take control and learn how to balance them. Food is the raw material, you are the scientist and your brain is the laboratory.

BALANCING THE NEUROTRANSMITTERS
AND FEELING GREAT

As you cruise through the rest of this chapter, take a brief look at what you're about to learn:

1. Endorphins: The Keys To Eternal Pleasure
2. Acetylcholine: Superstar Neurotransmitter of Memory and Thought
3. Norepinephrine: The Key To Staying Sharp And Alert
4. Dopamine/Serotonin: The Critical Neurotransmitter Axis
5. Nitric Oxide: Memory Enhancement and Powerful Erections

CONTROL YOUR BRAIN CHEMISTRY
AND CONTROL YOUR LIFE

The message of this chapter is simple: Food affects your brain chemistry, and your brain chemistry affects your mood. When your brain is balanced chemically, you will feel a sense of peace and calmness, whilst awakening your higher mind.

Sarah Leibowitz, Ph.D., one of the world's leading experts on the neurobiology of obesity, has demonstrated that various diets and various foods create very powerful changes in the brain.

The high fat/high carbohydrate 'junk food' diet alters the composition of the brain, stripping it of the neurotransmitters that foster a positive mood. This diet also dramatically increases the production of the hormones that cause overeating and bingeing. The brain of an obese person is chemically different from that of a thin person, and the habits that lead to obesity create a devastating downward spiral causing a biologically altered, inferior brain structure! The chain of events that lead to the downward spiral begins when the abuser creates a pleasurable association towards recreational/junk foods. Unfortunately, after the abuser has experienced the brief euphoric feeling that 'recreational food' supplies, they experience a debilitating 'physical low', caused by low blood sugar levels, unconsciously encouraging another fix.

Did you know that there are 40 million people in the U.S. reported as clinically depressed? The above conditions are all a result of a biologically altered brain, resulting from poor nutrition.

THE WORST CASE SCENARIO:
REFINED CARBOHYDRATES AND CRIME

Many of the foods served in jails include the following: sugar, coffee, white flour, margarine, mashed potatoes, quartered tomatoes, white bread, iceberg lettuce, pork chops, beef, and chicken.

To illustrate the power of food to control behaviour, a small study was carried out with inmates of a particular jail. It concluded that if you teach them to eat foods that help maintain stable blood sugar levels, only 20% return to crime, instead of the usual 80%. Researchers suggested that 90% of violent crimes are committed when the individual is suffering from low blood glucose (hypoglycaemia).

A brain deprived of its required fuel, shifts from higher cortical functions (conceptual, socially acceptable, knowing right from wrong) to lizard brain (fight or flight) functions. When the brain is in this state, even a minor stimulus can trigger off 'fight or flight' behaviour. Good nutrition protects the brain from entering 'fight or flight' mode, allowing it to function at a higher cortical level. Your brain is created daily from the food you eat, and your brain affects your behaviour. It's a basic law of behavioural biology!

1 - ENDORPHINS: THE KEYS TO PARADISE

Although endorphins are not technically neurotransmitters, their effects are similar. They were discovered in the 1970s and are your body's own opiates. When you think of opiates you probably think of drugs such as heroin, morphine and opium. But did you realise that the act of eating 'junk food' also supplies a hit of opiates to your brain?

People love to eat sweets and chocolate because they stimulate a short-lived endorphin 'high'. When someone injects heroin, they also stimulate their brain with a shot of opiates. So what's the difference? Dosage!

Think about it. Why is chocolate cake is a billion-pound industry? There's no logical reason to buy it. It's not nutritious. It makes you fat. It screws up your metabolism. And it's expensive. The only reason to buy it is because it feels so good to eat it!

In fact, the easiest way to make more endorphins in the short-term is by eating refined sugars and starches such as white flour breads, cereals, and pastas. But as you know these foods cause hormonal chaos on many levels.

DR ELLIOT BLASS TURNS UP THE HEAT

To highlight the power of recreational food, Dr Elliot Blass conducted some interesting experiments. His hypothesis was that sugar was somehow responsible for numbing pain in the same way endorphins do. He devised an experiment where rat pups placed their feet on a hot surface. In his research, he showed that after 11 seconds the rat pups became uncomfortable and jumped off. He then repeated the experiment, but gave the rat pups a sugar solution in advance. He couldn't believe what he saw! The rat pups didn't register the discomfort for 20seconds, doubling their pain tolerance. In the spirit of scientific research, Dr Blass wanted to know which neurochemical pathway was involved in numbing the pain. He devised a third experiment using the drug Naltrexone. Naltrexone is an opiate antagonist that's used in emergency rooms to bring heroine addicts out of a coma. Basically, Naltrexone only exerts its power on the endorphin system. So when Dr Blass gave the rat pups a dose of Naltrexone along with the sugar, there was no pain numbing effect. The endorphin stimulating effect of the sugar was nullified and their little paws were off the hot surface in 11 seconds again. The results were clear. Sugar creates pain tolerance by stimulating endorphins. Can you see why so many people are addicted to it?

WHY IS THERE SUCH A CURIOUS ATTRACTION BETWEEN HUMANS AND OPIATES?

Answer: Because opiates have a molecular structure similar to endorphin molecules, and the glucose receptor is closely associated with the endorphin system.

Although highly sophisticated, your brain was never designed to deal with sugar overload, but due to mass production of recreational convenience foods, sugar/carbohydrate addiction is now one of the most deadly addictions of all, along with smoking, alcoholism and drug abuse. Just as recreational drugs cause depression, low self-esteem, anxiety, and a myriad of other less than empowering states, the chronic use of food as a recreational drug also has this effect.

RECREATIONAL FOOD ABUSE CAUSES MORE DEATHS THAN RECREATIONAL DRUG ABUSE

In America 'junk food' is consumed at a frightening rate and 70% of all deaths in the U.S. can be linked to 'junk food' abuse. It is an addiction that is taking over the world. The addictive components of tea, coffee, chocolate and cocoa are all chemically related to 'speed' (amphetamine).

Even though cocaine and heroin (two of the most deadly drugs) are responsible for causing misery amongst many of their abusers, they don't account for anywhere near the same number of deaths associated with poor nutritional habits. Cocaine and heroin kill approximately 3000 people per year, 1500 each.

The problem with recreational convenience food is that it is often loaded with sugar, toxins and cooked fats. It causes massive increases in insulin, and simultaneous increases in body fat and toxicity. The endorphins that are released whilst eating these 'junk foods', prime the brain and create more cravings, until another shot of opiates hits the brain, encouraging the binge cycle. There aren't a lot of fat heroin addicts, but there are plenty of fat endorphin addicts. Food is the key to controlling your overall mood and emotions. Use it wisely.

ACCESSING A FLOOD OF MOOD ENHANCING NEUROCHEMICALS WITH MIND MACHINES

Another function of endorphins is to shield you from the psychological and physical effects of extreme stress. As stress mounts, your endorphins counteract some of the effects of the stress response. In an effort to alleviate stress and stimulate a quick endorphin 'boost', many people reach for recreational/junk food.

Do you want a better way to produce states of euphoria, energy, comfort, relaxation and joy, rather than turning to food? Mind machines may be the answer for you. I've used them to maintain balance when a hectic work schedule presents itself. If you are reading this book with the intention of losing unwanted fat, you need to break the habit of using recreational foods to activate your natural reward system. I recommend mind machines as a powerful alternative.

The habit of choosing food to alter your state is nothing but a calculated act of neurochemical self-adjustment. Just as a heroin addict is adjusting his or her neurochemical balance by consuming an endorphin substitute, many people use food to trigger the release of endorphins. These unconscious acts cause our brains to release the same neurochemicals associated with motherly love, happiness, comfort, and fulfilment, but as you know if you've read AGGRESSIVE HEALTH from cover to cover, there are many downsides.

When you use mind technology, you immediately produce rapid alterations in brain chemistry, restoring the natural balance of pleasure neurochemicals depleted by food or substance abuse. Simultaneously you strengthen and exercise the pleasure pathways within your brain. What a deal!

EUPHORIA IN THE WOMB

Your first experience of 'endorphin euphoria' was in your mother's womb. When she was pregnant she would have been producing levels of endorphins at least eight times higher than normal! If you were breastfed you would have benefited from the blissful effects of endorphins present in your mother's milk. Studies have shown that when babies are separated from their mothers, they display high levels of anxiety. If, however, the synthetic equivalent of endorphins is fed to them their anxiety disappears and they return to their blissful state. Endorphins alleviate anxiety and act as a substitute for motherly love and nourishment. Make sure you choose wisely where you get your next fix!

HOW TO BOOST ENDORPHINS NATURALLY

So, you've had enough of using artificial means to stimulate your brain. You want to produce more endorphins on a consistent basis using natural measures. The answer: Exercise. A mere thirty minutes or more of exercise will give you the same endorphin boost as a chocolate bar, but it will last all day, not just a few seconds. The best time to workout is in the morning, especially if you want to start your day on an endorphin high.

Endorphins have numerous roles within the body but essentially exist to bring you pleasure. Pleasure in the presence of pain, pleasure to alleviate stress, pleasure to reward you, pleasure to enhance or suppress memories and pleasure to determine what information you filter into your brain. If you want to learn massive amounts of information, then ensure you are in an environment that is incredibly pleasurable. It is a scientific fact that when your endorphins are flowing, information is more easily assimilated. Mind machines can cause endorphin levels to rise, which is why learning can be easier when you use the power of these machines. Endorphins encourage you to continue what you're doing; they stimulate interest, increase your focus, and help you develop laser-like concentration. Let's re-cap:

- Endorphins are critical in pain reduction, and are released in response to virtually any kind of significant physical or emotional stress.
- Endorphins exist to bring you pleasure. Pleasure in the presence of pain, pleasure to alleviate stress, pleasure to reward you, pleasure to enhance/suppress memories and pleasure to determine what information you filter into your brain.
- Dr Elliot Blass has shown that sugar stimulates endorphins but at the expense of wrecking your health and creating cycles of addiction. Many people are addicted for this reason. Be warned!
- People love to eat chocolate because it stimulates a short-lived endorphin 'high'. However, a mere thirty minutes or more of exercise will give you the same boost that will last all day, not just a matter of seconds. Workout in the morning and you'll feel great all day.
- The natural euphoric high that is associated with running is caused by an increased flow of endorphins in the brain.
- By using mind machines, you'll immediately begin to produce rapid alterations in brain chemistry, restoring the natural balance of pleasure neurochemicals depleted by food or substance abuse, whilst simultaneously strengthening and exercising the pleasure pathways within your brain. What a deal!
- Endorphins encourage you to continue what you're doing. They stimulate interest, focus, and concentration.
- Mind machines can cause endorphin levels to rise, which is why learning can be easier when you use the power of these machines.
- If you want to learn massive amounts of information, ensure you are in an environment that is incredibly pleasurable. People learn better when they are having fun, which translates this: People learn better when their endorphins are stimulated.
- Spend some time figuring out what you love, is it dancing, gymnastics, Bodyflow™, martial arts, scuba diving, clubbell® swinging, kettlebell swinging, surfing, mountain biking, reading, exercising, playing sports... you name it – If you love it – do it! There will be an endorphin reward waiting for you.
- Use mind machines to get your endorphin juices flowing and information will become more easily assimilated. And to enhance the process of information assimilation even more, embrace...

2 - THE ESSENTIAL MEMORY NUTRIENT – ACETYLCHOLINE

In the middle of the 20th Century, scientists discovered that acetylcholine is the most abundant neurotransmitter in the brain. Essential to higher mental processes such as learning and memory, acetylcholine has adopted the reputation of 'superstar neurotransmitter of memory and thought.' It is particularly concentrated in the hippocampus, the structure essential to the formation and recall of long-term memories. The power of this neurotransmitter is such that if you have a poor memory, but are too young to be suffering from memory impairment associated with old age, you've probably just a simple acetylcholine deficit. Acetylcholine helps neurons in the cortex retain the imprint of incoming information.

Even the confusion and loss of memory associated with Alzheimer's disease has now been linked in part to a lack of acetylcholine in certain areas of the brain. If however, acetylcholine is injected into those areas, or the subjects are given acetylcholine-boosting drugs, sufferers of the disease respond with dramatic gains in memory and other mental abilities.

WHAT ARE THESE SUBSTANCES THAT
INCREASE THE MEMORY MOLECULE?

Acetylcholine is produced within neurons by a complicated chemical process that requires oxygen, glucose, and the action of an enzyme, dependent on vitamins B5, C and choline (the primary ingredient of lecithin). The combination of B5, C and choline is incredibly effective in enhancing memory and mental performance. But don't let this confuse you...

WHETHER IT'S AN INCREASE IN MEMORY
OR A CLEARER STATE OF MIND, CHOLINE IS THE KEY

Fortunately the brain has the ability to absorb choline very rapidly and in times of stress, it has been proven that choline can provide an immediate boost to brain power. If you are studying or have a test or exam, a dose of choline is vital and will allow your brain to operate at its very best. Studies have shown that choline can also improve overall mental functioning and thought transmission, strengthening neurons in the memory centre of your brain. To illustrate this point, students at the Massachusetts Institute of Technology who took choline found they could learn longer lists of words and could remember better. Many people who take choline state that they have a clearer perception and feel that their overall mental functioning is enhanced. UC Berkeley researcher Mark Rosenzweig has shown a direct connection between acetylcholine and intelligence.

Acetylcholine also helps perform many functions outside the brain. For example if you read the Arnold Schwarzenegger Encyclopaedia of Body Building, you'll find that Arnold himself used lecithin (also rich in choline), in his early days of training, helping to build high levels of acetylcholine in his body and thus enhance the action of the nerve cells in his muscles to trigger muscle action. If it's good enough for Arnie then it's good enough for you! So what are the foods of choice if you want to build acetylcholine levels in your brain?

LOOK NO FURTHER THAN THE TWO ALMIGHTY SUPERFOODS: BEE POLLEN AND HEMP SEEDS

When you begin consuming bee pollen, you are getting an expceptional source of choline, via lecithin. Clinical evidence strongly indicates that lecithin is critical in preventing deterioration of your brain, by providing the raw materials necessary for the formation of acetylcholine. Usually it is recommended that you take vitamin C and vitamin B5 (pantothenic acid) with your lecithin, because these vitamins are needed to transform lecithin into acetylcholine, but in the case of bee pollen these vitamins are already present. Not only that, but with bee pollen you are getting a cocktail of 96 nutrients all in one hit. Dr Stephen Davies, a medical researcher, tested blood levels of B vitamins in thousands of people and found more than 7 in every 10 to be deficient. Use Bee pollen to your advantage today, superior brain health awaits.

HEMP SEEDS... THE REMARKABLE STORY CONTINUES...

Another all powerful brain food that will serve you for the rest of your life, is the hemp seed. The nutrients I want to focus on here are choline, inositol, lecithin.

- ✓ Choline is vital for nerve impulses from the brain through the nervous system. It also assists for liver and gall bladder function.
- ✓ Inositol is calming to the nervous system, promoting more harmony and balance. It also promotes hair growth, helps maintain optimal cholesterol levels and prevents artery hardening.
- ✓ Lecithin is a lipid found in the protective sheaths surrounding the brain and nervous system. Many people buy lecithin for its ability to breakdown fat, forgetting it also enhances liver activity, enzyme production and as we've already found, is a vital raw material for the production of acetylcholine.

AFA ALGEA IN E3LIVE HARMONISES BRAIN FUNCTION

The Central American University Report (1994) on malnourished grammar school children stated that academic results and exam scores improved tremendously after trials of wild blue-green algae were administered. E3Live has a unique energy that has an affinity to improving brain function. Clinical research shows that AFA algae balances EEG readings and improves central nervous functioning. In addition to consuming E3Live, eat more activated nuts and sprouted seeds in your daily nutritional routine. In the process of germination, the desirable phosphorus compounds such as lecithin increase dramatically. If you are an athlete...

HEMP IS BECOMING THE FOOD OF CHOICE FOR ATHLETES EVERYWHERE

When the blood profiles of marathon runners were studied, choline levels fluctuated dramatically. Researcher Richard Wurtman discovered that after 26 miles of running, choline drops by a staggering 40%. Studies also show that swimmers are able to swim for longer, without the perils of muscle fatigue, when they include choline rich foods such as hemp seeds, sprouted seeds and bee pollen into their diet.

MANIPULATE THE CHEMISTRY OF YOUR BRAIN
AND UNLEASH SUPER-INTELLIGENCE

As your diet changes, so does the chemistry of your brain, leaving it up to you to make the right choices. Treat acetylcholine as the foundation of your memory and brainpower and do all you can to eat foods that stimulate its production. Let's re-cap:

- Acetylcholine has adopted the reputation of 'superstar neurotransmitter of memory and thought'.
- Acetylcholine helps neurons in the cortex retain the imprint of incoming information.
- A simple acetylcholine deficit is often the answer if you have a poor memory, but too young to be suffering from memory impairment associated with old age.
- Even the confusion and loss of memory associated with Alzheimer's disease has now been linked to a lack of acetylcholine in certain areas of the brain. If however, acetylcholine is injected into those areas, or the subjects are given acetylcholine-boosting drugs, sufferers of the disease respond with dramatic gains in memory and other mental abilities.
- Keep brain levels of acetylcholine optimal and you'll help prevent memory loss and cognitive dysfunction.
- Studies of normal subjects show significant increases in scores on memory tests when given substances that increase the amount of acetylcholine in their brain.
- Acetylcholine is produced within neurons by a complicated chemical process that requires oxygen, glucose, and choline (the primary ingredient of lecithin).
- The combination of B5 and choline has proved effective in enhancing memory and mental performance.
- There is nothing difficult about restoring acetylcholine to normal levels, simply focus on sprouted nuts and seeds, such as hemp seeds and have a regular supply of bee pollen to hand. Clorophyll-based 'green drink' will supply about 2g of lecithin per serving. A recommended dose would be approximately 2-3g four times daily, for a total daily dosage of approximately 8-12g. Eat, juice and blend your greens and consume E3Live/wheatgrass juice daily.
- Fortunately the brain has the ability to absorb choline very rapidly and in times of stress, it has been proven that choline can provide an immediate boost to brain power. When studying or taking exams ensure you use these superfoods to your advantage. A simple dose will allow your brain to operate at peak levels of functioning, but what good is laser like memory if your mind is dull and listless?

3 – NOREPINEPHRINE:
THE KEY TO STAYING SHARP AND ALERT

Norepinephrine (NE) is a hormone that also functions as a neurotransmitter. It has an arousing, sharpening effect on the brain causing incredible alertness. NE is also vital in helping carry memories from short-term storage in the hippocampus to long-term storage in the neocortex.

Did you ever wonder why certain memories (especially ones that you experienced at moments of heightened arousal), remain vivid in your mind? That's NE in action. Whether it's great joy, intense fear, crisis, or love, when you're riding the wave of an adrenaline rush the memories are 'indelibly burned' into your memory. As mentioned earlier, however, too much norepinephrine can prevent the formation of new memories, and can interfere with rational thought and decision making, highlighting...

THE DANGERS AND EFFECTS OF THE DRUG 'SPEED'

NE plays a key role in memory and learning and the drug amphetamine (also known as speed) has a structure similar to NE. Although the drug is very dangerous with many side effects, students have often favoured it when cramming for exams. By eliminating the action of the adrenal glands and preventing the arousing effects, amphetamine stimulates a rapid increase in NE, enhancing the learning and memory processes. This unnatural state of intense mental alertness, allows large amounts of information to be absorbed and remembered (although many students use it to dance until dawn rather than cram for exams). But be warned, 'speed' can cause permanent brain damage and is often purchased illegally, having been mixed/cut with other toxic substances.

NE also governs your sleep patterns. Too much NE makes it almost impossible to fall asleep, which is why those who take 'speed' can often be found burning the midnight oil.

THE DANGERS OF THE DIET PILL ILLUSION

Did you know that many diet pills have been taken off the market because they contained amphetamine? The pills appeared to be useful to begin with because they stimulate NE which kills the appetite, causes insulin levels to drop, and fat to be burned as fuel. The only problem is that the body responds as if there is a famine and enters a survival/storage mode. The pills work well to cause an increase in metabolism, but at the expense of upsetting the body's natural rhythm. Drugs for weight loss are dangerous and unnecessary! If you are tempted to buy slimming pills, imagine yourself a year from now even fatter and more tired than you've ever been as you try to hold onto a life that is slipping away. I hope my point is clear, use food as your prescription and...

ACCESS YOUR OWN PURE NOREPINEPHRINE

Even though pure amphetamine is powerful, pure NE is superior in every way. Studies have concluded that when NE levels in the brain are reduced, memory and learning abilities drop dramatically. Cornell researchers found that by inhibiting the synthesis of NE in rats' brains, they interrupted their overall ability to remember for more than twenty-four hours.

Studies now show that if you increase NE levels in your brain, memory and learning ability increase dramatically. NE also allows the brain to return to a state of youthful flexibility and plasticity, allowing you to learn as much as you did when you were in your youth, a time when you were exposed to many forms of stimulation.

GIVE YOURSELF A MOOD BOOST –
INCREASE NOREPINEPHRINE IN YOUR BRAIN

NE is one of your primary natural happiness chemicals. With balanced levels in your brain, your mood will be heightened, you'll experience a more positive outlook on life. Insufficient levels of norepinephrine can cause depressed moods, an inability to concentrate, an inability to cope with stress, whilst preventing short-term memories from being stored as long-term memories. In addition, NE helps regulate your sex drive. When levels are low, the sexual urge diminishes dramatically.

The power of norepinephrine to elevate mood can be easily appreciated when you look at the life of a cocaine abuser. Cocaine is so powerful that even though the abuser may have a life of desperate misery, for the few minutes whilst they ride the NE 'high' caused by its brain altering effects – they'll be in a buoyant mood.

STIMULATE NOREPINEPHRINE THE EASY WAY

Exercise significantly increases norepinephrine production, improving appetite control, mood, sex drive and mental health. Ginkgo biloba has also received a great deal of publicity recently for its NE enhancing effects. NE tends to be depleted in certain areas of the brain in Alzheimer's patients, making Ginko a valuable supplement for prevention.

Ensure you lead a busy, confident, active, yet balanced lifestyle, full of love for what you are doing and the pleasure will be there for the taking. Let's re-cap:

- ◆ NE has an arousing, sharpening effect in the brain.
- ◆ NE plays a key role in memory and learning which is why students have been known to take the drug amphetamine (also known as 'speed') to cram for exams. It has a structure similar to NE.
- ◆ Many diet pills have been taken off the market because they contained amphetamine. Excessive NE kills the appetite indirectly, causing insulin levels to drop, allowing fat to be burned as fuel. The only problem is that the body goes into a survival state ensuring that anything that is eaten gets stored away in case

the artificial famine is repeated. Ultimately users gain more weight than they lost in the first place!

♦ Cornell researchers found that by inhibiting the synthesis of NE in rats' brains, they interrupted their overall ability to remember for more than twenty-four hours.

♦ If you increase NE levels in your brain you'll increase your memory and learning ability as your brain returns to a youthful state of flexibility and plasticity.

♦ NE is also one of your primary happiness chemicals. With balanced levels in your brain, your mood will be heightened and you'll experience more energy combined with a healthier outlook on life.

♦ Insufficient levels of norepinephrine can cause depressed moods, an inability to concentrate, an inability to cope with stress, and prevent the storage of long-term memories.

♦ NE also helps regulate sex drive. If levels of NE are too low, the sexual urge diminishes dramatically.

♦ The raw materials necessary for the production of norepinephrine are foods high in the amino acids phenylalanine and tyrosine. Hemp seeds are an excellent choice.

♦ Exercise significantly increases norepinephrine production, improving appetite control, mood, sex life and mental health. Now for the ultimate balancing act...

4 – THE CRITICAL NEUROTRANSMITTER AXIS: DOPAMINE AND SEROTONIN

Dopamine is partly responsible for creating mental energy and alertness. As you spark the fire of your brain's dopamine neurons, your outlook on the world will become more positive, lively and buoyant. When you exercise, increased levels of dopamine will give you the edge if you need to exercise longer.

The neurotransmitter serotonin is responsible for creating feelings of contentment and emotional control. With levels of serotonin balanced, you'll be free from the nagging temptations and cravings that plague so many people. You'll find it easy to say no to drugs, alcohol, binge eating and impulsive behaviour. These two neurotransmitters are part of a subtle balancing act.

SEROTONIN: THE MASTER WEIGHT-CONTROL DRUG

If you see a chocolate bar and automatically have to have it, pay attention! You may be suffering with low levels of serotonin.

The substance in your brain, partly responsible for carbohydrate cravings is MCH (melanin concentrating hormone). It is made in the hypothalamus and released in the frontal lobe, a part of the brain that makes decisions about what to eat. Since serotonin is the major neurotransmitter in the frontal lobe, when MCH is released, if levels of serotonin are too low, binge eating can prevail. In essence, too little serotonin may mean less control over your more animal-like impulses. Whatever you do, and whatever state of mind you are in…

TAKE CONTROL AND AVOID THE PERILS OF PROZAC

Emotions and moods are affected by serotonin, a lack of which can sometimes lead to depression. Take a look at the recreational food addicts. As the market place for these foods continues to expand, more and more people are becoming addicted to high carbohydrate foods that cause a transient increase in serotonin levels. The first by-product of excessive carbohydrate consumption is a corresponding increase in insulin levels, resulting in increased fat storage. But the worse is yet to come. If this spiral of addiction continues and insulin begins occupying the bloodstream morning, noon and night, the downward spiral becomes so devastating that the person begins to produce more 'bad' eicosanoids and begins to suffer from depression.

THE EICOSANOID LINK BETWEEN
SEROTONIN LEVELS AND DEPRESSION

Researchers discovered in 1983 that patients suffering with depression had two to three times more 'bad' eicosanoids in their spinal fluid, compared to those with normal mental health. The bad eicosanoid they singled out the most was PGE2. They also found elevated levels of it in their saliva. By balancing eicosanoids in your favour, and increasing the good ones such as PGE1 (a mood enhancer) you gain control at a level that no drug could ever achieve!

IS IT EASY TO SEE WHY DEPRESSION
IS REACHING EPIDEMIC LEVELS?

Anti-depressant drugs, like Prozac, are so powerful at elevating serotonin levels above normal, a bomb could explode and the user would still find it easy to remain relaxed. The downside is that the side effects rob the body of its biochemical integrity.

Prozac increases serotonin uptake in the brain, causing its users to feel an increased sense of well-being. The problem is it has potentially devastating side effects. It has been known to cause headaches, nausea, insomnia, and make its users anxious and jittery. It's also been known to cause heart seizures. A study from Harvard Medical School shows that 3.5% of the patients who took Prozac, became intensely violent and had a suicidal preoccupation after only 2-7 weeks.

As you can see, most drugs are used to suppress symptoms by inhibiting certain types of chemical reactions within the body. The problem is that when they bind to their targets, the cellular receptors, they don't have the same level of specificity as your own natural chemicals. What tends to happen is that they also interact with more cellular receptors than they should, which leads to devastating side effects. When you stimulate and balance your own internal chemistry naturally, you naturally engage your body's healing response.

If a life of disregard for your body has left you reaching for such drugs it's up to you to align yourself with the principles of AGGRESSIVE HEALTH and rebalance your biochemistry. What do I mean by balance? The re-establishment of neurotransmitter equilibrium and the core homeostatic processes that govern overall health.

CONSULT YOUR DOCTOR AND WAVE GOODBYE TO MANUFACTURED DRUGS

It doesn't take a genius to make the link between the number of people prescribed antidepressants who are also overweight and suffering from numerous illnesses. These drugs are fast becoming the nation's most popular mood enhancer. Too little serotonin can cause depression and violent behaviour. Too much serotonin can cause accelerated ageing, as insulin levels rise. Just like insulin and glucagon, serotonin and dopamine work in tandem. Ensure you keep the balance favourable.

RESTORE SEROTONIN LEVELS NATURALLY

Q: Should you devour as much carbohydrate as possible to restore serotonin levels?
A: No! Refined carbohydrates found in many convenience foods such as chocolate, crisps, breads, pastas and many snack foods are broken down quickly within your system and cause a rapid increase in blood sugar levels, which is a worse case scenario. Serotonin levels may rise, but the good feeling doesn't last, leaving its victim with a nagging sense of emotional malaise. If carbohydrates are used to enhance mood, gradually they become less and less stimulating and the user needs more to induce the 'good feeling'. Talk to an obese carbohydrate addict, and they'll tell you how much they can eat in one sitting!

The excessive levels of insulin cause an over production of bad eicosanoids (such as PGE2) which are strongly associated with depression. They also destroy the sensitivity of your insulin receptors and invite obesity, increasing your chance of almost every major illness in existence. Remember that most foods high in carbohydrate are also convenience foods high in sugar and rob your body of essential nutrients.

Q: Should you consume more serotonin?
A: No. Obviously you'd increase the amount of serotonin in your brain, but too much serotonin can cause platelet aggregation, increasing your chance of a heart attack.

Q: Should you supplement your diet with the precursor of serotonin, the amino acid tryptophan?
A: No. You can't buy tryptophan over the counter because it's banned! 38 people died of an adverse reaction to a contaminated batch of the product.

Q: Should you look to eat foods that are plentiful in the amino acid tryptophan?
A: Yes. Start with all your raw food favourites such as sprouted beans, activated nuts, such as almonds, hemp seeds etc. Pumpkin seeds are one of the best sources, as is

durian. If you are a meat eater, turkey is a great source as are most meats. If you're just after a snack, and want to unwind eat pumpkins seeds, almonds, chestnuts, peanuts, pecans, and walnuts and you'll feel more relaxed due to their high tryptophan content. Tryptophan is also the raw material and precursor of the sleep-inducing neurotransmitter melatonin.

Q: Is eating tryptophan foods all it takes?
A: Not entirely. The basics of AGGRESSIVE HEALTH are all critical. Superfoods rich in vitamin C and the B vitamins (especially B3 – niacin) help convert the amino acid tryptophan into serotonin – bee pollen is an excellent source of both. But just as important is the structure of your meals. Protein eaten on its own will help perk up your brain. The amino acid tyrosine will enter the brain and stimulate dopamine production.

ALL ABOARD! NEXT STOP – YOUR BRAIN CELLS!

Imagine a bus load of amino acids has just pulled up. If the tyrosine amino acids get off the bus and enter your brain cells, neuroactivity will speed up and you'll feel more sharp and alert. If more tryptophan amino acids get off, your brain will calm down and you'll feel more peaceful and tranquil. If you eat some carbohydrate with your protein, the corresponding rise in insulin keeps the tyrosine amino acids on the bus, allowing tryptophan to exit and enter the brain. Tryptophan will help you manufacture sleep inducing substances, such as serotonin and melatonin.

DOPAMINE: THE MASTER ENERGISER

Dopamine creates mental energy and alertness. The main function of dopamine is to help control physical movement. Levels of dopamine usually decrease with age, but with good dietary habits can easily be maintained.

If you see an elderly person struggle to co-ordinate a complex manoeuvre, you can assume they have low levels of dopamine in their brain. A lack of dopamine can cause a loss of co-ordination and muscular control and if the condition is left to worsen, muscular control diminishes and Parkinson's disease can often be the result.

If you are not yet convinced of the importance of maintaining your dopamine levels to ensure the serotonin-dopamine ratio is kept balanced, here are a few reasons to motivate you. High levels of dopamine:

- ✓ Increase your chance of achieving physical and mental longevity.
- ✓ Improve your overall mood and positive emotions.
- ✓ Increase your fat burning ability.
- ✓ Increase in your sex drive.
- ✓ Enhance your immunity.
- ✓ Improve your memory.
- ✓ Stimulate the pituitary gland to secrete growth hormone, giving you the greatest chance to burn fat, increase lean muscle mass and enhance mobility.

MANUFACTURING AND BOOSTING DOPAMINE

Dopamine and norepinephrine are manufactured in much the same way. The primary nutritional building blocks of both neurotransmitters are the amino acids tyrosine and phenylalanine. Remember the amino acid bus analogy and limit carbohydrate consumption if you want the most bang from your buck.

♦   The amino acid phenylalanine boosts the functioning of your brain and also suppresses the appetite. Good sources are almonds, avocados, lima beans, peanuts and seeds along with most protein rich foods.
♦   In studies where subjects were administered tyrosine, improvements were made in their ability to learn and assimilate information. Their ability to recall data improved and so did their reaction times. The tyrosine in sprouted hempseeds, almonds and avocados will help you concentrate. It can also be found in most protein rich foods.

FEED YOUR NEUROTRANSMITTERS
AND ELIMINATE STRESS AND DEPRESSION

When you are stressed, you begin to place high demands on your nutrient reserves. The same is true of your neurotransmitters because one of the responses to stress is that your brain's neurons are fired more frequently. If this is the case, it's up to you to include enough amino acids in your diet to regenerate your neurotransmitter status. Wheatgrass juice and E3Live are abundant in amino acids. Use them! If you want to engage in another activity that naturally increases dopamine then…

GET SWEATY TOGETHER: LOVERS OF SEX REJOICE

If you feel you are a little obsessed with sex, worry no more, everything is right about sex, as long as both parties are willing! Sex stimulates dopamine. In fact, people who have active sex lives have more powerful and better functioning immune systems and are less prone to a whole host of mental disorders. Although I don't want you to think of yourself as a 'dirty rat', research shows that when male rats have orgasms, a tremendous amount of dopamine is released into the synapses in their brain. Sex is a proven method of making more dopamine, which can lead to increased longevity and a life of vigour and well-being.

DON'T BE SAD, LET NATURE LOOK AFTER YOU

People are happier in the summer because they venture outside more, and literally 'see' more sunlight. When exposed to natural sunlight the brain produces more serotonin. And for those of you in live in less temperate climates, it isn't the absence of light in the winter that prevents you from 'getting enough' of this vital nutrient, it's just you may not be going outside as much. The light is still there in the winter but the cold months prevent people from venturing outside.

Seasonal affective disorder (SAD) is caused by a lack of natural sunlight, preventing sufficient serotonin from being manufactured, causing the unfortunate carbohydrate cravings that can so often lead to a downward spiral of ill health.

The answer is to eat an abundance of chlorophyll rich foods (for liquid sunshine), exercise outside, and use mind machines to your advantage. Bright light therapy and negative ion generators will also help anyone who suffers severely with this disorder. These methods are natural, they represent the best ways in which you can increase brain serotonin levels and decrease your craving for carbohydrates along with what you've discovered so far.

BECOMING 'ONE' WITH NATURE

Many people suffer from lack of sleep, natural light deprivation, and the perils of convenience food. These problems cause depletion of natural serotonin levels and can be linked to a simple artificial existence.

Look at the stress that exists in society today, excessive work, redundancies, failed marriages, the problems with drugs, alcohol and smoking, not to mention the never ending supply of convenience foods, all designed to strip your pockets of money and destroy your health. Are you surprised many people feel drawn towards the so-called 'happy pills' such as Prozac? With serotonin levels decreasing, if people don't get a prescription for an antidepressant, they often try to self medicate with food. The upshot is that whilst they add extra fat to their body, they suffer the problems associated with serotonin deprivation. Your serotonin levels influence whether or not you are depressed, prone to violence, irritable, impulsive or gluttonous. Some people even consider suicide! Even though there are hundreds of neurotransmitters in your brain, serotonin may be one of the most important.

BACK TO THE ALPHA-STIM FOR ULTIMATE STIMULATION

If you are substantially overweight, you will need to rely on other measures to improve the levels of serotonin in your brain. Begin with the Alpha Stim! It is incredibly powerful and has the capacity to restore neurotransmitter equilibrium. It is at the leading edge of mind technology and can also be used as a powerful pain healing device. You'll be able to purchase one at www.aggressivehealth.co.uk. Let's re-cap:

♦ The amino acid tyrosine is the main building block of dopamine. Dopamine is linked to mental energy, vigilance, and alertness. By firing the dopamine neurons in your brain you'll become more positive, more buoyant, and even more cheerful.

♦ In studies where subjects were administered tyrosine, improvements were made in concentration and learning ability. Their ability to recall data improved and so did their reaction times. Eat protein on an empty stomach and you'll feel the effects of tyrosine revving up your brain.

- If you want tyrosine to enter your brain rapidly, remember that it competes with other amino acids such as tryptophan to enter your brain. Tryptophan stimulates serotonin production. So eat your tyrosine foods first and avoid excessive carbohydrate consumption.
- Your emotions and moods are affected by serotonin, a lack of which can often lead to depression. To boost serotonin levels with food, eat your protein with some carbohydrates. The carbs stimulate insulin which drags the larger amino acids away leaving tryptophan to hop across the blood-brain barrier to make serotonin.
- MCH (melanin concentrating hormone) is produced in your brain and is one factor responsible for carbohydrate craving. It is made in the hypothalamus, but is released in the frontal lobe, a part of the brain that makes decisions about what to eat. Since serotonin is the major neurotransmitter in the frontal lobe, when MCH is released, if levels of serotonin are too low, binge eating can prevail.
- One of the responses to stress is that your brain's neurons are fired more frequently. You must have enough amino acids in your diet to regenerate critical neurotransmitters.
- Seasonal affective disorder (SAD) is caused by a lack of natural sunlight and prevents the manufacture of serotonin. Carbohydrate cravings are at their worst during this period, but can be eliminated with chlorophyll rich foods, the use of the mind machines, exercise (preferably outside), meditation, bright light therapy and negative ion generators. Call this the shotgun approach and you'll find it easy to succeed.
- If you want to unwind eat pumpkin seeds, durian, almonds, chestnuts, peanuts, pecans, and walnuts and you'll feel more relaxed due to their high tryptophan content. Turkey would be your food of choice if you were a lover of meat.
- If you want to concentrate choose brazil nuts, cashews, hazelnuts, macadamias, pine nuts, and pistachios. Remember to soak all of your nuts to activate them!

5 – NITRIC OXIDE AND MEMORY FORMATION

In 1998 the Nobel Prize in Medicine was awarded to Robert Furchgott, Ferid Murad, and Louis Ignarro for their research into the gaseous proto-hormone known as nitric oxide. Its role in memory formation is critical. When information gets stored in your short-term memory, nitric oxide is responsible for most of the reinforcement process allowing the memory to become properly encoded in long-term memory.

If you wish to keep your brain healthy until the final moments of your life and maintain the ability to translate short-term memories into stable long-term memories then continue to ensure you eat foods that are rich in the amino acid arginine that stimulate the production of nitric oxide.

In 1958 scientists from the Soviet Union made an important discovery. They found high levels of the fat absorbing amino acid arginine present in walnuts, pine nuts, pistachios, almonds, and peanuts.

Without enough arginine in your diet, you'll find it virtually impossible to make nitric oxide. Let's re-cap:

♦ The gaseous proto-hormone known as nitric oxide is critical for reinforcing memories stored in your short-term memory allowing them to become encoded in long-term memory.

♦ Arginine also stimulates the release of growth hormone from the pituitary gland, helping to stimulate muscle growth.

♦ Arginine-rich foods include soybeans, walnuts, pine nuts, pistachios, almonds, and peanuts. If you are a lover of meat, turkey would be the food of choice.

THE JOY OF SEXUAL LONGEVITY

Many factors are associated with age-associated sexual decline. Poor nutrition leads to poor hormonal communication, and when testosterone levels begin to decline, libido decreases in both sexes. At approximately age 50 testosterone levels gradually decrease, causing a simultaneous drop in sexual performance. However, one hormone is never responsible for the entire picture. Take a look at how various neurotransmitters affect sexual function.

♦ Dopamine is a key element in sexual desire and its power can be easily illustrated when you look at the results of the drug L-dopa on Parkinson's patients. The drug causes a rise in dopamine and almost immediately, patients are known to experience an increase in sex drive.

♦ Acetylcholine is important in controlling the blood flow to the genitals, in males and females. It is also a key factor in the sense of relaxation that has to be present for males to achieve erections and orgasms.

♦ Norepinephrine is the neurotransmitter that must be present in adequate amounts if you want to experience sexual arousal. If you've ever complained about being too tired to have sex, you may have simply been suffering from a norepinephrine deficit.

Nitric oxide is needed for penile erections, and for enhanced blood flow to the female genitalia. As you've just discovered, the amino acid arginine is responsible for the production of Nitric oxide. Look no further than walnuts, pine nuts, pistachios, almonds, and peanuts for more arginine. If you are a lover of meat, turkey would be the food of choice.

One supplement that will arouse your interest is Ginseng. For many years it has been used to enhance sexual vigour and an interesting experiment at Southern Illinois University illustrates this beautifully. Male rats given a diet that included ginseng took an average of just 14 seconds to initiate sexual contact with female rats (I like their style!), while male rats given no ginseng took an average of 100 seconds (I'm still suitably impressed – the term 'you dirty rat' has a whole new meaning).

E3LIVE AND COMPLETE PEACE OF MIND

Your brain comprises just 2% of your total body weight, but uses an enormous 20% of your body's energy resources. If there is the slightest break in the amino acid-peptide link, you may experience memory loss, mental fatigue or nervous disorders. The amino acid peptides are precursors of the all-important neurotransmitters, which carry messages from the brain to ordinary muscles, and from the organs back to the brain. For total nourishment and complete peace of mind use E3Live daily. The complete amino acid profile of AFA within E3Live assists in nourishing the brain and nervous system.

ARE YOU READY FOR THE CHALLENGE?

Recent research has shown that the mind and body have their own patterns of rest or alertness, with one predominant cycle that occurs approximately every 90 minutes, when the body stops externally oriented behaviour and takes about 15minutes to relax and replenish its energy. This is known as the ultradian rhythm. If you've ever found yourself daydreaming and feeling a little docile it was probably your body's natural stress control system kicking in.

By ignoring the relaxation response on a continual basis and overriding this ultradian rhythm, you could risk burnout and disease. Remember the salmon? Ensure you take a short break when it's time to relax and make use of the powerful mind machines! You'll feel a lot better than if you have a cup of coffee or push yourself to concentrate more.

♦ Use exercise and mind machines to stimulate your endorphins. You'll want to study more, learn more and will automatically become an information hungry machine!

♦ Use the power of raw greens and sprouted nuts and seeds to supply enough choline to produce acetylcholine.

♦ Exercise to increase the production of norepinephrine and dopamine. Also consume foods high in the amino acids tyrosine and phenylalanine. Hempseeds are an excellent choice as are most protein sources.

♦ If you want to unwind eat pumpkin seeds, durian, almonds, chestnuts, peanuts, pecans, and walnuts and you'll feel more relaxed due to their high tryptophan content, thus stimulating serotonin.

♦ If you want to concentrate choose brazil nuts, cashews, hazelnuts, macadamias, pine nuts, and pistachios. Remember to soak and sprout all nuts!

♦ Consume food high in the amino acid arginine to promote sexual vigour by stimulating nitric oxide. Look towards walnuts, pine nuts, pistachios, almonds, and peanuts for more arginine, and if you love meat choose turkey.

♦ Use Mind machines to re-establish neurotransmitter equilibrium and promote peak performance states of mind.

- ◆ Bee pollen is one of the many powerful superfoods rich in both B vitamins and vitamin C. In times of stress both are needed. Vitamin C will help you recover from adrenal stress from excessive work. Both B and C vitamins help support the conversion of the amino acid tryptophan found in protein into serotonin.
- ◆ One of the purposes of sleep is to re-establish neurotransmitter equilibrium. If you don't give your body enough building blocks to feed your neurotransmitters you'll need more sleep. AFA algae has a complete amino acid profile, delivering these building blocks.
- ◆ AFA found in E3Live improves children's academic performance – 1995, Sevulla et al, Univ. Centro Americana
- ◆ AFA found in E3Live improves Attention Deficit Disorder (ADD) – 1997 Jarratt, C, et al, The Centre for Family Wellness, Harvard, MA
- ◆ AFA found in E3Live reduces symptoms of Alzheimer's Disease – 1985, Cousens, Orthmedicine, Vol. 8, p.1-2

Superior nutrition specifically enhances our ability to excel as human beings – physically, mentally, emotionally and spiritually. Poor nutrition contributes to a "biologically altered brain" which functions at an inferior level.

As you've just learned, the picture of nutritional mastery is only as good as the quality of each stroke. By learning to manipulate your neurotransmitters with the applied use of food, you've really begun to master AGGRESSIVE HEALTH. It is a place where responsibility is as real as it gets. It doesn't necessarily mean you'll always be perfect, but you'll know why you feel the way you do at any given time. The aim of this chapter was to give you the key that opens the door to optimal brain function. By using the latest mind technology and the applied use of food to stimulate your brain, you'll become an information absorbing machine able to master many areas of your life.

Without energy, it's hard to achieve anything in life, but when your mind and body are working in perfect unison, anything is possible. It starts with AGGRESSIVE HEALTH and as far as I'm concerned everything else is simply an extension. AGGRESSIVE HEALTH makes you feel excellent. You don't need excessive amounts of money or drugs, you just need to understand how the combined power of peak performance nutrition, mind technology and exercise affects you.

The choice is yours. A brain that waits patiently, not knowing when it's going to get its full complement of essential nutrients, or a brain that is powerful and on purpose.

THE AGGRESSIVE HEALTH EVALUATION:
Do you eat with purpose?
Do you eat in a way that influences your mood?
Do you eat the necessary foods for the stimulation and balance of your neurotransmitters?
Do you eat enough protein and supply the essential amino acids necessary for a peak performance mind?

Everyone would prefer to die from natural causes rather than some debilitating disease. But what's the point of living to a 'ripe-old age' if your mind isn't also alive and vibrant. Without your 'marbles' you'd surely be lost...

CHAPTER 15

DISCOVER HOW EXERCISE IS THE GATEWAY TO SUPERIOR MENTAL HEALTH AND LONGEVITY

Studies from the Russian space program have found that young cosmonauts subjected to the forced inactivity of space flight, fall prey to depression. However, if they are put on a schedule of regular exercise, the depression is avoided.

With this information, why do physicians often prescribe anti-depressant drugs to their depressed patients when exercise appears to be a much better prescription?! What is it about exercise that causes the reversal of depression and the re-balancing of the body? The answer lies with a class of neurochemicals called catecholamines. When physicians prescribe drugs in an effort to raise the levels of these neurochemicals, horrific side effects are often the result.

Prozac has been known to cause headaches, nausea, insomnia, and make its users anxious/jittery. It's also been known to cause heart seizures. A study from Harvard Medical School shows that 3.5% of the patients who took Prozac, became intensely violent and had a suicidal preoccupation after only 2-7 weeks.

THE ONLY SIDE EFFECT OF EXERCISE IS EUPHORIA

Exercise is holistic. By engaging in physical activity, chemical messages are sent back and forth between your brain and various muscle groups. Part of this flow of biochemical information stimulates the production of catecholamines. Thus, whenever a doctor writes a prescription for an antidepressant, he is handing out a substitute for the body's own inner prescription, which is filled by exercise. The news that exercise offsets ageing has been well publicised, although its preventive effect on depression may not be as well known.

Exercise can also increase the production of the neurotransmitter norepinephrine and the 'feel good chemicals' endorphins – directly benefiting mood and often relieving depression. Depression is not only painful emotionally, but is destructive to memory. A number of studies have indicated that exercise is incredibly effective at dispelling depression and in many cases more effective than traditional therapies, including psychological counselling. Many problems associated with the mind and psyche can be overcome by controlling your biochemistry with correct nutrition and the application of exercise and movement.

RUN FOR YOUR LIFE!

Studies show that vigorous exercise can increase your brainpower, regardless of your current abilities. A young group of cross-country runners were tested for their overall cognitive ability during their 'off-season'. The results were recorded and compared with those taken at the end of the season. During this time they were running an average of at least thirty miles per week. By the end of the season, when tested, their cognitive ability had increased dramatically.

PLAY YOUR WAY TO GREATER INTELLIGENCE

An experiment with young, healthy monkeys also showed remarkable results. A large group was split into three:

♦ Group one was kept sedentary.
♦ Group two was given a running wheel.
♦ Group three was given an intricate series of ropes and bridges to play on.

Groups two and three grew more capillaries to their brain cells and showed an increase in their cognitive abilities, allowing their brains to utilise more oxygen and nutrients. The monkeys in group three with the complex play structures grew the largest number of dendritic connections, indicating that exercise is most valuable when combined with stimulating challenges.

KEEP IT SIMPLE FOR A HIGH PERFORMANCE MIND

Even a simple exercise program of 30 minutes of walking per day over a ten-week period has been showed to be particularly effective at improving memory. One study compared the memories of a group of elderly people. Half the group were sedentary, the other half were on a walking program. Over a period of several weeks the group that exercised showed significant improvement in memory skills, while the sedentary group remained the same.

THE NATURE OF YOUTH LEADS TO NATURAL BRILLIANCE

The simplest technique for supercharging your brain is movement. The less you move, the more likely you are to suffer from cognitive decline. Think about it, in the years when your brain was developing at lightning like speed, between the moment you were born and for the first few years of your life, you engaged in all sorts of movement. When was the last time you saw a baby being rocked in a chair or in their mothers arms? They crave movement! When was the last time you saw some kids spinning around and around until they fell over? Do you remember what it was like to roll down a grassy hill? As adults we do a number of things, activities at weekends, mountaineering, sky-diving, go-carting, dancing, sports, jet ski-ing, the list goes on. All these things require movement.

HAS YOUR LIFE BECOME MOTIONLESS?

The bottom line is simple: If you've fallen into a lifestyle that demands little movement, you're more likely to suffer from motion deprivation. If you spend most of the day sitting still, whilst your fingers tap, tap, tap away on a keyboard, only to go home and slouch in front of the television, it's time you made some changes. Start now by getting up and spinning around for a few moments: Clockwise to begin with then anticlockwise.

Movement stimulates the fluids of the inner ear, known as the vestibular system. This stimulation sends a flood of electrical impulses into your cerebellum and from there into the rest of the brain, including the pleasure and learning centres of the limbic system. Motion has amazing effects on your intelligence by directly stimulating learning.

Let's dig a little deeper so you fully understand why exercise will powerfully stimulate your brainpower. You've discovered what exercise does for your body but what about your brain?

NURTURE YOUR NATURAL NERVE GROWTH FACTOR

Mary was 76 years old and lay in her hospital bed somewhere between consciousness and unconsciousness. Alzheimer's had ravaged her mind. She didn't have a wisp of a memory, or any sense of personality. Fortunately, the doctors at the Karolinska Institute in Stockholm, Sweden, believed they could help her with a bold new innovative neurological treatment. With the support of her husband, the doctors began the experimental procedure that would hopefully save her from a life of 'nothingness'.

The treatment began with the surgeons drilling a small hole into her skull and inserting a catheter directly into her brain. They then began dripping a solution containing nerve growth factor into the catheter. The goal was to stimulate Mary's neurons to grow new dendritic branches and revive enough of her neurons to bring her brain back to life. Patiently they waited. Hours turned into days, and days turned into weeks, until finally a breakthrough.

Three weeks into the treatment and the doctors noticed something very significant, Mary's expressions started to became more lucid and gradually she became more aware of her surroundings.

The power of the treatment restored Mary's consciousness and within a short period of time she began to speak. One day, when her husband was at her bedside, she began to talk quietly to him about their life together. Her memories came flooding back. They both cried as they held each other in their arms. Nerve growth factor saved her. It's up to you to…

STIMULATE THE WONDER DRUG NATURALLY

Nerve growth factor (NGF) is a virtual wonder drug for the brain. It is similar to a brain hormone that stimulates the regeneration of the brain: brain-derived neurotropic factor (BDNF). NGF and BDNF are both produced most abundantly when the body is physically active. In all likelihood, these important brain chemicals were created by the evolutionary process to support the brain as it withstood physical challenges.

Everyone can produce nerve growth factor on a day to day basis by doing one thing: Exercise. Physical activity maintains a youthful brain that's vital, and regenerative throughout your entire life. Exercise is the key to the fountain of youth.

The greatest effects of exercise on both NGF and BDNF are in the most plastic areas of the brain, including the hippocampus (the brain's primary memory centre). This regional concentration accounts for much of the improvement in memory experienced by people who begin to exercise. NGF and BDNF, however, also support neurons throughout the brain, in the following ways:

- ♦ They transport BDNF to the forebrain cholinergic neurons.
- ♦ They 'rescue' damaged neurons from imminent death.
- ♦ They increase the production of the important neurotransmitters, acetylcholine and dopamine, and increase the number of dopamine receptors.
- ♦ They protect brain cells by increasing the activity of neuronal free-radical scavengers.

Even though cortisol, produced by stress, destroys BDNF, exercise can help to restore levels. Exercise also helps reduce cortisol secretion by controlling insulin levels.

BURN STRESS OUT OF YOUR BODY

The more you develop your cardiovascular system, the more you develop your ability to deal with stress. When you have a low resting heart rate, as a result of exercise, it prevents your adrenal glands from overreacting to stressors, and over-secreting cortisol. Exercise increases your immunity to disease by boosting the number of 'natural killer' cells, and by increasing your production of immunoglobin-A, an antibody that is one of your first lines of defence against infection.

Exercise protects your body against stress by burning off harmful stress chemicals. This is known as the tranquilliser effect and lasts for approximately four hours following exercise. It creates a virtual 'stress shield' during this time allowing you to ride the 'high' feeling great.

To achieve the tranquilliser effect, you must do just the right amount of exercise. In one study of joggers, those who jogged twenty-four miles per week, or about 30-45 minutes per day, experienced the tranquilliser effect the most. Those who jogged significantly less (fifteen miles per week), or significantly more (fifty-two miles per week), experienced less effect.

ENDORPHINS SWIM FREELY IN YOUR BODY AND BRAIN

Endorphins are at the heart of the tranquilliser effect. They are approximately 200 times more potent than morphine and increase approximately 500% during vigorous exercise. It only takes about fifteen to thirty minutes of exercise to stimulate their release and they remain active for about five hours – approximately the same length of time that the tranquilliser effect lasts. They are at their highest levels during the first thirty minutes after an exercise period.

In one classic study, a group of patients suffering with depression were split into three separate groups. One group was given psychotherapy for a limited number of weeks. Another group was given psychotherapy for as many weeks as the patients desired. The third group received no psychotherapy, but participated in a jogging program. At the end of the experiment, the patients in the jogging program had the lowest incidence of depression, while those in the unlimited psychotherapy program had the highest incidence.

In another study, patients suffering with depression jogged either five days a week, three days a week, or not at all. Those who jogged five days a week had significantly less depression at the end of the ten-week study. Those who jogged three days a week fared almost as well. Those who didn't jog didn't improve!

Exercise reduces depression for a number of reasons:
♦ It releases stimulating catecholamine neurotransmitters.
♦ It stimulates endorphin production.
♦ It increases oxygen flow to the brain.
♦ It helps remove neuronal debris.
♦ It stimulates the nervous system.
♦ It provides a powerful boost to self-esteem by increasing overall well-being.
♦ It improves body image and it increases feelings of personal power and responsibility.

Cognitive decline is often due to a lack of mental stimulation and a lack of physical movement. If you want to combine both and really set the wheels in motion, goto www.aggressivehealth.co.uk and purchase BodyFlow® by Scott Sonnon. Circular Strength Training™ will not only save your joints from a future of immobility, but will open the doorway to expressive movement, joint strength and more. Your body and brain has been programmed by evolution to require stimulation. Go for it!

ARE YOU READY FOR THE CHALLENGE?

I'm sure by now you've realised that exercise does more for your body and brain than you can ever imagine. Go and book a dance class, visit your local gym or maybe go for a snowboarding lesson/session! Whatever you choose to do, feel good about feeling good and remember all the reasons why exercise is going to enhance your life in every way. Here's a re-cap:

♦ Studies from the Russian space program have found that young cosmonauts subjected to the forced inactivity of space flight fall prey to depression, but when put on a schedule of regular exercise, this depression is avoided. Remember to use your rebounder.

♦ A number of studies have indicated that exercise is incredibly effective at dispelling depression and in many cases more effective than traditional therapies, including psychological counselling.

♦ Exercise protects your body against stress by burning off harmful stress chemicals. When you have a low resting heart rate, as a result of exercise, it prevents your adrenal glands from overreacting to stressors, and over-secreting cortisol. In fact, approximately four hours following exercise, people experience a tranquilliser effect that diminishes their physical response to stress. Remnants of the tranquilliser effect may remain for up to twenty-four hours.

♦ Endorphins, which are 200 times more potent than morphine, increase approximately 500% during vigorous exercise. After they are released, they remain active for about five hours – approximately the same length of time that the tranquilliser effect lasts.

♦ A group of cross-country runners were tested for cognitive ability during their off season, and again at the end of the season. They scored significantly higher after running at least thirty miles per week.

♦ Even a simple exercise program of 30 minutes walking per day over a ten-week period has been showed to be particularly effective at improving memory.

♦ Exercise is essential for optimal brain function. It supplies the brain with nerve growth factor, it reduces stress and it enhances neuronal metabolism.

♦ Nerve growth factor (NGF) is a virtual wonder drug for the brain. It is similar to a brain hormone that also stimulates regeneration of the brain: brain-derived neurotropic factor (BDNF). NGF and BDNF are both produced most abundantly when the body is physically active.

♦ Exercise increases your immunity to disease by boosting your immune system's number of 'natural killer' cells, and by increasing your production of immunoglobin-A, an antibody that is one of your first lines of defence against infection.

So there you have it, exercise increases the brain's uptake of oxygen and glucose. It speeds the removal of necrotic debris from brain cells. It enhances the production of various neurotransmitters such as norepinephrine and dopamine, and increases the availability of brain-related enzymes, such as Co-enzyme Q-10. It increases the output of endorphins. It decreases cortisol output leading to less perceived stress in any situation. It has a tranquillising effect on the brain decreasing any chance of depression. It helps lower blood pressure by helping to control insulin levels. It helps stabilise blood sugar levels (thereby helping to stabilise mood and energy) again by assisting in the control of insulin. Exercise also burns calories, increases muscle mass, and strengthens bones. So the question becomes, can you be bothered? If your answer isn't a resounding YES, read this chapter until it is!

THE AGGRESSIVE HEALTH EVALUATION:
Are you using exercise to enhance your mind as well as your body?

PART FOUR

EMBRACE AN UNLIMITED FUTURE AND PREPARE TO CREATE MIRACLES EVERY STEP OF THE WAY

CHAPTER 16

SQUEEZE EVERYTHING OUT OF LIFE AND PREPARE TO SHARE YOUR WISDOM WITH YOUR GREAT, GREAT GRANDCHILDREN

If someone offered you a magical pill that could guarantee all the above and more, would you say, "No thanks, I'd prefer to die from some crippling disease." The answer is obvious!

Even though most people would choose to avoid a crippling disease, you still hear the common catchphrase, "I don't want to live a long life, who wants to live for a long time if they are going to be senile and need looking after?" Or, "Everybody dies of something, sooner or later, so you might as well die from something that makes you feel good." But just stop for a minute. If you think that being alive for a shorter period of time will mean you'll remain mobile and fully functional until you pass away – Think again. Whether you die at 55 or 155, one thing is for certain, you are more likely to die from a disabling illness early on in life than in later life.

If you have the genetic potential to live between 120 and 140 years of age, there can only be one conclusion. To die any earlier means you must have engaged in daily habits or rituals that accelerated the ageing process, causing you to die prematurely.

Take a look at the suffering endured by victims of cancer, crippling strokes, or Alzheimer's disease. These horrific scenes cause people to see sense, not stupidity. What is my point? As usual it's simple. If you don't concern yourself with taking care of things now, you'll never reach your genetic potential. If you don't reach your genetic potential then the likelihood of you dying from a killer disease increases dramatically. It's better to die later than sooner, in peace, not in pain. And it's better to die as yourself, rather than a poor, brain-destroyed victim of Alzheimer's.

It's up to you to see the world the way it is and then make it the way you want it. Use the principles to make your life as perfect as possible and prepare to remain youthful in a world that seems to age faster than necessary.

REACHING OUT FOR THE MAXIMUM

When I found out that the likely maximum lifespan of a human being is in the region of 120 to 150 years (or above), I was curious to say the least. I wanted to know everything that could allow me to reach this maximum. Out of a range of possibilities, there exists a magic formula that dramatically lengthens the life span in animals. This magic formula is likely to work for humans because it's been tested on almost every species alive to date. If you want to reach your genetic potential and live a totally vivacious life, it's time you learnt about …

THE GREAT CALORIE RESTRICTION EXPERIMENTS

University of California expert on ageing, Dr. Roy Walford, has reported that cutting down on food consumption is the only method that retards the ageing process, extending the maximum life-span of warm-blooded animals. You may be thinking that you are too old to begin applying this principle, but animal studies indicate a possible 10-20% increase in life span by reducing calories, starting as late as middle age. Even though experts use the terms 'calorie restriction', 'underfeeding', or even 'under nutrition' I prefer to use another term that is more in line with the principles of AGGRESSIVE HEALTH. The term I use is 'An Optimal Minimum'.

The definition for 'An Optimal Minimum' is eating as much of every nutrient your body needs, at any given time. If you are exercising or under stress you may need more that someone who is only doing 15mins exercise per day living relatively stress free. The problem with the dietary habits of western civilisation is that they are built around high calorie, nutrient deficient foods that lack any real 'life-force'. With an optimum minimum, calories are restricted, but not at the expense of vital nutrients or high vibrational raw foods.

Calorie restriction promotes longevity by providing a number of physiological advantages.

- It places less strain on the organs of digestion and assimilation.
- It produces fewer free radicals.
- It boosts levels of antioxidant enzymes by as much as 400%.
- It increases immune system strength by up to 300%.
- It lowers blood insulin levels and cholesterol.
- It increases glucose tolerance and lowers blood pressure.

For example, studies have shown that 'optimum minimum' eating has achieved a remarkable 300% life-extension with fish and a 60% increase in lifespan with rats. Rhesus monkeys on a calorie-restricted diet have leaner bodies, lower blood pressure, more optimal cholesterol levels, lower blood glucose and lower fasting insulin than the same animals, fed a higher level of calories. Communication between hormones is also enhanced due to less waste build-up, in and around cells.

Melatonin and DHEA normally decrease during ageing but begin to rise when calorie restriction/optimal minimum eating prevails.

BECOMING OLDER AND WISER
IN A WORLD OF MENTAL DETERIORATION

Dr Walford also indicated that as well as maximising lifespan, calorie restriction can prevent the brain from deteriorating. His experiments indicate that caloric restriction prevents the decline of the dopamine receptors in the brain cells of animals. If this can be carried over to humans, it would mean that the action of one of the most important neurotransmitters could be enhanced. It isn't unusual for dopamine to decline in the elderly, causing restricted bodily movement, including Parkinson's disease.

Another one of Dr. Walford's experiments indicated that the function of the dendrites within brain cells is also improved when calories are restricted. Again, if this applied to humans, it would be a major breakthrough in longevity. The ability to grow new dendrites is one of the most important aspects of brain plasticity. In recent years, researchers have found that new dendritic connections can be forged up until the very last moments of life, allowing your brain to regenerate as long as you're alive. Anything that might stimulate this regeneration is obviously valuable, but remember that…

THERE ALWAYS EXISTS A BARE MINIMUM

Although this may come as no surprise, there is one thing you must remember once you've decided to restrict the calories in your diet. No matter how much you restrict your calorie intake, you must ensure you consume adequate amounts of raw greens and their juices along with wheatgrass juice and AFA algae. Hemp seeds and flax should play a vital role in your diet to supply an abundance of amino acids, and for some people animal protein is key. You must also consume adequate amounts of raw plant fats to meet your daily requirement of essential fatty acids, and ensure you get your carbohydrates from raw foods such as vegetables and sprouted nuts, seeds, beans, and lentils along with a few select fruits. By eating raw foods you'll include an abundance of micronutrients from vitamins and minerals to phytochemicals, enzymes and antioxidants. Your colon must also be clean to allow the maximum absorption of nutrients. Have you invested the cleanse I talk about to eliminate mucoid plaque and booked a series of colonics yet?

CUT CALORIES BY 40%
AND WATCH YOUR BODY RETURN TO YOUTH

As long as you utilise every other principle in this book, if you eat an 'optimal minimum' and cut your calorie intake by 40%, you can expect to increase your maximum life span, the functionality of your neurotransmitter receptors, your learning ability, your immune system function, your kidney function and the length of female fertility.

You can also expect to decrease your body fat percentage, your loss of bone mass, your blood glucose levels, your insulin levels, your chance of cancer, your chance of autoimmune disease, your blood lipid levels, your chance of heart disease and your chance of diabetes.

PUT THE SHOVEL DOWN AND STOP FILLING YOUR FACE!

There are many ways to look at why calorie restriction works, maybe it's not that calorie restriction actually provides these benefits, but that gluttony promotes the decrease in longevity. When you look around and see what most people shovel into their bodies, is it any wonder many people die so prematurely? The body can only handle so much waste before it weakens and breaks down.

Dietary restriction experiments in animals have been going on for at least 60 years. Everything from primitive single-cell pond animals to small mammals (such as rats and mice) have been successfully tested on. Just imagine what happens when you combine all these principles together…

SAVE THE ELDERLY FROM AN EARLY GRAVE

In the 1960s, a team of scientists in Spain reported an experiment with two groups of elderly people in a nursing home. One group ate their usual diet, whilst the next group restricted their calorie intake whilst increasing their intake of nutrients. After three years, the second group had experienced 50% less illness and half the rate of death compared to the first.

THE THREE PIVOTAL POINTS
OF 'OPTIMAL MINIMUM' EATING

By eating an 'optimal minimum' you can slow ageing right down and produce amazing results. Here are three very powerful reasons why:

PIVOTAL POINT NO. 1 – By overexposing yourself to free radical attack, you simply accelerate the ageing process. One of the easiest ways to do this is to eat too many calories.

According to Dr. Lawrence E. Lamb, M.D., "The repair of cell membranes in animals on restricted caloric intake even suggests the possibility that calorie limitation could help reverse earlier changes caused by oxidants."

Longevity, or the risk of mortality, correlates very well with blood levels, or dietary intakes of vitamin C, vitamin E, vitamin A and beta-carotene. A recent study published in the American Journal of Clinical Nutrition followed 11,178 people between the ages of 67 and 105 over ten years. The overall risk of death was reduced by 42% for those who took supplements of both vitamins C and E.

PIVOTAL POINT NO.2 – 'Optimum minimum' eating increases the production of protective enzymes. These are as follows:

1. Superoxide dimutase (SOD), known to reduce the superoxide free radicals to hydrogen peroxide.
2. Glutathione peroxidase, known to reduce hydrogen peroxide to water.
3. Glutathione catalase, known to also reduce hydrogen peroxide to water.

By eating an 'optimum minimum' you also increase your production of melatonin, another efficient scavenger of hydroxyl free radicals, the true villains that promote cellular damage.

Do you remember what you learned about wheatgrass juice in chapter 2? Wheatgrass is a superior food source of a Superoxide dimutase (SOD). Laboratory trials and clinical tests have proven SOD is a safe and effective enzyme that protects us from cell damage. Most cellular damage is caused by superoxides, infection, ageing, radiation, and poisoning by bad food, air, or drugs. Wheatgrass juice, along with E3Live should never be underestimated. Use them.

PIVOTAL POINT NO. 3 – Reduce calories by eating an 'optimum minimum' and you take the most important step towards slowing the ageing process. When you reduce calories you reduce insulin production, promoting a more favourable balance between itself and glucagon, whilst encouraging a more favourable eicosanoid balance, optimising hormonal communication throughout your body.

When you reduce insulin secretion, you automatically stabilise blood glucose levels and minimise the stimulation of cortisol. Excess cortisol inhibits the formation of eicosanoids and kills cortisol-sensitive cells in the brain and the thymus. An example of a community that abide by these principles are…

THE HUNZAS, A COMMUNITY OF CENTENARIANS

Let me introduce you to the Hunzas, a community that live in the Mountain Peaks of the Himalayas, where the borders of Kashmir, China, India and Afghanistan converge. They have a population of only 30,000, but a reputation that has been spread far and wide around the world. They have an amazing record of producing centenarians, many living up to ages of 145 years.

If you were to visit them you'd realise they know nothing of disease and are endowed with remarkably high levels of health and vibrancy. I bet you never even realised that there is a community on this planet where cancer and heart disease is unheard of. What about arthritis, varicose veins, constipation, stomach ulcers or appendicitis? No chance! Even mumps, measles and chicken pox are just meaningless words to these people. So before I share with you some secrets of this amazing community, take a look at the reputation of the Hunzas:

♦ The Hunzas possess boundless energy/enthusiasm and are very serene.
♦ At one hundred years old, a Hunza is considered neither old nor elderly.

◆ They consider physical and intellectual maturity to be at its highest when they've been alive for 100 years.

◆ It is not uncommon for Hunza men to father children at the age of 80.

◆ Hunza women at the age of 80 look no different from the most youthfully slim and vibrant 40-year-olds we see in our society. Hunza women remain slim, supple and graceful, and maintain excellent posture.

◆ The Hunzas have no idea what it means to be obese. Cellulite is unknown to them.

◆ Hunza men have been seen carrying what we'd consider backbreaking loads, up steep mountain paths, at the age of 100.

Their first belief is simple: The food you eat is your best medicine. Dr MacCarrisson put their belief to the test. He created an experiment using 3 groups of mice, each eating a different diet.

1. The first group, nourished exclusively on Hunza food, flourished and enjoyed spectacular health.
2. The second group was fed a diet similar to that of the people of neighbouring Kashmir. They developed a number of diseases.
3. The third group received a typical British diet, and quickly developed all the symptoms of neurathenia (nervous weakness, exhaustion and irritability).

IF YOU ARE WAITING FOR THE SECRET, IT CAN BE SUMMED UP IN ONE WORD: FRUGALITY

They eat only two meals a day. They rise at 5a.m. but don't eat their first meal until 12 noon. Hunza food is completely natural, containing no chemical additives and by eating small portions, they show a high degree of vitality and enthusiasm. Their preferred fruits and vegetables include potatoes, string beans, peas, carrots, turnip, squash, spinach, lettuce, apples, pears, peaches, apricots, cherries and blackberries. They eat many nuts such as walnuts, hazelnuts, almonds, beechnuts etc. Nuts often constitute an entire meal or are eaten with fruit, or mixed into salad. Almonds are eaten whole, or used to make oil through a process that has been passed from generation to generation. When they do eat meat, which is quite rare, small portions are eaten, chicken being their most common source.

Much of the water the Hunzas drink comes from glaciers, and carries colloidal minerals. A high raw diet in alignment with the principles of AGGRESSIVE HEALTH will supply an abundance of colloidal minerals.

SURVIVING THE WINTER WITH SPROUT POWER

In his book Healthy Hunzas, John Tobe reports that the Hunzas use the power of sprouts to survive the long, cold winters, in the Himalayan mountains. Sprouts provide them with vital nutrients, and when winter turns to spring and food supplies are low, the Hunzas rely on sprouts as a source of vitamins, enzymes, and energy.

HARNESSING THE PRINCIPLES OF THE HUNZAS

In addition to daily physical exercise, the Hunzas practice certain basic yoga techniques, notably yogic breathing. Yogic breathing is very slow, deep and rhythmic, and makes use of the entire thoracic cavity.

Relaxation is the key to health and the Hunzas, both young and old, practice it regularly. You can do the same and spread 'powernaps' throughout your day. I tend to use short 10-minute sessions on my Proteus light/sound machine and generally get amazing results. Many mind machines can train you to reach deep states of relaxation very quickly.

Rather than work in quick bursts, the Hunzas know they can work much longer if they are not tense and take regular breaks. They enter a state of deep relaxation and focus inwards, listening to the silence of their soul.

THE HUNZAS MAINTAIN A POWERFUL MIND

One thing that has been proven by modern medicine is that when the mind becomes dull – due to a lack of curiosity or interest, it begins to deteriorate, and when the mind deteriorates, the body does as well, resulting in muscular, cellular and circulatory degeneration. The difference with the Hunzas is that they rejoice at the thought of getting old because to them, age equals wisdom and maturity. When they are older they are a greater value to society.

Hunzas prefer to remain physically active for as long as possible. They follow the principle that 'to live' means 'to move'. If you want to adopt the mindset of a Hunza start by thinking that your youth (the first stage in life), ends at around 50, next comes the middle years, which last until 80 and finally comes the age of plenitude, the best years of your life!

Hunza people live everyday as if their whole life were ahead of them. In some respects they are like children – happy in the present moment, not worried about the future.

ARE YOU USING THE POWER OF WILD GREENS
TO MAXIMISE YOUR POTENTIAL?
THE DAGASTANIS ARE...

In the Caucasus Mountains of southern Russia, and on the coast of the Caspian Sea, live the inhabitants of the Dagestan republic. Out of the two million residents of this province, the oldest recorded Dagestani lived to a ripe old age of 146, with many reaching ages between 120-130 years. Their diet consists of a plethora of wild grasses and weeds. Chickweed, shepherd's purse, rose hips, camomile, lambs quarters, thistle, thyme, sorrel, yellow dock, vetch, daisy, clover, wild marjoram, oregano, amaranth, mustard, garlic, and the grasses of wheat, barley, and oats make up the mainstay of their diet. With the young leaves they create mouth-watering salads and with the older more fibrous ones they create health-giving soups and stews. Even seeds are used to make tea, breads and pancakes after being crushed into a powder.

Intrigued at their amazing health, researchers from the Caspian medical college examined 154 alpine residents. 130 lived at altitudes of 6400 ft above sea level, whilst 24 lived on flat lands. The age range of the group was between 85 and 116 years and in an effort to learn the secrets of this group, the researchers moved into their homes for 10 – 12 days. They bombarded them with questions, and tests, weighing them, whilst examining their dietary/lifestyle habits.

Those who seem to be maximising their longevity have the most consistent habits. They start their day by waking between 5am and 6am and rather than eat a 'hearty' breakfast, they drink nothing but tea made from weeds and grasses. This tea is also drunk before and after meals for increasing appetite and improving digestion. Then between 9am and 10am they eat a light breakfast. The 90-year-olds ate the most green 'chlorophyll' rich foods, but even the children included these health-giving foods in their diet.

DEAD NUTRITIONISTS LEAD BY EXAMPLE!

In their quest for the secret of eternal youth, many nutritionists have written books on the subject of longevity, certain in their assumption of what constitutes perfect health. Those who are old may give you valuable tips. Those who are dead, lead by example! Nathan Pritikin, Professor Arnold Ehret, Dr Norman Walker and Paul Bragg all have two things in common. Firstly they are dead! Secondly they all wrote nutritional books claiming they could lead you down the path to health and longevity. So, who lived the longest? Let's take a look.

The Pritikin Program for Diet and Exercise, was a popular book during the 1970s. Nathan Pritikin popularised a diet that consisted of mostly complex carbohydrates and minimal cholesterol, fat and protein. He died of leukaemia at the pinnacle of his success at age 69, from the complications surrounding an experimental medical treatment.

Ehret had a different focus. He specialised in long fasts and a diet rich in fruit and green leafy vegetables. Everyone thought he was in exceptional health. Unfortunately he focused more on fruit than fresh raw greens and in 1922 at age 56 he died from a fractured skull after falling backwards and hitting his head! Can you imagine what the condition of his bones must have been like! This is a warning! Ensure you don't dissolve your bones away by not eating enough calcium rich raw foods – skull fractures very rarely cause death!

Norman Walker was famous in the USA for his electrical juicers. Not only did he advise eating a diet high in fruit and vegetables, but he also recommended a variety of juice cocktails. One of my favourite books, 'Colon health', written by Norman Walker highlights the importance of having a series of regular colonics. This man was a genius! His remarkable recovery from a so-called 'terminal illness' in his thirties gave him a great foundation of health on which to build. The foundation must have been strong as he lived to 109! He was vital and alive up until the morning of his death, where he was found dead in his study.

Paul Bragg (1881-1976) paved the way for many of today's health educators. He promoted a lifestyle of deep breathing, water fasts, organic foods, drinking water, juicing, exercise and listening to your body. Ravaged by tuberculosis as a teenager, Paul Bragg developed his own approach to health that had its foundation built on a diet of raw living foods. Bragg was an awesome athlete and a true role model for the power of diet, movement and rest. Bragg died in an unfortunate accident, doing what he loved – surfing. Can you imagine riding the waves when you're 95? One of the things that made Paul Bragg different was his emphasis on enzyme therapy for exceptional health.

Whether you call it common sense, need scientific proof, or need a first hand example of a dead raw foodist – a diet high in raw, electrically charged, nutrient rich food along with enzymes is the only way to truly succeed. When raw greens, raw plant fats, fruits, sprouts, salads and vegetables are correctly used and understood exceptional health is the result. In chapter 2 you discovered the power of greens, and I hope that message has remained strong throughout this book. Vegetables supply nutrients in concentrations not found in fruit, especially calcium. Take Norman Walker's example to heart, and become an example yourself! An abundance of greens per day, juiced, blended or eaten raw will help guarantee strong bones and scintillating health!

ARE YOU READY FOR THE CHALLENGE?

Your training is nearly complete, and the AGGRESSIVE HEALTH 'black belt' is just around the corner, but remember, like any martial art, the black belt is only the beginning. With an abundance of energy and enthusiasm for life, you can achieve anything you desire. The only question is: Where have you set the limits? The same is true of this chapter. You have the potential to live pain free and full of vitality well into your hundreds and beyond! Use what you know and the gateway to success will open itself very wide. Here's a re-cap that'll remind you why 'optimal minimum' eating is the ultimate goal:

♦ If you have the potential to live between 120 and 140 years old there can only be one conclusion. To die any earlier means you must have engaged in daily habits or rituals that over time caused you to accelerate the ageing process. Do you want to suffer with cancer, be crippled by a stroke, or ravaged by Alzheimer's?

♦ University of California expert on ageing, Dr. Roy Walford, has reported that calorie restriction is the only method that retards ageing and extends the maximum life span of warm-blooded animals. Animal studies indicate a possible 10-20% increase in life span by cutting down on calories, starting as late as middle age.

♦ Calorie restriction promotes longevity by providing a number of physiological advantages: It places less strain on the organs of digestion and assimilation, it produces fewer free radicals, it boosts levels of antioxidant enzymes by as much as 400%, it increases immune system strength by up to 300% and most importantly of all, lowers blood insulin levels.

♦ Melatonin and DHEA normally decrease during ageing but begin to rise with calorie restriction.

- Studies with fish have achieved a remarkable 300% increase in life-extension. Studies with rats have produced a 60% increase in life-extension. Rhesus monkeys on a calorie-restricted diet have leaner bodies and lower blood pressure, cholesterol, blood glucose and fasting insulin (see next chapter for explanation) than the same animals fed a higher level of calories.

- Dr Walford indicated that calorie restriction could prevent your brain from deteriorating during the ageing process. Caloric restriction prevents the decline of the dopamine receptors in the brain cells of animals, enhancing one of the most important neurotransmitters.

- Another one of Dr. Walford's experiments indicated that the function of dendrites within the brain cells also improved by restricting calories in animals.

- If you eat an 'optimal minimum' and cut your calorie intake by 40%, you can expect to increase your maximum life span, the functionality of your neurotransmitter receptors, your learning ability, your immune system function, your kidney function and the length of your female fertility. You can also expect to decrease your body fat percentage, your loss of bone mass, your blood glucose levels, your insulin levels, your chance of cancer, your chance of autoimmune disease, your blood lipid levels, your chance of heart disease and your chance of diabetes.

- 'Optimum minimum' eating increases the production of superoxide dimutase, glutathione peroxidase and glutathione catalase – three very powerful protective enzymes.

- By using the principle of 'optimal minimum' eating, you can begin to think like a Hunza. Their perception of life is as follows: The first stage of life, called the age of youth, ends at around 50, next comes the middle years, which last until 80 and finally comes the age of plenitude, the best years of their life!

- Healthy ageing is having a good quality of life and quantity of life. The ideal is to die as young as possible as late as possible.

- Over a 40-year period, if you sleep one hour less per day, you gain 15 extra days each year, totalling 1.7 years over the course of 40 years. In that time you could master anything. Think about it!

The concept of treating food as if it were a drug began some 2500 years ago when Hippocrates said, "Let food be your medicine, and let medicine be your food."

THE AGGRESSIVE HEALTH EVALUATION:
Are you extending your life by *happily* eating an 'optimal minimum'?
Have you mastered each principle enough to utilise these fine distinctions?

You may have lost unwanted body fat, increased your lean body mass, enhanced every aspect of your mental health, and feel superior in every way, but don't let your progress stop there! To highlight the power of AGGRESSIVE HEALTH endeavour to find out what changes have taken place at the cellular level.

CHAPTER 17

FORGET THE PLACEBO EFFECT! LET SCIENCE SEE HOW POWERFUL AGGRESSIVE HEALTH REALLY IS – GET TESTED

If you've had enough of swimming in the sea of confusion and are ready to leap out and make a powerful shift in your understanding of health – read on. This is a real opportunity for you to discover the secrets behind the engine room of AGGRESSIVE HEALTH. So let's begin.

WHY DIDN'T GOD GIVE US WARNING LIGHTS?

Do you remember the last time you were driving your car and the oil light came on? What did you do? If you're like most people, you pulled into the garage, purchased some oil, popped the bonnet and filled her up. Do you remember the last time you had an electrolyte overload? Did you look down and see your nipples flashing? Of course not. What about the last time you were low on water? Did your fingernails start to glow? You may think these are ridiculous suggestions, but if people had a variety of warning lights that alerted them to the fact that their health was deteriorating there would be a lot less suffering in the world. Imagine how useful it would be to get a clear picture of your core homeostatic processes. Imagine being able to use this data to your advantage so you could create a more perfect diet for YOU, optimising YOUR health. There are many approaches and tests available today, but at the forefront of the wellness revolution is biological terrain testing. For more information contact www.biomedx.com.

Bioterrain testing assesses your biological individuality and highlights any imbalances that prevent you from experiencing optimal health. Think back to a time when you weren't feeling your best. Can you imagine how delighted you'd be if you knew why you were feeling this way? Imagine if your imbalances were exposed and presented to you in a clear, concise manner along with a simple plan to restore balance and harmony. Rather than looking at obvious symptoms, and making generalizations based on data gathered from the masses, biological terrain testing targets YOU and YOUR imbalances.

THE MISSING LINK TO DISEASE FREE LIVING

If you've embraced the principles of AGGRESSIVE HEALTH there's a high likelihood you feel fantastic and without knowing it you may raised your zeta potential and unconsciously driven all of your core homeostatic processes into the ideal zone. Zeta potential is a term used to discuss the electrical charge around a colloidal particle. Surprisingly, zeta potential isn't a subject discussed at medical school; so don't trot down to your doctors for a detailed explanation. Zeta potential is critical to your health and the ignorance surrounding it may account for the billions of people suffering the ravages of disease. Two important points that will capture your attention are as follows:

When zeta potential is raised so is your ability to
1)   suspend toxins for elimination and
2)   suspend nutrients for absorption and transportation to your cells.

"Let's have some more of that!" I hear you cry. But guess what? If you engage in habits that lower zeta potential, you may as well throw in the towel! As zeta potential drops, so does any chance of exceptional health.

Dr. T.C. MCDANIEL FINDS HIS OWN SOLUTION TO PVCs

Dr T.C. McDaniel, author of 'Disease Reprieve – Living Into The Golden Years' was 56 years old and experiencing many cardiovascular complications. His heart was constantly skipping beats and nobody (not even the finest heart specialists) could figure out why. He was left to find his own solution. Fortunately he stumbled across the concept of zeta potential. What he discovered was that as zeta potential begins to fall, the blood begins to thicken and sludge, but as zeta potential begins to rise the blood begins to flow more freely. Dr McDaniel went on to learn that blood is a suspension of anions, cations and non-ions and if he could manipulate the ratios of these three electrically charged particles he could raise zeta potential and create amazing results. So what did Dr T.C..McDaniel do to help improve his condition? I'll come to that shortly.

ZETA POTENTIAL IN EVERY DAY LIFE

When you flush dirty water down the drain, have you ever wondered how treatment plants purify the water before it is returned to your house? In order to filter out pollutants, the treatment facility pours in highly cationic substances like aluminium sulphate that pulls the waste together like a magnet. As the waste gathers together it increases in weight and eventually collects at the bottom of the holding tank, leaving the clean water to continue on its journey. In simple terms, cations are positively charged particles that bring things together. In the example above the cationic substance pulls the waste together making it so heavy it falls out of harms way allowing the water to arrive cleanly at your door. An anionic substance would just disperse the dirt and the water would never get clean.

WHY DO YOU WASH YOUR HANDS WITH SOAP AND WATER?

In continuing the example, if you were to rush to the sink to wash your hands, why would you use 'soap and water' rather than just 'water'? Well, by adding soap you make the water 'wetter'. The soap changes the electrical properties of the water because of its anionic nature. When you use the anionic soap and change the electrical properties of the water, the combination disperses particles easier than water alone and you end up with squeaky clean hands.

Enzymes are powerful for many reasons, but one of the reasons you rarely hear about is their ability to cause dispersion. They are anionic in nature, highlighting their power. This is another reason why Vitalzym has such a powerful effect on the blood (see page 73) and why animal protein (cationic in nature) can cause problems if eaten in excess.

So there you have it – cationic substances are positively charged and pull things together (coagulators), anionic substances are negatively charged and disperse things. In your blood, the terrain is a mix of cationic, anionic and non-ionic substances. The key is in the ratio. Too many cationic substances such as animal protein, and zeta potential drops! Too much sugar and alcohol and you increase the non-ionic load (interfering with ionic mobility) causing zeta potential to drop. Increase the ratio of anionic substances and you begin to encourage more flow as zeta potential rises.

BACK TO THE STORY!
WHAT DID Dr MCDANIEL DO WHEN HE FIGURED ALL THIS OUT?

He created his own 'anionic surfactant' to disperse the excessive cations, he drank more pure water, eliminated the bad cations from his diet and his PVCs (premature ventricular contractions) disappeared. Question: Why haven't you been told this before? Because information like this could bankrupt pharmaceutical giants almost overnight. Be warned – there's money in 'them there' pills!

BRINGING YOUR CORE-HOMEOSTATIC SYSTEMS
BACK INTO FINE BALANCE

Do you know what your electrolyte status is and how it affects your overall health? Are you forcing your kidneys to work overtime to dilute your urine? Does your saliva highlight a lymphatic system that's lost its flow? How is your overall anion to cation ratio in your body affecting your overall health? Are you winning the war against free radical attack? Is your capacity to develop the energy making molecule ATP at its peak? Are your cells communicating properly on a biochemical level? Is the permeability of your cell membranes balanced allowing optimal exchange of nutrients and waste? Are you effectively metabolising fats and sugars or are you stuck in one particular oxidising pathway? Do you have efficient protein digestion, a healthy balance of soluble and insoluble ureas along with efficient potassium uptake (which effects the thyroid and ultimately effects fat metabolism)? Have you created an internal terrain that optimises hormone, receptor site and enzyme function? Do you regularly eat foods that build up your body's pH buffers for emergencies?

As you can see, biological terrain testing deals with so many of the body's homeostatic processes, the results build an unrivalled picture of health. With this 'hard data' it is easy to make targeted suggestions on how to bring the balance back, rather than just general advice.

Ultimately, the principles of AGGRESSIVE HEALTH allow you to purify your body, allowing life energy to flow more freely through you. Life energy is a term I use, but it is refered to in many different ways by many different cultures. Indians call it Prana, Chinese Chi, Japanese Ki, Hawaiians Mana, Tibetans Tumo and Orgone energy by the Reich. Biological terrain testing is by far the most comprehensive protocol for assessing health, but if you are unable to book an appointment...

THE BRUTAL TRUTH IS ONLY A BLOOD TEST AWAY

Your blood represents the brutal truth about your health. It can't lie, it can't deceive and it can't misinform. I believe the further you are away from the principles of AGGRESSIVE HEALTH, the closer you are towards chronic disease and accelerated ageing! If the following values apply to you then you are hyperinsulinemic, ageing faster than normal and putting your health at risk.

♦   Your triglycerides are greater than 200mg/dL.
♦   Your HDL cholesterol less than 35mg/dL.
♦   Your fasting insulin greater than 15 units/ml.
♦   Your glycosylated haemoglobin greater than 9 %.
♦   Your fasting-triglyceride:HDL cholesterol ratio is greater than 4.

ACCELERATED AGEING LEADS TO ACCELERATED DEATH: TAKE YOUR FOOT OFF THE INSULIN ACCELERATOR AND SLOW DOWN THE AGEING PROCESS

As you age, various biological markers of ageing change within your body as you get closer to your last day on earth. Take a look at what happens to the biological markers as you age:

♦   Insulin resistance increases.
♦   Systolic Blood Pressure increases.
♦   Percentage body fat and lipid ratios increase.
♦   Glucose tolerance decreases.
♦   Aerobic capacity decreases.
♦   Muscle mass and strength decreases.
♦   Temperature regulation decreases in efficiency.
♦   Immune function diminishes.

The list of physiological changes can all be related to excessive levels of the hormone insulin! Take your foot off the ageing accelerator by eating foods that maintain optimal hormonal control. The more you focus on the habits of success the easier you'll find it to remain in control.

THE MYSTERY OF AWARENESS UNCOVERED

Isn't it amazing that in two years, 98% of the atoms in your body will have been exchanged for new ones? It may sound absurd, but 24 months from now you could have totally rebuilt your body.
　　　Ageing is a natural process, but it's worth noting that there are some organisms that never age, such as single-celled amoebas, algae, and protozoa. Parts of you also remain ageless – your emotions, ego, personality type, IQ, and other mental characteristics, as well as vast portions of your DNA. Physically, it makes no sense to say that the water and minerals in your body are ageing, for what is 'old water' or 'old salt'? These components alone make up 70% of your body. The honeybee at certain times of the year can shift its hormones and completely reverse its age. In the human body, shifts in hormones may not be as dramatic, but there is enough latitude that on any given day, your hormone profile may be younger than the day, month, or even year before. The last place you can exert influence over your age is in your mind…

SHIFT YOUR MENTAL STATE AND ADD YEARS TO YOUR LIFE

When someone shifts their awareness they can have a dramatic effect on their own physiology. It's as simple as placing your attention on memories that you really enjoyed, past triumphs or exciting times in your life. When you think about your first love, you trigger a cascade of hormones associated to that experience. If you consistently focus on a time when you succeeded at something you'll continually feel the emotion of success and your whole biochemistry will confirm this.

TURNING BACK THE HANDS OF TIME

To illustrate this principle, a psychologist, Ellen Langer and her colleagues at Harvard conducted an experiment in 1979 in an effort to reverse the biological age of a group of men. The men in the group were all over 75 years of age and in good health. Her theory was that by manipulating their environment, she could get them to experience life as it was twenty years ago.

They met at a country resort for 1 week, knowing they'd be subject to innumerable tests both physically and mentally. Each one came alone, with no reminders of any year past 1959, no newspapers, photos, tapes or CDs, or anything that would take their focus off of 1959.

At the resort, every last effort was made to ensure their life would be similar to the one they lived 20 years ago. Whenever they picked up a paper or magazine, it would be from the year 1959. The music played was from 1959. Every piece of furniture was from 1959. In fact, every last little trinket was from 1959. One of the rules of the week was that the men had to fully associate to the experience of being in the year 1959. Every conversation, movement, gesture, catchphrase, thought and feeling had to be related to their life in 1959 and to make this easier the entire environment was set up as if they'd gone back in time. ID photos were given to each subject, with pictures taken from 1959. They referred to all current affairs as if it was 1959 and talked about their jobs as if they were still in employment.

Langer and her team used this time to measure each and every marker of biological age. They measured physical strength, posture, perception, cognition, and short-term memory, along with thresholds of hearing, sight, and taste.

The experiment by the Harvard team gave each man a chance to alter his self-image, hypothesising that the shift in self-awareness would directly influence the ageing process.

Whether you call it play-acting or not, the results were remarkable! Everything about their life improved. Their memories became sharper, their manual dexterity improved, their mobility improved and they became more self-sufficient. They cooked their own meals, cleaned up after themselves and totally adopted the role of a 55-year-old. One week produced the following results:

♦   Their faces looked younger by an average of three years.
♦   Their fingers lengthened (fingers usually shorten with age).
♦   Their joints regained flexibility.
♦   Their posture straightened out.
♦   Their muscle strength increased.
♦   Their hearing sense and vision improved remarkably.
♦   Their intelligence increased.

Although a landmark in the study of ageing, Professor Langer attributed the success of the study to three factors:

1. The group behaved as if they were younger. Could you also do this?
2. They were treated like 55 year olds, rather than 75 year olds (like at home).
3. They had to follow complex procedures as part of their daily routine. Could you also increase your level of stimulation? Maybe you could start playing a musical instrument, or rekindle your enjoyment of art, such as painting. Maybe you could engage in various sports endeavours or even just begin to challenge your mind with crossword puzzles? The options are endless.

THE REMARKABLE RESULTS OF TIME TRAVEL

By becoming inner time travellers, Langer was able to create an environment that allowed the men to travel back in time by 20 years. The most exciting result was that their whole physiology followed. Stop for a minute now and consider all the ways you could creatively manipulate your mind to allow these changes to occur. Remember the more vivid your participation, the closer you will come to duplicating the body chemistry of youth.

Stimulate your mind today and re-access old pathways of youth, making them new again, and again, until you feel the energy radiate and reverberate throughout your entire body and out into the world. It's up to you to change your inner experience and travel back in time using the biochemistry of memory as your vehicle.

VISUALISATION:
ANOTHER VEHICLE TO ENHANCE HEALTH

There's now scientific proof that visualisation works. Researchers using high tech equipment have shown that when you 'see' pictures, or 'hear' music in your mind, parts of your brain are stimulated and send messages to your endocrine and nervous system. Mental imagery actually triggers physical responses in your body.

Your imagination is very powerful. Have you ever been lying in bed at night and thought you heard a door open downstairs? Did your heart start pounding as you broke out into a sweat, wondering whether there was an intruder or not? If there was an intruder, I apologise for bringing the memory to the forefront of your mind. But if there wasn't an intruder, you can see how the threat was all in your imagination.

In the 1970s, Dr Carl Simonton, a cancer specialist at the University of Oregon, conducted a study in which he found that 30 out of 159 terminal cancer patients went into complete remission whilst using guided imagery to combat their cancers. Another 22% experienced a decrease in the size of their tumours, and even those who died lived twice as long as they'd been expected to live. This is powerful news and hopefully will ignite you desire to study N.L.P. and hypnosis which teaches you how to consciously take control of your mind for greater success.

ENJOY YOUR LEARNING CURVE
AND KEEP COMING BACK TO BASICS

I'm sure you're amazed at how many wonderful ideas and concepts you've learned throughout AGGRESSIVE HEALTH, but how many are you going to implement into your life? Remember, there will be times when you make mistakes and find it challenging, but this isn't a big deal, so don't treat it like one. Lighten up – It's all well and fine wanting to be perfect over night, but it's not necessarily the best route to take. Develop your own learning curve and you'll build references for your exciting future.

THE ULTIMATE CHALLENGE

Optimal nutrition is an excellent gateway to a rich, more fullfilling life, but health is more than just nutrition. You aren't just a bundle of cells crying out for nutrients, you are a spiritual being. For you to tap into your limitless potential, you need to be 'alive' and 'vibrating' with energy! Your bioelectrical nature must be fed with foods that have 'high vibrations' allowing your energy to grow. Green leafy vegetables, raw plant fats, fruits, vegetables, sprouts and wheatgrass juice accelerate the electrical activity inside every cell. A diet of bread, potatoes, meats, canned vegetables, and other refined 'recreational' foods doesn't!

Many people think they can supply all the nutrients necessary for peak performance by taking a standard multi-vitamin and mineral formula, but how can these kinds of supplements add life and energy to your body? A vitamin pill won't sprout up and grow into a healthy living plant! Vitamin supplements may be useful to balance an existing problem, but live raw foods create unshakeable health! Raw foods are a virtual goldmine of every conceivable nutrient needed for life. Your cells reach out for these kinds of charged nutrients with an irresistible magnetism.

I PRAY YOU CONTINUE TO DREAM
AND ACT ON THOSE DREAMS

We have journeyed a long way together. How much further you go will be down to you! AGGRESSIVE HEALTH has shared with you the necessary tools and insights to radically change your life. But what you do from here is entirely your decision. When you put this book down, you can do what many people do and completely forget what you've learned and wonder why you can't get control of your life, or you can make it your personal mission to use AGGRESSIVE HEALTH for what it was meant to be: a guide to living an extra-ordinary life. Make your decision wisely!

A QUICK REVIEW TO CATAPULT YOU INTO ACTION

Let's review the key concepts of AGGRESSIVE HEALTH that make it such a revolutionary approach to nutrition and peak performance. You know that food has more effect on your body than any prescription drug and that it's your responsibility to find your own preferred fuel mix (the ideal ratio of protein, carbohydrate and fat). You know that your No.1 priority is building a diet based around raw, 'living' foods and nutrient rich superfoods (see appendix 1). You've learned how to make the most effective use of chlorophyll-rich green leafy vegetables. Whether you juice, blend or eat more of them, or focus on a daily shot of wheatgrass juice and AFA algae, they are critical to the overall picture.

You've learned about the importance of sprouted beans, activated nuts/seeds and how they can transfer their 'life-force' directly to you. You've discovered that in cultures where the incidence of cancer is low, B17 intake is high. Apricot kernels, wheatgrass juice and mung beans are all critical foods in this category, as are seeds of the common fruit.

You've learned that you have a unique requirement for fat, but regardless of what it is, you now know how to select the finest fats for exceptional health. Ground flax seeds, hemp seeds, hemp oil, olive oil, coconut butter and avocados are all to be experimented with to get the balance right for you.

You've learned that detoxification is a process that can be accelerated when you systematically cleanse the three tubes of detoxification. You've also learnt that mucoid plaque can rob you of your health if not eliminated. You know that colonic hydrotherapy is critical, especially if you've been eating a diet full of 'nutritionally suicidal foods'.

Finally, section one offered you a prescription for aerobic exercise that'll help you increase your fitness and longevity, whilst speeding up the detoxification process by as much as 800%.

Next you learned how to trigger the biological switches that kick-start fat metabolism and how protein selection is critical if you are to determine your ultimate fuel mix. You then discovered the power of the super-hormones: eicosanoids. You've learned how to keep the eicosanoid production pathway functioning optimally by keeping delta 6 desaturase active, delta 5 desaturase inactive and by keeping insulin and glucagon balanced.

You've learned how to sculpt your body with 'the tools of the AGGRESSIVE HEALTH trade' simultaneously unleashing a cascade of youth enhancing hormones.

You've learned that stress is a powerful destroyer of health, and that the stress hormone cortisol is directly linked to high blood-insulin levels. You've learned how the hormones related to stress, nutrition and exercise all inter-relate and how Transcendental Meditation and mind-machines can help control and eliminate the stress response, whilst conditioning peak performance states of mind. You've also learned that stimulation and an enriched environment is the only way to maintain a powerful brain long into your future and that movement/exercise is a critical nutrient for increasing mental health and longevity.

You've discovered which foods to select if you want to create neurotransmitter equilibrium, and finally you've discovered how to maximise your lifespan by encompassing the principle of eating an 'optimal minimum'.

There is too much talk of balance in today's society. In my opinion, it's just a word that gets people off the hook. Lead a balanced lifestyle? What does that mean?

Think more in terms of cycles. Cycles of exercise, rest and nutrition. Cycles of eating for optimal health and cycles of eating for pleasure. Cycles of hard training and cycles of easy training. Cycles of acidity and cycles of alkalinity. Cycles of activity to stimulate your brain and body and cycles of rest and deep, profound relaxation encouraging harmonious brain states. Once you learn your ultimate fuel mix, you can cycle between high protein and low protein, high carb and low carb, ultimately fine tuning your instinct.

I BID YOU FAREWELL AND PRAY
THAT YOU EMBRACE THE GIFT OF LIFE

I don't expect you to master this book in a day or even a week. Give yourself time. Some things we've discussed will come more easily to you than others. Remember, life has a processional effect. As you make changes in the direction of perfect health, you'll learn, grow and open the doorway for more change. The tiny changes you make, over time, usually make the biggest difference.

Treat this book as a motivating force that helps you choose a different direction in life. Imagine what would have happened if you hadn't changed your eating habits. Imagine where you'd be five, ten, fifteen years from now. By changing your eating habits by only 1 degree you take a different path in life. As you travel along this path, the change will be imperceptible to begin with, but in a few years or a decade from now, the path chosen will be completely different from the one you were on, until there's no similarity at all.

This is what AGGRESSIVE HEALTH can do for you. If you learn to appreciate the power of raw food and use it to your advantage the difference you'll experience in the coming few weeks, months and years will be phenomenal. Whether you do what I do and go for the 'shot gun' approach (where you use as many of the principles as possible) or whether you make tiny changes over time, you've taken responsibility and a step in the right direction. Every action you take has an equal and opposite reaction leading you towards your ultimate destination.

My last questions to you are simple. Where are you now in your life and where are you going? Where will you be five years from now or ten years from now if you follow your current path? Are you doing what you love with people who inspire you? Or, in your own opinion, are you living a mediocre existence? Be honest and take a good look at yourself. You have the capability to be and do whatever you choose. The choices you make in life take you in a specific direction. Remember, the best way to predict the future is to get a clear idea of what's happening now.

The 21st Century Vitruvian man represents the true essence of AGGRESSIVE HEALTH – peak performance nutrition, 21st Century advances in Mind Technology, along with the finest tools to reshape, strengthen and evolve your body into whatever you desire. Every time you see the cover of AGGRESSIVE HEALTH, be reminded of who you are and who you can become.

MY FINAL MESSAGE TO YOU, MY FRIEND

If you can help yourself and go on to help others with this information then I congratulate you. Helping other people achieve success and fulfil their dreams is one of the greatest gifts life can give you. I challenge you to take action and use what you've learned. Make your life a masterpiece and join the elite group of people who don't just talk the talk, but walk the walk. Become a model for excellence.

For now, I thank you for your commitment and for reading AGGRESSIVE HEALTH to the end. All that you've learned has helped me in my life and hopefully will help you in yours. I hope I've inspired you to the point where you continue to look for human excellence everywhere you turn. Let AGGRESSIVE HEALTH be the stepping-stone that propels you to great things, in life and in love.

THE ULTIMATE AGGRESSIVE HEALTH EVALUATION:
Have you mastered the principles of AGGRESSIVE HEALTH so that every day you feel stronger, healthier and more vibrant as you reclaim your energy and charge at life?

APPENDIX

AGGRESSIVE HEALTH SUPERFOODS
Contact www.aggressivehealth.co.uk for more details

SEA VEGETABLES – kelp, arame, kombu and hijiki are all high in sodium alginate, an exceptional chelator for pulling radioactive toxins from the body.

SPROUTED FOODS – deceptively powerful in creating exceptional health – read about them in chapter 3. They are the cheapest superfoods available.

BEE POLLEN – high in minerals, vitamins and live enzymes. Pound for Pound, bee pollen is the highest protein food, higher than meat or diary. Clinically, bee pollen has been shown to significantly reduce the side effects of chemotherapy. It is also high in lecithin, critical for brain/nervous system health. Note: Note all bee pollen is created equally – contact us for more details.

VITALZYM – In tests conducted to find a fibrinolytic enzyme to go along with their up coming natural cancer therapy, the University of Southern California, through the Apex Research Inst. tested 70 of the proteolytic enzyme products available today for enzymatic action. Of the 70, Vitalzym ranked #1. With a mighty 1500mg of active ingredients Vitalzym is effective in the fight against inflammation, fibrosis or scar tissue, autoimmune conditions, viruses and toxins in the blood. Systemic enzymes are the foundation that makes all your other vitamin and mineral supplements work. We have roughly 3000 enzymes in our bodies and over 7000 enzymic reactions. As we age enzyme levels plummet. Vitalyzm can bridge the gap and help you hold onto your youth.

GREENS FOR LIFE – Greens for life contains over 4000mg certified organic Barley Juice Powder per serving. It has a powerful 100:1 Fruits and Greens extract made of 27 different fruits and vegetables. High doses of chlorella and Spirulina deliver large amounts of essential nutrients to help eliminate heavy metals and other toxic pollutants. Greens For Life contains all the essential amino acids and a micro-encapsulated Lactospore™ culture for maintaining intestinal health and improved digestion.

WHEATGRASS JUICE – and other grass juices – read about these in chapter 2. When you begin growing and juicing these juices you are getting the best quality superfood possible. Home grown juices beat every other superfood hands down.

KLAMATH LAKE BLUE/GREEN ALGAE – read about high quality blue green algae in chapter 2.

MANGOSTEEN JUICE - In 2001, a single pharmacological study from a European university indicated the following pharmacological properties of mangosteen's xanthones: antidepressant, anti-tuberculosis, anti-microbial (bacteria and fungus), anti viral, anti-leukemic, anti-tumour, anti-ulcer and anti-diabetic effects. A mangosteen xanthone directly inhibits the cyclooxygenase enzyme, thus interrupting the chain of events resulting in inflammation. One single mangosteen xanthone outperformed four existing chemo drugs. It scores 17,000 on the ORAC test (oxygen radical absorbance capacity) one ounce is 30times more powerful than an ounce of fruit and veg – making this a powerful free radical scavenger.

NONI JUICE – With a history of helping people with Allergies, arthritis, asthma, fibromyalgia, depression, diabetes, Types 1 and 2, digestion, energy, heart disease, high Blood pressure, HIV, increased alertness, multiple sclerosis, pain, headaches, skin and hair problems, sexual enhancement, sleep, stress. This superfood is worth investigating further.

RAW CHOCOLATE - Cacao is high in magnesium and the beauty mineral sulfur. Magnesium is great for women during their monthly cycle and sulfur builds strong nails, hair, beautiful, shiny skin, detoxifies the liver, and supports healthy pancreas functioning. Anecdotal reports indicate that cacao detoxifies mercury because it is so high sulfur. Monoamine oxidase enzyme inhibitors (MAO inhibitors) produce favourable results when consumed by allowing more serotonin and other neurotransmitters to circulate in the brain. Phenylethylamine (PEA) found in chocolate is an adrenal-related chemical that is also created within the brain and released when we are in love. PEA also plays a role in increasing focus and alertness. A neurotransmitter called anandamide, known as "The Bliss Chemical" is released while we are feeling great and can be found in this superfood.

MACA - Maca contains high amounts of vitamins, minerals, enzymes and all the essential amino acids. It has about 10% bioavailable calcium and about 12-14% bioavailable protein. It contains nearly 60 phytochemicals. Athletes use maca to boost energy, stamina and performance. Men use maca to increase erectile tissue response. It has been hailed Nature's Viagra! Maca is mineral dense, helps stimulate the pituitary and balance hormonal production.

APRICOT KERNALS - Apricot kernels contain amygdalin, which is also known as vitamin B17. B17 attacks cancer cells, making this an excellent superfood to boost B17 profile in your body. The Hunzas who have an almost non-existent history of cancer in their society have high levels of amygdalin (vitamin B17) in their diet.

MSM – methylsulfonylmethane, is a safe, natural, side-effect-free remedy for many types of pain and inflammation conditions. It has been used successfully with degenerative arthritis, chronic back pain, chronic headache, muscle pain, fibromyalgia, tendonitis and bursitis, carpal tunnel syndrome, TMJ, allergies and more. A true superfood.

GOJI BERRIES/GOJI JUICE – Goji berries contain up to 21 trace minerals (zinc, iron, copper, calcium, germanium, selenium, and phosphorus) and are the richest source of carotenoids, including beta-carotene (more beta carotene than carrots), of all known foods or plants on earth! They contain 500 times the amount of vitamin C, by weight, than oranges making them second only to camu camu berries as the richest vitamin C source on earth. Goji berries contain vitamins B1, B2, B6, and vitamin E.

MESQUITE MEAL – This high protein meal contains good quantities of calcium, magnesium, potassium, iron and zinc, and is rich in the amino acid lysine. The nutrients in mesquite are absorbed slowly due to the high fibre content. The digestive time for mesquite is to 4 to 6 hours unlike wheat that digests in 1 to 2 hours. These factors result in a food that maintains a constant blood sugar for a sustained time and as a result prevents hunger. Here is a food that supports the diabetic's diet and helps maintain a healthy insulin system in those not affected with blood sugar problem.

ALOE VERA - Used by people to help eliminate arthritis, bowel disease, and other ailments such as asthma and irritable bowel syndrome. It has a reputation for boosting the immune system of cancer and AIDS sufferers. It contains over 75 known ingredients and can help the assimilation of other nutrients when taken together.

CELL FOOD - Cellfood Concentrate is a completely natural and effective way to give the body the oxygen, minerals, enzymes and amino acids needed to maintain health. In a six month double blind trial on endurance athletes; the study completed at the Institute for Sport Research at the University of Pretoria in South Africa showed an increase in VO2 max, an increase in haemoglobin saturation, enhanced performance and recovery times.

URINE THERAPY - Once your diet is full of the right foods and you are engaging in the habits that lead to exceptional health, urine therapy can be more powerful than anything else.
"In successfully treating allergies with this substance, other conditions were also coincidentally relieved such as multiple sclerosis, colitis, hypertension, lupus, rheumatoid arthritis, hepatitis, hyperactivity, diabetes, herpes zoster, mononucleosis and so on…" Dr. N.P. Dunne, M.D., Allergy Specialist
For more information buy Your Own Perfect Medicine by Martha Christy.

CREATIVITY – V – MONOTONY
WHAT'S THE BEST APPROACH TO AGGRESSIVE HEALTH?

Ironically, both are as important as each other. Each of us has about ten favourite meals. What are yours? Do they build health or do they destroy health? It's your mission to get creative, eliminate your old favourites and replace them with 10 new meals that are in alignment with the principles of AGGRESSIVE HEALTH. It is then and only then, you can use monotony to your advantage by not complicating your food choices. You'll have predictable yet enjoyable meals that serve your unassailable health. Too much diversity means you'll struggle to stick to any plan. It's your responsibility to find out what works for you. Don't expect to see an AGGRESSIVE HEALTH cookbook – it's up to you to create the recipes that deliver results!

ORDER FORM

1-6 COPIES OF AGGRESSIVE HEALTH - £13 PER COPY

7-11 COPIES OF AGGRESSIVE HEALTH - £12 PER COPY

12 COPIES OR OVER - £10 PER COPY

Shipping will vary depending on quantity – get a quote from
www.aggressivehealth.co.uk

Total Amount Enclosed £/$_____

SHIP TO:

Name _____

Address_____

_____

Post Code _____ Country _____

Email address _____

Phone Number _____

Send cheque, money order or bankers draft to contact details found at
www.aggressivehealth.co.uk or alternatively – order online.

Vitälzym – Systemic Enzyme Support

In tests conducted to find a fibrinolytic enzyme to go along with their up coming natural cancer therapy, the University of Southern California, through the Apex Research Inst. tested 70 of the proteolytic enzyme products available today for enzymatic action. Of the 70, Vitalzym ranked #1.

With a mighty 1500mg of active ingredients Vitalzym is effective in the fight against inflammation, fibrosis or scar tissue, autoimmune conditions, viruses and toxins in the blood. Systemic enzymes are the foundation that makes all your other vitamin and mineral supplements work. We have roughly 3000 enzymes in our bodies and over 7000 enzymic reactions. As we age enzyme levels plummet. Vitalyzm can bridge the gap and help you hold onto your youth. Ask for your FREE CD at

www.aggressivehealth.co.uk

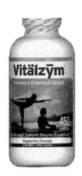
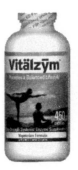

GREENS FOR LIFE

"Who Else Wants To Turbo Charge Their Life With The Tastiest, Most Potent Green Superfood Available"

- A 100% natural formula containing an abundance of vitamins, minerals, anti-oxidants, amino acids and enzymes
- Restores the acid/alkaline balance of the body and helps maintain a neutral pH-balance for optimal health
- Contains over 4000 mg of 10:1 Barley Grass extract per daily portion.

www.aggressivehealth.co.uk

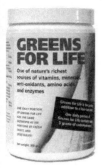

Discount Voucher

Thank-you for purchasing Aggressive Health. Please send this voucher (or email me the code GFL-AG-1000) with your cheque to the contact details found at www.aggressivehealth.co.uk for the following discounts.

£8 off 300g container = £27 (RRP £35)

Postage is FREE with this Voucher

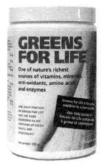

Live Blood Analysis Voucher

£15

OFF

Thank-you for purchasing Aggressive Health. Please use this voucher to receive £15 discount when you book a live blood consultation.

For more information contact www.aggressivehealth.co.uk

Bioterrain Analysis Voucher

£25

OFF

Thank-you for purchasing Aggressive Health. Please use this voucher to receive £25 discount when you book for a biological terrain consultation.

For more information contact www.aggressivehealth.co.uk

INDEX